Current Research in Medical Imaging

Current Research in Medical Imaging

Editor: Catheriene Blevins

AMERICAN
MEDICAL PUBLISHERS
www.americanmedicalpublishers.com

AMERICAN
MEDICAL PUBLISHERS
www.americanmedicalpublishers.com

Cataloging-in-Publication Data

Current research in medical imaging / edited by Catheriene Blevins.
p. cm.
Includes bibliographical references and index.
ISBN 978-1-63927-648-6
1. Diagnostic imaging. 2. Diagnostic imaging--Research.
3. Imaging systems in medicine. I. Blevins, Catheriene.
RC78.7.D53 C87 2023
616.075 4--dc23

American Medical Publishers,
41 Flatbush Avenue,
1st Floor, New York,
NY 11217, USA

ISBN 978-1-63927-648-6 (Hardback)

Contents

Preface

Medical imaging is the technique of producing images of the internal parts of the body. It facilitates medical intervention and clinical analysis, along with providing a visual representation of the functioning of tissues and organs. It reveals the internal structures that are covered by bones and skin, and helps in diagnosing and treating various diseases. Medical imaging makes use of various radiological and organic imaging techniques that utilize electromagnetic energies, sonography, isotope, magnetic, and thermal imaging. There are various types of medical imaging that are utilized currently for health care, including radiography, ultrasound, tomography, magnetic resonance imaging, photoacoustic imaging and echocardiography. Medical imaging is developing at a fast pace due to various developments in the techniques of image processing, including recognition, analysis and enhancement of images. Technological advancements that will contribute in presenting in depth visualization at the cell level are the future of medical imaging. This book contains some path-breaking studies on medical imaging. There has been rapid progress in this field and its applications are finding their way across multiple areas of medicine. This book will serve as a valuable source of reference for graduate and post graduate students.

Significant researches are present in this book. Intensive efforts have been employed by authors to make this book an outstanding discourse. This book contains the enlightening chapters which have been written on the basis of significant researches done by the experts.

Finally, I would also like to thank all the members involved in this book for being a team and meeting all the deadlines for the submission of their respective works. I would also like to thank my friends and family for being supportive in my efforts.

Editor

1

Molecular Imaging of Pulmonary Inflammation and Infection

Chiara Giraudo [1,*,†], Laura Evangelista [2,†], Anna Sara Fraia [1], Amalia Lupi [1], Emilio Quaia [1], Diego Cecchin [2,3] and Massimiliano Casali [4]

1 Department of Medicine-DIMED,Institute of Radiology, University of Padova, 35100 Padova, Italy; annasara.fraia@gmail.com (A.S.F.); amalialupi88@gmail.com (A.L.); emilio.quaia@unipd.it (E.Q.)
2 Nuclear Medicine Unit, Department of Medicine-DIMED, University of Padova, 35128 Padova, Italy; laura.evangelista@unipd.it (L.E.); cecchin.diego@unipd.it (D.C.)
3 Padova Neuroscience Center (PNC), University of Padova, 35131 Padova, Italy
4 Azienda Unità Sanitaria Locale–IRCCS di Reggio Emilia, 42121 Reggio Emilia, Italy; massimiliano.casali@ausl.re.it
* Correspondence: chiara.giraudo@unipd.it
† These authors contributed equally to this work.

Abstract: Infectious and inflammatory pulmonary diseases are a leading cause of morbidity and mortality worldwide. Although infrequently used in this setting, molecular imaging may significantly contribute to their diagnosis using techniques like single photon emission tomography (SPET), positron emission tomography (PET) with computed tomography (CT) or magnetic resonance imaging (MRI) with the support of specific or unspecific radiopharmaceutical agents. ^{18}F-Fluorodeoxyglucose (^{18}F-FDG), mostly applied in oncological imaging, can also detect cells actively involved in infectious and inflammatory conditions, even if with a low specificity. SPET with nonspecific (e.g., ^{67}Gallium-citrate (^{67}Ga citrate)) and specific tracers (e.g., white blood cells radiolabeled with ^{111}Indium-oxine (^{111}In) or ^{99m}Technetium (^{99m}Tc)) showed interesting results for many inflammatory lung diseases. However, ^{67}Ga citrate is unfavorable by a radioprotection point of view while radiolabeled white blood cells scan implies complex laboratory settings and labeling procedures. Radiolabeled antibiotics (e.g., ciprofloxacin) have been recently tested, although they seem to be quite unspecific and cause antibiotic resistance. New radiolabeled agents like antimicrobic peptides, binding to bacterial cell membranes, seem very promising. Thus, the aim of this narrative review is to provide a comprehensive overview about techniques, including PET/MRI, and tracers that can guide the clinicians in the appropriate diagnostic pathway of infectious and inflammatory pulmonary diseases.

Keywords: lung; inflammation; infection; PET; SPET; PET/CT; PET/MRI

1. Introduction

Infectious and inflammatory pulmonary diseases are a leading cause of morbidity and mortality worldwide. In the United States, lung infections represent the eighth most common cause of death, with an incidence of up to 7 cases per 1000 people per year and are associated with a very high hospitalization rate [1,2]. In Europe, the annual incidence of pneumonia ranges between 1.08 and 1.7 per 1000 people per year [3], with increased mortality rate especially in elderly patients [4].

In addition to pulmonary infections, inflammatory lung diseases are very frequent, such as interstitial lung diseases [5]. Considering the significant burden of such diseases, a prompt diagnosis and early treatment represent the primary goals.

Despite the key role of radiological imaging in detecting and localizing infections or inflammations, since different diseases may cause similar patterns, morphological imaging might be not sufficient to reach the correct diagnosis. Thus, molecular imaging, adding information about the functional activity of the detected lesions, may significantly contribute to both the diagnostic process and the response to treatment. Single photon emission tomography (SPET), and positron emission tomography (PET) or PET/computed tomography (CT) and magnetic resonance imaging (MRI) are very sensitive in detecting the functional/metabolic activity of infectious or inflammatory areas, thus resulting in the useful monitoring of disease activity, mainly after treatment [6].

The aim of this narrative review is to provide a comprehensive overview about techniques and tracers that can guide the clinicians in the appropriate diagnostic pathway.

For the sake of clarity, we divided the argument in three macro areas related to the used tracers: SPET/CT, PET/CT and PET/MRI. Furthermore, two tables, Tables 1 and 2, summarizing the main techniques and tracers that can be used for the assessment of benign lung diseases have been included.

Table 1. Tracers, techniques and targets.

Tracer	Technique	Target
18F-FDG	PET	Neutrophils, lymphocytes, eosinophils and macrophages
67Ga/68Ga citrate	SPECT/PET	Neutrophils and leukocytes
99mTc-leukocites	SPECT	Leukocytes
111In/68Ga-Somatostatic receptors	SPECT/PET	Lymphocytes, monocytes and macrophages (also fibroblasts)
11C-PK11195	PET	Monocities and neutrophils

FDG: fluorodeoxyglucose; PET: positron emission tomography; SPECT: single photon emission tomography;Ga: Gallium; In: Indium; 11C: 11Choline.

Table 2. Clinical indications and main radiopharmaceutical agents for the assessment of various benign lung diseases.

Tracer	Disease	Clinical Indication
Radiolabeled WBC	Pneumonia	-
	Pleural and lung infections	Diagnosis
	Mycobacterial infections	Diagnosis
^{67}Ga-citrate	Pulmonary infections	-
	Pneumonia*	-
	Tuberculosis	Diagnosis, evaluation of response to therapy, active vs. nonactive disease
	Sarcoidosis	Diagnosis
FDG	Pulmonary fibrosis	-
	Tuberculosis	-
	Sarcoidosis and extrapulmonary involvement	Diagnosis, evaluation of response to therapy, biopsy guide

WBC=white blood cell; FDG=fluorodeoxyglucose; *especially in immunocompromised patients; Ga: Gallium.

2. SPET and SPET/CT

Several clinical studies, demonstrated that in patients with opacities detected at x-ray or CT, ^{67}Gallium-citrate (^{67}Ga-citrate), ^{111}In-oxine (^{111}In) or ^{99m}Tc hexamethyl propyleneamine-oxime (HMPAO)-labelled autologous leukocytes (white-blood-cell, WBC) scintigraphy may contribute to reach the correct diagnosis of infection or inflammation [7,8].

Despite the successful application of planar scintigraphy or SPET for inflammatory and infectious lung diseases, such techniques are affected by poor spatial resolution [9]. This limit has been partially overcome by the introduction of SPET/CT, allowing not only a precise anatomical localization of the lesions but also a more precise distinction between areas of physiological uptake and infections [10–12]. SPET/CT demonstrated a high sensitivity, up to 85% in inflammatory disease, especially when labelled WBC are used [13].

The use of radiolabeled WBC, ^{67}Ga-citrate and other SPECT tracers will be discussed in the next three paragraphs.

2.1. Radiolabeled WBC

Radiolabelled leukocytes, marked in vitro and reintroduced into the circulation, provide an accurate map of the distribution of labelled WBC within the lung, allowing a robust assessment of pulmonary diseases [14,15]. The characteristics of the uptake depend on chemotaxis, number and types of labelled cells, and the prevalent cellular component involved in the inflammatory response [16].

Since most of the labelled leukocytes are neutrophils and it is well known that bacterial infections cause an immune response mediated by such cells, SPET/CT with radiolabeled WBCs is very sensitive in identifying this type of infections. Nevertheless, it has to be considered that different ranges of accuracy are reported in the literature. For instance, in a series of 13 patients, a full correspondence between the focal uptake at SPET/CT and the clinical and instrumental evidence of infection was achieved [17]. On the contrary, Cook et al. obtained an agreement only in 14 out of 27 cases of pneumonia [18]. Finally, two studies on larger populations showed that ^{111}In-WBC SPET/CT has a sensitivity of 94% and a specificity of 64% in detecting pleural and lung infections [14], while it reported a negative predictive value equal to 99% in excluding pulmonary infections in immunocompromised patients [19].

Pulmonary application of SPET and SPET/CT with radiolabeled WBC have been used in animal models for several other diseases. For example, Audi et al. demonstrated in a murine model that ^{99m}Tc-HMPAO-WBC uptake occurs 24 h after hyperoxia-induced lung injury and such tracer might be then used as preclinical marker or during follow-up [20].

Despite the current high diagnostic value of SPET/CT and its further promising areas of application, specific challenges have to be considered. First, a recent study involving 20 patients with active bronchiectasis who underwent ^{99m}Tc-HMPAO-WBC scan showed that a segmental or lobar uptake might be due labelled leukocytes concentrated in pulmonary bronchiectasis filled of secretions rather than to pneumonia [21]. Second, an accurate interpretation and adequate correlation with clinical findings are necessary. Furthermore, from a technical point of view it is mandatory to distinguish the pathological uptake occurring 4 h after injection of the labelled tracer from the early normal diffuse pulmonary activity (i.e., background activity).

Finally, it has been shown that radiolabeled WBCs have a lower diagnostic value for opportunistic infections (e.g., *Pneumocystis carinii*) and/or mycobacterial infections and sarcoidosis [22,23]. For such diseases, ^{67}Ga-citrate has provided better results [24], although in recent years it has been extensively replaced by ^{18}F-fluorodeoxyglucose (^{18}F-FDG)-PET/CT.

2.2. Gallium-67 Citrate

^{67}Ga-citrate is an analogue of ferric iron that, after intravenous injection, dissociates from the citrate and binds to the plasmatic transferrin in the circulating blood. Into the extracellular space, the ^{67}Ga complex binds with strong avidity to the lactoferrin and the siderophores, which are predominantly released by activated neutrophils and bacteria, thus causing its accumulation in areas affected by infections [25,26]. Nevertheless, considering the intense ^{67}Ga-citrate uptake also in presence of agranulocytes, it has to be considered that, similarly to ^{18}F-FDG, it is also absorbed by cells with an increased glucose metabolic rate [27]. For this reason, to detect opportunistic pulmonary infections and differentiate infections from Kaposi sarcoma or lymphomas in immunocompromised patients, the use of ^{67}Ga-citrate combined with thallium-201 chloride (^{201}Tl) has been proposed. In HIV patients with pneumonia due to *Pneumocystis carinii*, a diffuse homogenous pulmonary uptake occurs with ^{67}Ga-citrate albeit not with ^{201}Tl. On the contrary, Kaposi sarcoma shows pathologic uptake with ^{201}Tl but not with ^{67}Ga-citrate. Pulmonary lesions due to lymphoma demonstrate metabolic activity with both tracers [28].

Considering lung infections, patients affected by tuberculosis usually show pulmonary parenchymal and nodal pathologic uptake of ^{67}Ga-citrate. Although ^{18}F-FDG PET is the most widely used molecular imaging technique to assess this infection [29], ^{67}Ga-citrate seems to have high sensitivity (83%–100%) in detecting active and inactive lesions, avoiding potential pitfalls due to malignancies, granulomatous disease, and aspergillosis [30–38]. The ^{67}Ga-citrate uptake is related to activated foamy macrophages, granuloma progression and load of Mycobacterium tuberculosis both in the affected pulmonary sites and in the sputum. Late in 1976, Siemens et al demonstrated a correlation between ^{67}Ga-citrate uptake and disease activity in 192 out of 197 patients with active tuberculosis. A progressive decrease of the metabolic activity has been also shown after three to nine months of treatment. Since none of the examined patients with inactive tuberculosis showed pathologic ^{67}Ga-citrate uptake, it has been demonstrated that such tracer is accurate in differentiating active disease from fibrosis [30]. However, controversial results have been obtained some years later by Walsh et al. who reported 27% of specificity and 69% of positive predictive value of ^{67}Ga-citrate for detecting active foci of tuberculosis [32]. Furthermore, Goswami et al. pointed out that ongoing treatments may reduce the sensitivity of ^{67}Ga-citrate in tuberculotic patients [39]. It has also been demonstrated that in active pulmonary tuberculosis, ^{67}Ga-citrate uptake correlates with the acid-fast bacilli load in the sputum [40]. According to such evidence, ^{67}Ga-citrate has been suggested as an indicator of activated macrophages and bacterial load, guiding the prompt isolation and treatment of patients with active pulmonary disease. Recently, the association of ^{67}Ga-citrate with ^{111}In, using a novel dual-isotope radiolabeling approach conjugated with vaccines was successfully used in a preclinical animal model to assess the efficacy of a mucosal vaccines for tuberculosis [41].

Rizzato et al. in a multicenter European study [42] demonstrated that ^{67}Ga-citrate scintigraphy is more sensitive than chest X-rays for sarcoidosis and that its uptake correlates with the level of angiotensin-converting enzyme (ACE). The typical signs of sarcoidosis at ^{67}Ga-citrate imaging are the so-called *lambda* and *panda* signs. These aspects are due to the predominant uptake of the right-sided paratracheal lymph nodes and to the symmetrical uptake in the lacrimal and parotid glands, respectively. Nevertheless, these signs have a poor diagnostic sensitivity in biopsy-proven sarcoidosis patients [43–45] and the panda sign may occur in several other diseases (e.g., HIV, lymphomas and Sjogren's syndrome).

SPET with ^{67}Ga-citrate has been applied for inflammatory disorders evolving in pulmonary fibrosis (e.g., idiopathic pulmonary fibrosis (IPF), lymphoid interstitial pneumonitis), for inhalational and occupational pulmonary diseases, (e.g., asbestosis, berylliosis, coal worker pneumoconiosis), collagen vascular diseases (e.g., systemic lupus erythematosus and systemic sclerosis), and other noninfectious inflammatory disease, including pulmonary alveolar proteinosis, eosinophilic pneumonia, Wegener's granulomatosis, and eosinophilic granuloma [46–59].

Despite the above-mentioned advantages, ^{67}Ga-citrate is affected by several limits, such as an adverse dosimetry, long acquisition times, high number of false positives and risk of artifacts. For instance, it requires long intervals (24-72 hours) between the radiopharmaceutical injection and the acquisition [60]. Therefore, its role in clinical practice has progressively reduced, which has created space for the development of new radiopharmaceuticals.

2.3. Other SPET/CT Tracers

In addition to the use of radiolabeled WBC and ^{67}Ga-citrate, several other molecules have been tested for investigating lung inflammatory and infectious disease by SPET/CT, in humans and in preclinical settings.

In tuberculosis or simil-tuberculotic syndromes, ^{99m}Tc-methoxyisobutylisonitrile (MIBI) [61,62] and ^{99m}Tc(V)-dimercaptosuccinic acid (DMSA) [63] have been successfully used for pulmonary and extrapulmonary involvement. In 1995, Gulaldi et al. also suggested that a ^{99m}Tc-DMSA scanning could represent a valid alternative to ^{67}Ga-citrate [64].

Based on the expression of somatostatin receptors in the granulomatous lesions, ^{99m}Tc-EDDA-tricine-HYNIC-Tyr3-octreotate has been used as radiotracer for distinguishing between active and inactive tuberculotic lesions [65]. In 2017, Montiero et al. suggested that in pulmonary and extra-pulmonary granulomatous infections SPET/CT with radiotracer as ^{99m}Tc-EDDA-HYNIC-TOC or ^{111}In-DTPA-octreotide may successfully differentiate active infectious lesions detected on CT from residual scar tissue [66]. As for tuberculosis, radiolabeled analogues of somatostatin, like ^{111}In pentetreotide, have been applied for pulmonary and extra thoracic lesions due to sarcoidosis. Kwekkeboom et al. detected a pathologic uptake at SPET in 97% of 46 patients with sarcoid lesions seen on a chest X-ray [67]. Several authors comparing ^{67}Ga-citrate with different tracers demonstrated for instance that somatostatin receptor analogues and ^{18}F-FDG may even perform better than ^{67}Ga-citrate for pulmonary and extrapulmonary lesions [68–71].

A recent retrospective cross-sectional study evaluated the role of ^{99m}Tc-ethambutol SPET/CT in detecting both pulmonary and extra-pulmonary tuberculotic infections, demonstrating, also in pediatric patients, high sensitivity and positive predictive value (both >90%) [72].

Foss et al. using a murine model of pulmonary tuberculosis localized areas of infection by a monoclonal antibody for tissue-bound C3 deposits [73].

In interstitial lung diseases, Zheng et al recently used the collagen-targeting agent ^{99m}Tc-CBP1495, in in-vitro and ex-vivo experiments, to assess lung fibrosis [74], being the fibrosis characterized by the pathological accumulation of collagen in the extracellular matrix.

Several preclinical studies addressed the role of different radiolabeled agents selectively binding to antibiotics (e.g., ciprofloxacin, sparfloxacin, enroflaxacin, ceftizoxime, ethambutol, fluconazole) not only for diagnosing infections and inflammatory processes, but also to distinguish one from the other and even differentiate bacterial infection from lesions caused by other pathogens [75,76]. However, some biases related to animal selection and index test, actually limit their transfer from preclinical models to humans [77].

More recently, antimicrobial peptides (AMPs) labeled with isotopes both for SPET (^{99m}Tc) and PET imaging (^{68}Ga) have grown as more specific agents to localize infections since they specifically bind to bacterial cell membranes. In particular, ubiquicidin (UBI 29-41) has shown encouraging results in human clinical trials [78]. The use of this new category of agents is, to date, mainly limited to the preclinical phase, without strong evidence in the humans and therefore the introduction in the clinical practice seems interesting but far.

Perfusion and ventilation scintigraphy have been used also for chronic obstructive pulmonary disease (COPD) and asthma, both characterized by inflammation and bronchial obstruction. Perfusion scintigraphy is performed using radiolabeled macroaggregate particles, whereas ventilation scintigraphy is conducted by micron-sized, and submicron-sized aerosols (99mTc-labeled DTPA and 99mTc-labeled clusters of carbon particles [Technegas], respectively) or inert radioactive gases (133Xe and 81mKr).

Already in 1997, SPECT with Technegas was successfully applied on healthy volunteers to investigate airway closure [79]. Since then, several studies have explored its use for asthmatic patients. For instance, Farrow et al. demonstrated a significant correlation between severe airway hyperresponsiveness and airway closure at ventilation SPECT/CT [80]. Recently, the same group of researchers examining 14 patients with asthma showed that the ventilation is reduced in areas affected by bronchoconstriction and that the degree of such decrease can be predicted by acinar ventilation heterogeneity [81]. Overall, the role of ventilation scintigraphy for asthma can be considered complementary to functional tests and this technique can be useful for the assessment of the extension of pulmonary involvement, and for monitoring the response to treatment.

Technegas provided very interesting results also for diagnosing and grading the severity of COPD [82]. Using 99mTc-labeled DTPA, the distinction between nonsmoker COPD and asthmatic patients has been achieved in a cohort of 84 patients [Karakavus_83]. In particular, the muco-ciliary clearance, assessed by 99mTc-DTPA in terms of T $\frac{1}{2}$, was significantly higher in patients with asthma than in nonsmoking COPD patients [83].

3. PET and PET/CT

PET and PET/CT are mainly used in the oncological field even if it is well known that they play a significant role also for inflammatory and infectious diseases [84–89]. Several tracers have been applied for both techniques even if ^{18}F-FDG is the most commonly used in clinical practice. The use of ^{18}F-FDG and other PET tracers will be discussed in the next two paragraphs.

3.1. ^{18}F-FDG

^{18}F-FDG is very sensitive for detecting infections and inflammations because the activated inflammatory cells increase the expression of glucose transporters (GLUT 1, GLUT 3). Moreover, cytokines and grow factors released in inflammatory sites increase the affinity of glucose transporters for the deoxyglucose. ^{18}F-FDG uptake is proportional to the cellular metabolic rate [84,89] and binds to the majority of infection and inflammation cells such as neutrophils, lymphocytes, eosinophil and macrophages (Figure 1).

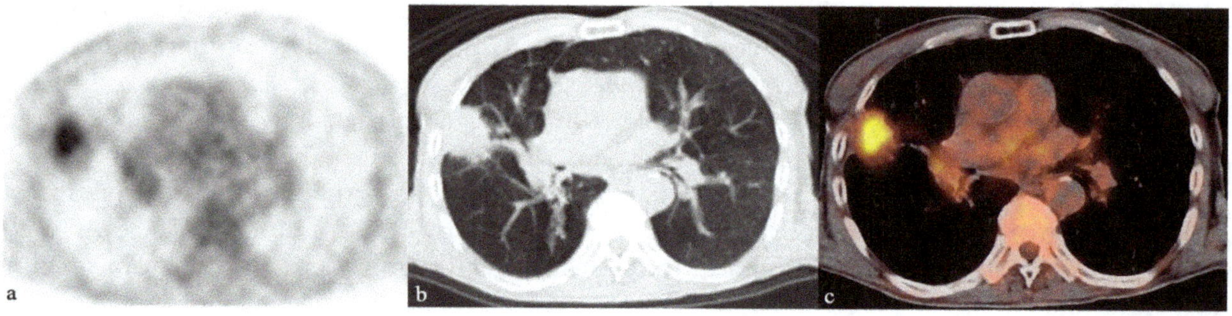

Figure 1. A 79-year-old male affected by pneumonia due to *Pseudomonas aeruginosa* who was examined by ^{18}F-FDG-PET/CT. The ^{18}F-FDG-PET (**a**), axial CT (**b**), and fused image (**c**) of the ^{18}F-FDG-PET/CT scan demonstrate the pulmonary consolidation, with high tracer uptake, in the middle lobe due to the infection.

In pulmonary infections ^{18}F-FDG-PET/CT has been applied for tuberculosis even if it is characterized by low specificity [90]. Semiquantitative measurements (i.e., standardized uptake values) have not proven to reliably distinguish between infection and pulmonary neoplastic lesions [91–94].

Several studies reported the use of ^{18}F-FDG-PET for monitoring aspergillosis [95] and evaluating the efficacy of chemotherapy in echinococcosis [96]. Indeed, by conventional radiology, parasite viability cannot be assessed, while the detection of metabolic activity with PET may guide the treatment to prevent relapses [97,98]. Bleeker-Rovers et al. demonstrated that the decrease of ^{18}F-FDG uptake in PET/CT scan can be applied to determine the success of antifungal therapy for lung abscess due to Candida [99].

In patients affected by sarcoidosis, ^{18}F-FDG-PET and PET/CT can play an important role for assessing reversible granuloma, detecting occult diseases, evaluating treatment response and even indicating the most suitable site for biopsy [100,101]. In particular in stage IV that is characterized by fibrosis and mass-like lesions, ^{18}F-FDG uptake of reversible granulomas plays a key role in the diagnostic and therapeutic approach [102,103].

To date, only a small number of subjects with either chronic obstructive pulmonary disease or cystic fibrosis have been evaluated with ^{18}F-FDG-PET or PET/CT, but the available data suggest that ^{18}F-FDG-PET can quantify lung inflammation levels and may thus be a useful biomarker of inflammatory cell activity. ^{18}F-FDG uptake may also serve as a biomarker for treatment response to antibiotic therapy, showing a rapid reduction of ^{18}F-FDG uptake in patients with acute exacerbations [104,105].

Finally, ^{18}F-FDG-PET/CT, combining morphological and anatomical information, is very useful in assessing the extent of extrapulmonary involvement [106].

The high metabolic rate associated with acute and chronic inflammatory lung diseases, makes ^{18}F-FDG especially suitable for assessing and even quantifying the activity of different diffuse or focal inflammatory pulmonary diseases (e.g., smoking-related disease, asthma, cystic fibrosis, organizing pneumonia, IPF, non-specific interstitial pneumonia) [107,108] (Figure 2). ^{18}F-FDG uptake can be detected when neutrophils are activated and sequestered within the lungs before their trans-endothelial migration into airways. For this reason, ^{18}F-FDG -based techniques can be applied for diagnosing acute lung injury or acute rejection of lung graft [109].

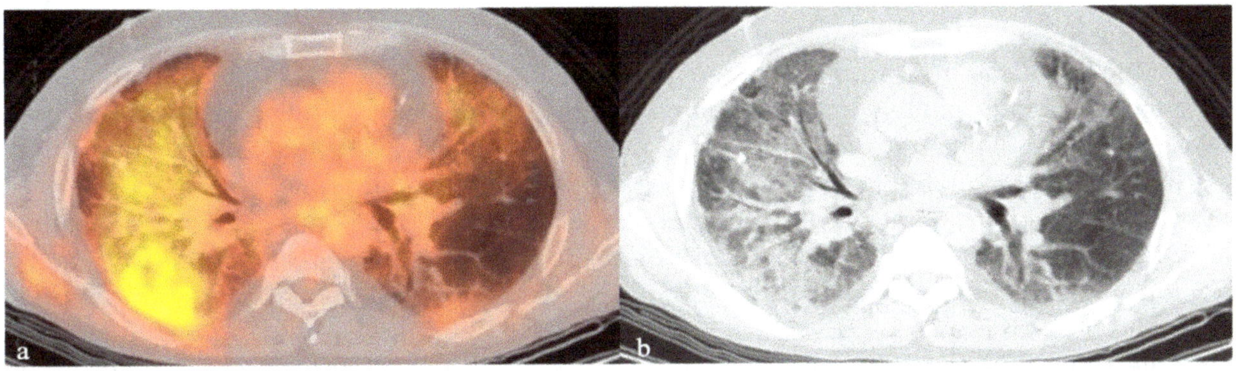

Figure 2. A 60-year-old male with end-stage interstitial lung disease examined by ^{18}F-FDG-PET/CT, which demonstrates the high metabolism (**a**) of the affected pulmonary areas (**b**).

In particular, regarding COPD, a very recent article demonstrated in this group of patients a significant correlation between the metabolic activity of respiratory muscles at ^{18}F-FDG-PET/CT and pulmonary function tests [110]. Such evidence unveils a new field of application of this technique.

Furthermore, the oxidative stress, as determinant inflammation factor, may cause pathologic uptake in case of acute rejection or bronchiolitis obliterans after lung transplant as well as for acute lung injury and acute respiratory distress syndrome [111,112].

3.2. Other PET/CT Tracers

Besides ^{18}F-FDG, other tracers have been tested for pulmonary PET and PET/CT imaging. For instance, ^{11}C-choline, ^{18}F-fluoroethylcholine (^{18}F-FEC), 30-deoxy-30-(^{18}F) fluoro-L-thymidine (^{18}F-FLT), ^{68}Ga-citrate, ^{68}Ga-peptides, (^{18}F) sodium fluoride (^{18}F-NaF), and radiolabeled anti-tuberculosis drugs. In particular, ^{11}C- choline and ^{18}F-FEC being analogues of lipids are incorporated into the wall of the Mycobacterium. ^{11}C-Choline has also been applied to differentiate lung cancer from active tuberculosis but with controversial results [113–115].

^{18}F-FLT has been tested in a small number of patients affected by sarcoidosis, showing a lower performance than ^{18}F-FDG for the identification of extra-cardiac lesions [116].

It has been also demonstrated a correspondence between the increased uptake of ^{68}Ga-peptides, such as ^{68}Ga-DOTANOC, in areas of peripheral and subpleural abnormalities detected at high-resolution CT in patients with IPF. The association of ^{18}F-FDG and ^{68}Ga-DOTATOC PET/CT examinations could also provide a combined information about ongoing inflammation and fibroblastic process [117].

^{18}F-NaF has been successfully applied in a murine model to detect microcalcifications not detectable at CT in mice with chronic tuberculosis [118], but clinical results are still missing.

Regarding inflammatory diseases, a recent study introduced radiolabeled fluciclatide, an arginine-glycine-aspartic acid peptide, for assessing the angiogenesis and myofibroblast differentiation that characterize the development of pulmonary fibrosis [119].

As several preclinical studies suggested, a radiotracer based on inducible nitric oxide synthase could be useful to study human lung disease but its applicability in clinical settings still needs to be further validated [120,121]. Nevertheless, Huang et al. had already successfully applied one-hour dynamic ^{18}F-NOS PET/CT for endotoxin-induced lung inflammation in healthy volunteers [122].

As for SPET, a number of PET studies are ongoing concerning the labelling and initial clinical use of AMPs [123–125] mainly labeled with ^{68}Ga. Although preliminary AMPs seems very promising in differentiating inflammation and infection.

3.3. Magnetic Resonance Imaging (MRI) and PET/MRI

MRI is a well-established technique especially suitable for the assessment of soft tissues and characterized by the extraordinary advantage, among others, of using nonionizing radiofrequency electromagnetic radiations [126,127].

Unfortunately, MRI is not the first choice for pulmonary imaging because of the low proton density of the lungs and the occurrence of movement artifacts due to heartbeats and breathing. Novel imaging techniques like parallel imaging, shared echo-technique, and rotating phase encoding permit to at least partially overcome such limitations. Nevertheless, the lack of clear indications and the necessity of protocols tailored to specific diseases still reduce its application.

Regarding the protocols, a recent review about pediatric chest MRI suggested that fast breath-hold T1 and T2-weighted (T1w and T2w, respectively) images and free breathing steady state free precession sequences provide adequate anatomical and pathological information with a short scan time. Furthermore, it has been shown that respiratory triggered T2-weighted sequences can replace breath-hold sequences in patients with respiratory difficulties or infant, while short tau inversion recovery (STIR) can enhance differences in the signal intensity of pathological areas [126].

Applying the appropriate protocol, despite the above-mentioned limits, MRI demonstrated to be accurate for the assessment of pulmonary infections in animal models as well as in clinical settings [128–134]. Nowadays, it is well known that areas of high signal intensity on T2w images reflect the presence of intra-alveolar fluid whereas consolidation are hyperintense on T2w images and isointense on T1w images after gadolinium. Abscesses, additionally to the hyperintensity seen on T2w, show restricted diffusion at Diffusion Weighted Imaging (DWI) and rim enhancement; this latter finding is usually absent in case of necrosis. Simple pleural effusion is hyperintense on T2w and hypointense on T1w images, while in case of empyema the pleura appears thickened, shows septa, enhancement and restricted diffusion [129,135–138].

Some typical CT signs of pulmonary diseases have a direct correspondence on MRI. For instance, Ekinci et al. using T2w balanced fast field echo, T1w turbo spin-echo (TSE), and T2w TSE sequences in the axial and coronal planes, detected the reverse halo sign in immunocompromised patients affected by pneumonia [139]. The same authors, nevertheless highlighted that an accurate diagnosis of tree-in-bud nodules, centrilobular nodules, halo sign and nodules overall, especially if very small, is still challenging at MRI [139].

Ozcan et al. demonstrated that using a radial acquisition method (i.e., BLADE sequence) a higher sensitivity for nodules, ground-glass opacities and consolidation, compared to half-Fourier acquisition single-shot turbo spin-echo, volumetric interpolated breath-hold examination and Fast low angle shot magnetic resonance imaging [140] can be achieved and spectral adiabatic inversion recovery and high resolution isotropic volume examination after contrast are suitable for the evaluation of invasive fungal infection [141]. Moreover, other useful tools such as intravoxel incoherent motion–derived parameters and apparent diffusion coefficient, can be applied for diagnostic purposes, allowing for example the prediction of the treatment response to fungal infection [142].

MRI allows also a distinction between malignant tumors and tuberculomas, having the latter a significantly lower signal intensity on T2w [143,144]. Chung et al. suggested the use of volume-interpolated three-dimensional gradient echo T1w for diagnosing Mycobacterium avium complex pneumonia since it not only allows a robust evaluation of pulmonary nodules and masses but increases the contrast and minimizes the acquisition time and partial volume averaging [145].

Considering other infectious diseases, MRI still has a low specificity for aspergillosis in the early stage, but its diagnostic value is higher in the later stages of the diseases since it well demonstrated the target sign with rim enhancement [146,147].

Considering pulmonary inflammatory diseases, fluid-sensitive sequences are very useful in demonstrating active processes [148] and overall MRI allows the characterization of the extent of the diseases and the differentiation between acute inflammation and fibrosis [149–153].

For instance, in interstitial lung diseases, which are characterized by inflammation and fibrotic remodeling [154], the development of quantitative MRI techniques could help distinguishing between the two components evaluating the differences in relaxation time [155–157]. Similarly, it has been shown that ground glass opacities, reticulation and honeycombing have different T2 relaxation values and that T2 values significantly increase with fibrosis. Thus, T2 mapping could play a role in monitoring interstitial lung diseases [158,159]. Moreover, in patients affected by non-specific interstitial pneumonia the T2 relaxation significantly differs between active and stable fibrotic patients [160]. The injection of gadolinium may contribute to the diagnostic process of inflammatory diseases, since the endothelial injury allows the extravascular flow of contrast medium [161].

For the assessment of fibrosis, a gadolinium-based probe targeted to type I collagen (e.g., EP-3533) was successfully applied for diagnosing early disease and monitoring lung fibrosis in an animal model [162,163].

MRI was increasingly applied also in patients with asthma, demonstrating the occurrence of segmental lung edema and being a robust method for monitoring the response to treatment. [164–167]. Furthermore, it has been shown that hyperpolarized gases allow the evaluation of functional changes in distal small airways of asthmatic patients. In particular, using an isotope of helium (i.e., 3HE), hyperpolarized through a circularly polarized laser light and administered as inhalation contrast media, lung airspaces can be assessed, and ventilation defects diagnosed since they appear as signal voids [168–174].

In specific clinical conditions like cystic fibrosis, MRI can be even preferable than CT, despite the lack of details, given the risk associated with long term radiation exposure associated with multiple CT scans. MRI has already proven to be reliable in the evaluation of structural changes like bronchiectasis, wall thickening, mucus plugging, and infiltrates [126,171–173] and novel sequences such as ultrashort or zero echo time and multiparametric-functional imaging are expected to provide additional information (Figure 3). Furthermore, scores based on Diffusion weighted imaging demonstrated to strongly correlate with the severity of the disease and the amount of mucus [174] as well as of being associated with symptoms scores, spirometry measurements and inflammation during disease's exacerbation [164,175,176]. Hyperpolarized gases such as 129Xe showed inhomogeneous ventilation patterns with areas of lacking ventilation in such patients [177].

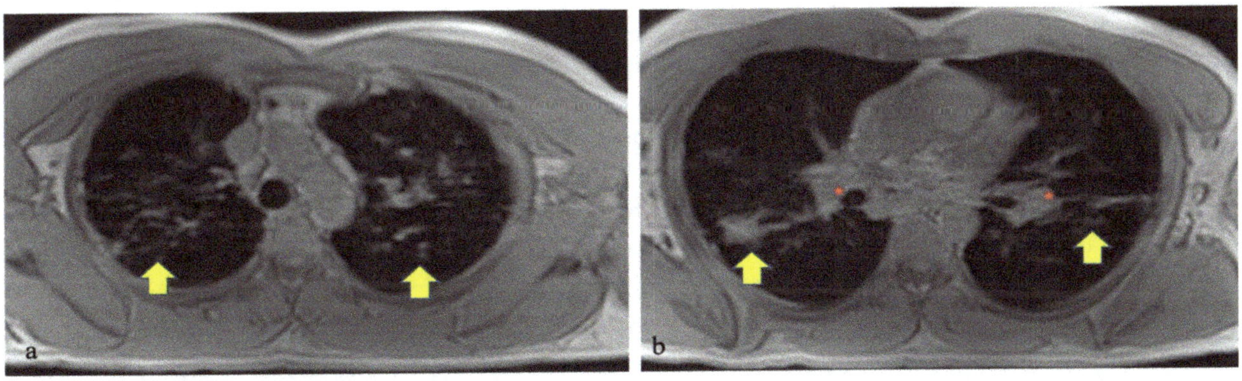

Figure 3. Short echo-time of the lungs showing multiple pulmonary nodules and enlarged hilar lymph nodes (respectively, yellow arrows and red asterisks in (**a**) and (**b**)) in a 40-year-old male patient affected by sarcoidosis.

According to the recent above-mentioned evidence, MRI is progressively becoming a valid radiation-free alternative that will increasingly be applied in the next years, taking full advantage of all technological progresses and of the expanding use of hybrid techniques, such as PET/MRI [129,138,178–184] (Figure 4).

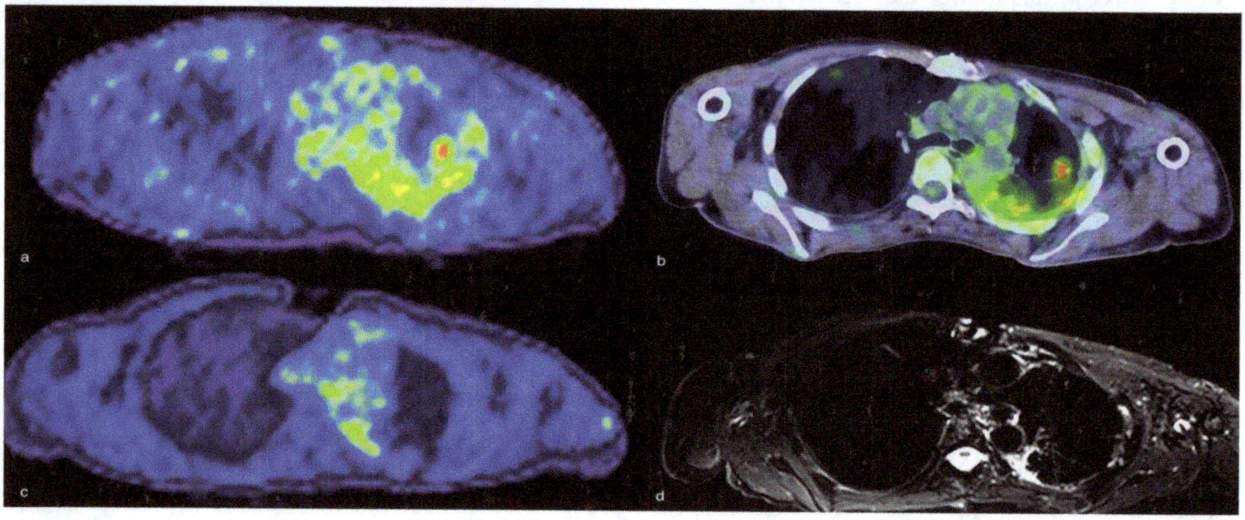

Figure 4. ^{18}F-FDG-PET (**a**) and fused axial ^{18}F-FDG-PET/CT (**b**) demonstrating a pulmonary infection with high metabolic activity in the left upper lobe which then decreased after treatment with antibiotics at ^{18}F-FDG-PET/MR (fused axial image in (**c**) and axial STIR in (**d**).

Indeed, PET/MRI, providing simultaneous metabolic and functional information, is a robust technique with a broad spectrum of applications especially in the oncological field. Also for pulmonary imaging, it has been successfully applied for the assessment of primary and metastatic lesions [185–190]. Regarding infectious diseases, in a recent study, ^{18}F-FDG-PET/MR showed a similar performance than PET/CT in detecting pulmonary lesions due to tuberculosis [191]. Nevertheless, further research, including multicenter research trials, is needed for establishing the role of this diagnostic tool for inflammatory and infectious lung diseases.

4. Future Perspectives

The upcoming technical progress in molecular imaging and the transposition into clinical settings of the knowledge gained in experimental preclinical studies are expected to change our perspectives and introduce new diagnostic tools for pulmonary imaging [127,180].

For instance, we may expect the application of ^{19}F markers, such as perfluorcarbon compounds, which allow to track stem and immune cells. Indeed, in experimental disease models, it has been demonstrated that taking advantage of the negligible ^{19}F background signal, inflammation can be assessed [192,193].

Furthermore, fluorescence and bioluminescence, using the optical properties of tissues originated from biochemical reactions and biological processes, through the use of fluorochromes, reporter genes and optical contrast agents, will favor even greater versatility in nuclear imaging, although to date clinical applications for optical imaging are still missing [194,195].

5. Conclusions

In conclusion, molecular imaging could potentially play a key role for inflammatory and infectious pulmonary diseases. SPET and SPET/CT using radiolabeled WBC allow for the characterization of pneumonia, while tuberculosis and inflammatory disease have been historically assessed using ^{67}Ga-citrate. However, for radioprotection reasons and worldwide availability, ^{67}Ga-citrate will be presumably abandoned. ^{18}F-FDG-PET/CT, providing information about the glucose metabolism, is highly reliable to detect active lesions for several types of lung diseases like tuberculosis, sarcoidosis and inflammatory disease in general, but the low specificity represents an important limitation. We could hypothesize that radiolabeled (probably with ^{68}Ga) AMPs, specifically binding to bacterial cell membranes could, in the future, be used as a second line after ^{18}F-FDG to increase specificity of the diagnostic process. In addition, we expect an increasing application of MRI and PET/MRI in this setting.

Author Contributions: Conceptualization: C.G., E.Q., D.C. Data curation: L.E., D.C., M.C. Investigation: C.G., A.S.F., A.L. Writing—Draft Preparation: C.G., A.S.F., A.L., L.E. Writing—Review & Editing: L.E., C.G., D.C., E.Q., M.C. All authors have read and agreed to the published version of the manuscript.

Acknowledgments: We acknowledge the support from the study group on infectious diseases of the Italian Association of Nuclear Medicine (AIMN).

References

1. Marrie, T.J.; Huang, J.D. Epidemiology of community-acquired pneumonia in Edmonton, Alberta: an emergency department-based study. *Can. Respir. J.* **2005**, *12*, 139–142. [CrossRef] [PubMed]
2. Ramirez, J.A.; Wiemken, T.L.; Peyrani, P.; Arnold, F.W.; Kelley, R.; Mattingly, W.A.; Nakamatsu, R.; Pena, S.; Guinn, B.E.; Furmanek, S.P.; et al. Adults Hospitalized With Pneumonia in the United States: Incidence, Epidemiology, and Mortality. *Clin. Infect. Dis.* **2017**, *65*, 1806–1812. [CrossRef] [PubMed]
3. Torres, A.; Peetermans, W.E.; Viegi, G.; Blasi, F. Risk factors for community-acquired pneumonia in adults in Europe: a literature review. *Thorax* **2013**, *68*, 1057–1065. [CrossRef] [PubMed]
4. Trotter, C.L.; Stuart, J.M.; George, R.; Miller, E. Increasing hospital admissions for pneumonia, England. *Emerg. Infect. Dis.* **2008**, *14*, 727–733. [CrossRef] [PubMed]
5. Navaratnam, V.; Fleming, K.M.; West, J.; Smith, C.J.; Jenkins, R.G.; Fogarty, A.; Hubbars, R.B. The rising incidence of idiopathic pulmonary fibrosis in the UK. *Thorax* **2011**, *66*, 462–467. [CrossRef]
6. Dimastromatteo, J.; Charles, E.J.; Laubach, L.E. Molecular imaging of pulmonary diseases. *Resp. Res.* **2018**, *19*, 1–17. [CrossRef]
7. Kao, C.H.; Wang, S.J.; Liao, S.Q.; Lin, W.Y.; Hsu, C.Y. Usefulness of gallium-67-citrate scans in patients with acute disseminated tuberculosis and comparison with chest x-rays. *J. Nucl. Med.* **1993**, *34*, 1918–1921.
8. Forstrom, L.A.; Loken, M.K.; Cook, A.; Chandler, R.; McCullough, J. In-111-labeled leukocytes in the diagnosis of rejection and cytomegalovirus infection in renal transplant patients. *Clin. Nucl. Med.* **1981**, *6*, 146–149. [CrossRef]
9. Bar-Shalom, R.; Yefremov, N.; Guralnik, L.; Keidar, Z.; Engel, A.; Nitecki, S.; Israel, O. SPET/CT using 67Ga and 111In-labeled leukocyte scintigraphy for diagnosis of infection. *J. Nucl. Med.* **2006**, *47*, 587–594.
10. Ingui, C.J.; Shah, N.P.; Oates, M.E. Infection scintigraphy: added value of single-photon emission computed tomography/computed tomography fusion compared with traditional analysis. *J. Comput. Assist. Tomogr.* **2007**, *31*, 375–380. [CrossRef]
11. Grubstein, A.; Bernstine, H.; Steinmetz, A.P. Chest CT and gallium-67 SPET scintigraphy scan co-registration in a post-heart transplantation patient with unresolved fever. *Isr. Med. Assoc. J.* **2007**, *9*, 827–828. [PubMed]
12. Bajaj, S.K.; Seitz, J.P.; Qing, F. Diagnosis of acute bacterial prostatitis by Ga-67 scintigraphy and SPET-CT. *Clin. Nucl. Med.* **2008**, *33*, 813–815. [CrossRef] [PubMed]
13. Schuster, D.M.; Alazraki, N. Gallium and other agents in diseases of the lung. *Semin. Nucl. Med.* **2002**, *32*, 193–211. [CrossRef] [PubMed]
14. Segall, G.M.; McDougall, I.R. Diagnostic vale of lung uptake of indium-111 oxine-labeled white blood cells. *Am. J. Roentgenol.* **1986**, *147*, 601–606. [CrossRef] [PubMed]
15. Love, C.; Opoku-Agyemang, P.; Tomas, M.B.; Pugliese, P.V.; Bhargava, K.K.; Palestro, C.J. Pulmonary Activity on Labeled Leukocyte Images: Physiologic, Pathologic, and Imaging Correlation. *Radiographics* **2002**, *22*, 1385–1393. [CrossRef] [PubMed]

16. Signore, A.; Jamar, F.; Israel, O.; Buscombe, J.; Martin-Comin, J.; Lazzeri, E. Clinical indications, image acquisition and data interpretation for white blood cells and anti-granulocyte monoclonal antibody scintigraphy: An EANM procedural guideline. *Eur. J. Nucl. Med. Mol. Imaging.* **2018**, *10*, 1816–1831. [CrossRef] [PubMed]

17. McAfee, J.G.; Samin, A. In-111 labeled leukocytes: A review of problems in image interpretation. *Radiology* **1985**, *155*, 221–229. [CrossRef]

18. Cook, P.S.; Datz, F.L.; Disbro, M.A.; Alazraki, N.P.; Taylor, A.T. Pulmonary uptake in indium-111 leukocyte imaging: clinical significance in patients with suSPETed occult infections. *Radiology* **1984**, *150*, 557–561. [CrossRef]

19. Love, C.; Tomas, M.B.; Palestro, C.J. Pulmonary activity on labelled leukocyte images: Patterns of uptake and their significance. *Nucl. Med. Commun.* **2002**, *23*, 559–563. [CrossRef]

20. Audi, S.H.; Clough, A.V.; Haworth, S.T.; Medhora, M.; Ranji, M.; Densmore, J.C.; Jacobs, E.R. 99MTc-Hexamethylpropyleneamine Oxime Imaging for Early Detection of Acute Lung Injury in Rats Exposed to Hyperoxia or Lipopolysaccharide Treatment. *Shock* **2016**, *46*, 420–430. [CrossRef]

21. Altiay, G.; Çermik, T.F. 99mTc-HMPAO labelled white blood cell scintigraphy in the diagnosis and monitoring of response of the therapy in patients with active bronchiectasis. *Rev. Esp. Med. Nucl. Imagen. Mol.* **2012**, *31*, 9–14. [PubMed]

22. Fineman, D.; Palestro, C.J.; Kim, C.K.; Needle, L.B.; Vallabhajosula, S.; Solomon, R.W.; Goldsmith, S.J. Detection of abnormalities in febrile AIDS patients with In-111-labeled leukocyte and GA-67 scintigraphy. *Radiology* **1989**, *170*, 677–680. [CrossRef] [PubMed]

23. Palestro, C.J.; Schultz, B.L.; Horowitz, M.; Swyer, A.J. Indium-111-leukocyte and gallium-67 imaging in acute sarcoidosis: Report of two patients. *J. Nucl. Med.* **1992**, *33*, 2027–2029. [PubMed]

24. Lavender, J.P.; Lowe, J.; Barker, J.R.; Burn, J.I.; Chaudhri, M.A. Gallium 67 citrate scanning in neoplastic and inflammatory lesions. *Br. J. Radiol.* **1971**, *44*, 361–366. [CrossRef] [PubMed]

25. Hoffer, P.B.; Huberty, J.; Khazan-Bushi, H. The association of 67Ga and lactoferrin. *J. Nucl. Med.* **1977**, *18*, 713–717. [PubMed]

26. Tsan, M.F.; Chen, W.Y.; Scheffel, U.; Menon, S.; Wagner, H. Mechanism of gallium localization in inflammatory lesions. *J. Nucl. Med.* **1977**, *18*, 619.

27. Higashi, T.; Kobayashi, M.; Wakao, H.; Jinbu, Y. The relationship between 67Ga accumulation and ATP metabolism in tumor cells in vitro. *Eur. J. Nucl. Med.* **1989**, *15*, 152–156. [CrossRef] [PubMed]

28. Turoglu, T.H.; Akisik, M.F.; Naddag, S.Y.; Omar, W.S.; Kempf, J.S.; Abdel-Dayem, H.M. Tumor and Infection Localization in AIDS Patients: Ga-67 and Tl-201 Findings. *Clin. Nucl. Med.* **1998**, *23*, 446–459. [CrossRef]

29. Gambhir, S.; Ravina, M.; Rangan, K.; Dixit, M.; Barai, S.; Bomanji, J.; International Atomic Energy Agency Extra-pulmonary TB Consortium. Imaging in extrapulmonary tuberculosis. *Int. J. Infect. Dis.* **2017**, *56*, 237–247. [CrossRef]

30. Siemsen, J.K.; Grebe, S.F.; Sargent, E.N.; Wentz, D. Gallium-67 scintigraphy of pulmonary diseases as a complement to radiography. *Radiology* **1976**, *118*, 371–375. [CrossRef]

31. Siemsen, J.K.; Grebe, S.F.; Waxman, A.D. The use of gallium-67 in pulmonary disorders. *Semin. Nucl. Med.* **1978**, *8*, 235–249. [CrossRef]

32. Walsh, T.J.; Bekerman, C.; Chausow, A.; Szidon, P. The value of gallium-67 scanning in pulmonary tuberculosis. *Am. Rev. Respir. Dis.* **1985**, *132*, 746–747. [PubMed]

33. Santin, M.; Podzamczer, D.; Ricart, I.; Mascaro, J.; Ramon, J.M.; Dominguez, A.; Rufi, G.; Gudiol, F. Utility of the gallium-67 citrate scan for the early diagnosis of tuberculosis in patients infected with the human immunodeficiency virus. *Clin. Infect. Dis.* **1995**, *20*, 652–656. [CrossRef] [PubMed]

34. Goldfarb, C.R.; Colp, C.; Ongseng, F.; Finestone, H.; Havas, J. Gallium scanning in the 'new' tuberculosis. *Clin. Nucl. Med.* **1997**, *22*, 470–474. [CrossRef] [PubMed]

35. Lai, F.M.; Liam, C.K.; Paramsothy, M.; George, J. The role of 67gallium scintigraphy and high resolution computed tomography as predictors of disease activity in sputum smear-negative pulmonary tuberculosis. *Int. J. Tuberc. Lung. Dis.* **1997**, *1*, 563–569.

36. Utsunomiya, K.; Narabayashi, I.; Nishigaki, H.; Tsujimoto, K.; Kariyone, S.; Ohnishi, S. Clinical significance of thallium-201 and gallium-67 scintigraphy in pulmonary tuberculosis. *Eur. J. Nucl. Med.* **1997**, *24*, 252–257.

37. Ergün, P.; Turay, U.Y.; Ortapamuk, H.; Biber, C.; Keyf, I.A.; Çayan, C.; Erdoğan, Y. The role of gallium-67 scintigraphy and high resolution computed tomography as predictors of disease activity in sputum smear negative pulmonary tuberculosis. *Turk. Respir. J.* **2003**, *4*, 123–126.
38. Sultana, S.; Buscombe, J.R.; Hilson, A.J. In pyrexia resulting from occult tuberculosis Ga-67 citrate is still more sensitive than newer agents such as Tc-99m selusomab. *Clin. Nucl. Med.* **2005**, *30*, 414–415. [CrossRef]
39. Goswami, G.K.; Jana, S.; Santiago, J.F.; Buyukdereli, G.; Salem, S.S.; Heiba, B.; Abdel-Dayem, H.M. Discrepancy between Ga-67 citrate and F-I8 fluorodeoxyglucose positron emission tomographic scans in pulmonary infection. *Clin. Nucl. Med.* **2000**, *25*, 490–491. [CrossRef]
40. Hsu, C.C.; Huang, Y.C.; Chuang, Y.W.; Lee, T.L.; Yeh, J.J. Association between gallium-67 uptake by lung foci and sputum smear status in patients with pulmonary tuberculosis. *Nucl. Med. Commun.* **2012**, *33*, 941–946. [CrossRef]
41. Thakur, A.; Rodriguez-Rodriguez, C.; Saatchi, K.; Rose, F.; Esposito, T.; Nosrati, Z.; Andersen, P.; Christensen, D.; Hafeli, U.O.; Foged, C. Dual-Isotope SPET/CT Imaging of the Tuberculosis Subunit Vaccine H56/CAF01: Induction of Strong Systemic and Mucosal IgA and T-Cell Responses in Mice Upon Subcutaneous Prime and Intrapulmonary Boost Immunization. *Front Immunol.* **2018**, *30*, 2825.
42. Rizzato, G.; Blasi, A. A European survey on the usefulness of 67Ga lung scans in assessing sarcoidosis. Experience in 14 research centers in seven different countries. *Ann. N. Y. Acad. Sci.* **1986**, *465*, 463–478. [CrossRef] [PubMed]
43. Israel, H.L.; Albertine, K.H.; Park, C.H. Whole-body gallium 67 scans. Role in diagnosis of sarcoidosis. *Am. Rev. Respir. Dis.* **1991**, *144*, 1182–1186. [CrossRef] [PubMed]
44. Sulavik, S.B.; Spencer, R.P.; Weed, D.A.; Shapiro, H.R.; Shiue, H.R.; Castriotta, R.J. Recognition of distinctive patterns of gallium-67 distribution in sarcoidosis. *J. Nucl. Med.* **1990**, *31*, 1909–1914. [PubMed]
45. Sulavik, S.B.; Spencer, R.P.; Palestro, C.J.; Swyer, A.J.; Teirstein, A.S.; Goldsmith, S.J. Specificity and sensitivity of distinctive chest radiographic and/or 67Ga images in the noninvasive diagnosis of sarcoidosis. *Chest* **1993**, *103*, 403–409. [CrossRef] [PubMed]
46. Gelb, A.F.; Dreisen, R.B.; Epstein, J.D.; Silverthorne, J.D.; Bickel, Y.; Fields, M.; Border, W.A.; Taylor, C.R. Immune complexes, gallium lung scans, and bronchoalveolar lavage in idiopathic interstitial pneumonitis-fibrosis. *Chest* **1983**, *84*, 148–153. [CrossRef]
47. Baughman, R.P.; Fernandez, M. Radionuclide imaging in interstitial lung disease. *Curr. Opin. Pulm. Med.* **1996**, *2*, 376–379. [CrossRef]
48. Schiff, R.G.; Kabat, L.; Kamani, N. Gallium scanning in lymphoid interstitial pneumonitis of children with AIDS. *J. Nucl. Med.* **1987**, *28*, 1915–1919.
49. Nimkin, K.; Oates, E. Gallium-67 lung uptake in extrinsic hypersensitivity pneumonitis. *Clin. Nucl. Med.* **1989**, *14*, 451–452. [CrossRef]
50. Brown, D.G.; Aguirre, A.; Weaver, A. 67Gallium scanning in talc-induced pulmonary granulomatosis. *Chest* **1980**, *77*, 561–565. [CrossRef]
51. Hayes, A.A.; Thickbroom, G.W.; Guelfi, G.R.; Musk, A.W.; van der Schaaf, A.A. Computer quantitation of gallium 67 lung uptake in crocidolite (blue asbestos) workers of Western Australia. *Eur. J. Nucl. Med.* **1990**, *16*, 855–858. [CrossRef] [PubMed]
52. Deseran, M.W.; Colletti, P.M.; Ratto, D.; Ansari, A.N.; Siegel, M.E. Chronic berylliosis. Demonstration by gallium-67 imaging and magnetic resonance imaging. *Clin. Nucl. Med.* **1988**, *13*, 509–511. [CrossRef] [PubMed]
53. Kanner, R.E.; Barkman, H.W.; Rom, W.N.; Taylor, A.T., Jr. Gallium-67 citrate imaging in underground coal miners. *Am. J. Ind. Med.* **1985**, *8*, 49–55. [CrossRef] [PubMed]
54. Lin, R.Y. Severe spirometric defects in systemic lupus erythematosus. A possible role for bronchoalveolar lavage and gallium scanning. *Clin. Rheumatol.* **1987**, *6*, 276–281. [CrossRef] [PubMed]
55. Baron, M.; Feiglin, D.; Hyland, R.; Urowitz, M.B.; Shiff, B. 67Gallium scans in progressive systemic sclerosis. *Arthritis Rheum.* **1983**, *26*, 969–974. [CrossRef]
56. Yeh, S.D.; White, D.A.; Stuver-Pepe, D.E.; Caravelli, J.F.; Van Uitert, C.; Benua, R.S. Abnormal gallium scintigraphy in pulmonary alveolar proteinosis (PAP). *Clin. Nucl. Med.* **1987**, *12*, 294–297. [CrossRef]
57. Morals, J.; Carrier, L.; Gariepy, G.; Le Bel, L.; Chartrand, R.; Picard, D. Gallium-67 pulmonary uptake in eosinophilic pneumonia. *Clin. Nucl. Med.* **1988**, *13*, 41–43.

58. Alpert, L.I. Pulmonary uptake of gallium-67 in Wegener's granulomatusis. *Clin. Nucl. Med.* **1980**, *5*, 53–54. [CrossRef]
59. Javaheri, S.; Levine, B.W.; McKusick, K.A. Serial 67Ga lung scanning in pulmonary eosinophilic granuloma. *Thorax* **1979**, *34*, 822–823. [CrossRef]
60. Seabold, J.E.; Palestro, C.J.; Brown, M.L.; Datz, F.L.; Forstrom, L.A.; Greenspan, B.S.; McAfee, J.G.; Schauwecker, D.S.; Royal, H.D. Procedure guideline for gallium scintigraphy in inflammation. Society of Nuclear Medicine. *J. Nucl. Med.* **1997**, *38*, 994–997.
61. Raziei, G.; Masjedi, M.R.; Fotouhi, F.; Asli, N.I.; Shafiei, B.; Javadi, H.; Assadi, M. The role of 99mTc-MIBI scintigraphy in the management of patients with pulmonary tuberculosis. *Eur. Rev. Med. Pharm. Sci.* **2012**, *16*, 622–629.
62. Ahmadihosseini, H.; Sadeghi, R.; Zakavi, R.; Kakhki, V.R.; Kakhki, A.H. Application of technetium-99m-sestamibi in differentiation of active from inactive pulmonary tuberculosis using a single photon emission computed tomography method. *Nucl. Med. Commun.* **2008**, *29*, 690–694. [CrossRef] [PubMed]
63. Sun, S.S.; Kao, C.H. Demonstration of skeletal tuberculosis with Tc-99m (V) DMSA scintigraphy and a negative Ga-67 scan. *Clin. Nucl. Med.* **2002**, *27*, 539. [CrossRef] [PubMed]
64. Gulaldi, N.C.; Bayhan, H.; Ercan, M.T.; Kiber, M.; Oztürk, B.; Oğretensoy, M.; Bekdik, C.F. The visualization of pulmonary tuberculosis with Tc-99m (V) DMSA and Tc-99m citrate in comparison to Ga-67 citrate. *Clin. Nucl. Med.* **1995**, *20*, 1012–1014. [CrossRef]
65. Ahmadihosseini, H.; Abedib, J.; Ghodsi Rad, M.A.; Zakavi, S.R.; Knoll, P.; Mirzaeic, S.; Sadeghi, R. Diagnostic utility of 99mTc-EDDA-tricine-HYNIC-Tyr3-octreotate SPET for differentiation of active from inactive pulmonary tuberculosis. *Nucl. Med. Commun.* **2014**, *35*, 1262–1267. [CrossRef]
66. Monteiro, P.H.S.; de Souza, T.F.; Moretti, M.L.; Resende, M.R.; Mengatti, J.; de Lima, M.D.C.L.; Santos, A.O.; Ramos, C.D. SPET/CT with radiolabeled somatostatin analogues in the evaluation of systemic granulomatous infections. *Radiol. Bras.* **2017**, *50*, 378–382. [CrossRef]
67. Kwekkeboom, D.J.; Krenning, E.P.; Kho, G.S.; Breman, W.A.; Van Hagen, P.M. Somatostatin receptor imaging in patients with sarcoidosis. *Eur. J. Nucl. Med.* **1998**, *25*, 1284–1292. [CrossRef]
68. Lebtahi, R.; Crestani, B.; Belmatoug, N.; Daou, D.; Genin, R.; Dombret, M.C.; Palazzo, E.; Faraggi, M.; Aubier, M.; Le Guludec, D. Somatostatin receptor scintigraphy and gallium scintigraphy in patients with sarcoidosis. *J. Nucl. Med.* **2001**, *42*, 21–26.
69. Nishiyama, Y.; Yamamoto, Y.; Fukunaga, K.; Takinami, H.; Iwado, Y.; Satoh, K.; Ohkawa, M. Comparative evaluation of 18F-FDG PET and 67Ga scintigraphy in patients with sarcoidosis. *J. Nucl. Med.* **2006**, *47*, 1571–1576.
70. Prager, E.; Wehrschuetz, M.; Bisail, B.; Woltsche, M.; Schwarz, T.; Lanz, H.; Sorantin, E.; Aigner, R.M. Comparison of 18F-FDG and 67Ga-citrate in sarcoidosis imaging. *Nuklearmedizin* **2008**, *47*, 18–23.
71. Keijsers, R.G.; Grutters, J.C.; Thomeer, M.; Du Bois, R.M.; Van Buul, M.M.; Lavalaye, J.; Van Den Bosch, J.M.; Verzijlbergen, F.J. Imaging the inflammatory activity of sarcoidosis: sensitivity and inter observer agreement of 67Ga imaging and 18F-FDG PET. *Q. J. Nucl. Med. Mol. Imaging* **2011**, *55*, 66–71. [PubMed]
72. Kartamihardja, A.H.S.; Kurniawati, Y.; Gunawan, R. Diagnostic value of 99mTc-ethambutol scintigraphy in tuberculosis: compared to microbiological and histopathological tests. *Ann. Nucl. Med.* **2018**, *32*, 60–68. [CrossRef] [PubMed]
73. Foss, C.A.; Kulik, L.; Ordonez, A.A.; Jain, S.K.; Michael Holers, V.; Thurman, J.M.; Pomper, M.G. SPET/CT Imaging of Mycobacterium tuberculosis Infection with [125I]anti-C3d mAb. *Mol. Imaging Biol.* **2019**, *21*, 473–481. [CrossRef] [PubMed]
74. Zheng, L.; Ding, X.; Liu, K.; Feng, S.; Tang, B.; Li, Q.; Huang, D.; Yang, S. Molecular imaging of fibrosis using a novel collagen-binding peptide labelled with 99mTc on SPET/CT. *Amino Acids* **2017**, *49*, 89–101. [CrossRef]
75. Britton, K.E.; Wareham, D.W.; Das, S.S.; Solanki, K.K.; Amaral, H.; Bhatnagar, A.; Katamihardja, A.H.S.; Malamitsi, J.; Moustafa, H.M.; Soroa, V.E.; et al. Imaging bacterial infection with (99m)Tc-ciprofloxacin (Infecton). *J. Clin. Pathol.* **2002**, *55*, 817–823. [CrossRef]
76. Vinjamuri, S.; Hall, A.V.; Solanki, K.K.; Bomanji, J.B.; Siraj, Q.; O'Shaughnessy, E.M.; Das, S.S.; Britton, K.E. Comparison of99mTc-Infecton imaging with radiolabelled white-cell imaging in the evaluation of bacterial infection. *Lancet* **1996**, *347*, 233–235. [CrossRef]

77. Auletta, S.; Varani, M.; Horvat, R.; Galli, F.; Signore, A.; Hess, S. PET Radiopharmaceuticals for Specific Bacteria Imaging: A Systematic Review. *J. Clin. Med.* **2019**, *8*, 197. [CrossRef]
78. Akhtar, M.S.; Imran, M.B.; Nadeem, M.A.; Shahid, A. Antimicrobial Peptides as Infection Imaging Agents: Better Than Radiolabeled Antibiotics. *Int. J. Pept.* **2012**, *2012*, 1–19. [CrossRef]
79. King, G.G.; Eberl, S.; Salome, C.M.; Meikle, S.R.; Woolcock, A.J. Airway closure measured by a technegas bolus and SPECT. *Am. J. Respir. Crit. Care Med.* **1997**, *155*, 682–688. [CrossRef]
80. Farrow, C.E.; Salome, C.M.; Harris, B.E.; Bailey, D.L.; Bailey, E.; Berend, N.; Young, I.H.; King, G.G. Airway closure on imaging relates to airway hyperresponsiveness and peripheral airway disease in asthma. *J. Appl. Physiol.* **2012**, *113*, 958–966. [CrossRef]
81. Farrow, C.E.; Salome, C.M.; Harris, B.E.; Bailey, D.L.; Berend, N.; King, G.G. Peripheral ventilation heterogeneity determines the extent of bronchoconstriction in asthma. *J. Appl. Physiol.* **2017**, *123*, 1188–1194. [CrossRef] [PubMed]
82. Bajc, M.; Chen, Y.; Wang, J.; Li, X.Y.; Shen, W.M.; Wang, C.Z.; Huang, H.; Lindqvist, A.; He, X.Y. Identifying the heterogeneity of COPD by V/P SPECT: a new tool for improving the diagnosis of parenchymal defects and grading the severity of small airways disease. *Int. J. Chron. Obs. Pulmon. Dis.* **2017**, *12*, 1579–1587. [CrossRef] [PubMed]
83. Karacavus, S.; Intepe, Y.S. The role of Tc-99m DTPA aerosol scintigraphy in the differential diagnosis of COPD and asthma. *Clin. Respir. J.* **2015**, *9*, 189–195. [CrossRef] [PubMed]
84. Mochizuki, T.; Tsukamoto, E.; Kuge, Y.; Kanegae, K.; Zhao, S.; Hikosaka, K.; Hikosaka, M.; Hikosaka, M.; Tamaki, N. FDG uptake and glucose transporter subtype expressions in experimental tumor and inflammation models. *J. Nucl. Med.* **2001**, *42*, 1551–1555.
85. Kubota, R.; Yamada, S.; Kubota, K.; Ishiwata, K.; Tamahashi, N.; Ido, T. Intratumoral distribution of fluorine-18-fluorodeoxyglucose in vivo: high accumulation in macrophages and granulation tissues studied by microautoradiography. *J. Nucl. Med.* **1992**, *33*, 1972–1980.
86. Bell, G.I.; Burant, C.F.; Takeda, J.; Gould, G.W. Structure and function of mammalian facilitative sugar transporters. *J. Biol. Chem.* **1993**, *268*, 19161–19164.
87. Pauwels, E.K.; Ribeiro, M.J.; Stoot, J.H.; McCready, V.R.; Bourguignon, M.; Mazière, B. FDG accumulation and tumor biology. *Nucl. Med. Biol.* **1998**, *25*, 317–322. [CrossRef]
88. Zhuang, H.; Alavi, A. 18-fluorodeoxyglucose positron emission tomographic imaging in the detection and monitoring of infection and inflammation. *Semin. Nucl. Med.* **2002**, *32*, 47–59. [CrossRef]
89. Paik, J.Y.; Lee, K.H.; Choe, Y.S.; Choi, Y.; Kim, B.T. Augmented 18F-FDG uptake in activated monocytes occurs during the priming process and involves tyrosine kinases and protein kinase C. *J. Nucl. Med.* **2004**, *45*, 124–128.
90. Chang, J.M.; Lee, H.J.; Goo, J.M.; Lee, H.Y.; Lee, J.J.; Chung, J.K.; Im, J.G. False positive and false negative FDG-PET scans in various thoracic diseases. *Korean J. Radiol.* **2006**, *7*, 57–69. [CrossRef]
91. Sathekge, M.M.; Maes, A.; Pottel, H.; Stoltz, A.; van de Wiele, C. Dual time-point FDG PET-CT for differentiating benign from malignant solitary pulmonary nodules in a TB endemic area. *S. Afr. Med. J.* **2010**, *100*, 598–601. [CrossRef] [PubMed]
92. Chen, C.J.; Lee, B.F.; Yao, W.J.; Cheng, L.; Wu, P.S.; Chu, C.L.; Chiu, N.T. Dual-phase 18F-FDG PET in the diagnosis of pulmonary nodules with an initial standard uptake value less than 2.5. *Am. J. Roentgenol.* **2008**, *191*, 475–479. [CrossRef] [PubMed]
93. Kaneko, K.; Sadashima, E.; Irie, K.; Hayashi, A.; Masunari, S.; Yoshida, T.; Omagari, J. Assessment of FDG retention differences between the FDG-avid benign pulmonary lesion and primary lung cancer using dual-time-point FDG-PET imaging. *Ann. Nucl. Med.* **2013**, *27*, 329–339. [CrossRef] [PubMed]
94. Heysell, S.K.; Thomas, T.A.; Sifri, C.D.; Rehm, P.K.; Houpt, E.R. 18-Fluorodeoxyglucose positron emission tomography for tuberculosis diagnosis and management: A case series. *BMC Pulm. Med.* **2013**, *21*, 13–14. [CrossRef]
95. Franzius, C.; Biermann, M.; Hülskamp, G.; Frosch, M.; Roth, J.; Sciuk, J.; Schober, O. Therapy monitoring in aspergillosis using F-18 FDG positron emission tomography. *Clin. Nucl. Med.* **2001**, *26*, 232–233. [CrossRef]
96. Reuter, S.; Schirrmeister, H.; Kratzer, W.; Dreweck, C.; Reske, S.N.; Kern, P. Pericystic metabolic activity in alveolar echinococcosis: assessment and follow-up by positron emission tomography. *Clin. Infect. Dis.* **1999**, *29*, 1157–1163. [CrossRef]

97. Reuter, S.; Buck, A.; Manfras, B.; Kratzer, W.; Seitz, H.M.; Darge, K.; Reske, S.N.; Kern, P. Structured treatment interruption in patients with alveolar echinococcosis. *Hepatology* **2004**, *39*, 509–517. [CrossRef]
98. Stumpe, K.D.; Renner-Schneiter, E.C.; Kuenzle, A.K.; Grimm, F.; Kadry, Z.; Clavein, P.A.; Deplazes, P.; von Schulthess, G.K.; Muellhaupt, B.; Amman, R.W.; et al. F-18-fluorodeoxyglucose (FDG) positron-emission tomography of Echinococcus multilocularis liver lesions: proSPETive evaluation of its value for diagnosis and follow-up during benzimidazole therapy. *Infect.* **2007**, *35*, 11–18. [CrossRef]
99. Bleeker-Rovers, C.P.; Warris, A.; Drenth, J.P.; Corstens, F.H.; Oyen, W.J.; Kullberg, B.J. Diagnosis of Candida lung abscesses by 18F-fluorodeoxyglucose positron emission tomography. *Clin. Microbiol. Infect.* **2005**, *11*, 493–495. [CrossRef]
100. Glaudemans, A.W.; de Vries, E.F.; Galli, F.; Dierckx, R.A.; Slart, R.H.; Signore, A. The use of (18)F-FDG-PET/CT for diagnosis and treatment monitoring of inflammatory and infectious diseases. *Clin. Dev. Immunol.* **2013**, *2013*, 623036. [CrossRef]
101. Mostard, R.L.; van Kroonenburgh, M.J.; Drent, M. The role of the PET scan in the management of sarcoidosis. *Curr. Opin. Pulm. Med.* **2013**, *19*, 538–544. [CrossRef] [PubMed]
102. Teirstein, A.S.; Machac, J.; Almeida, O.; Lu, P.; Padilla, M.L.; Iannuzzi, M.C. Results of 188 whole-body fluorodeoxyglucose positron emission tomography scans in 137 patients with sarcoidosis. *Chest* **2007**, *132*, 1949–1953. [CrossRef] [PubMed]
103. Coker, R.K. Management strategies for pulmonary sarcoidosis. *Clin. Risk. Manag.* **2009**, *5*, 575–584. [CrossRef] [PubMed]
104. Klein, M.; Cohen-Cymberknoh, M.; Armoni, S.; Shoseyov, D.; Chisin, R.; Orevi, M.; Freedman, N.; Kerem, E. 18F-fluorodeoxyglucose-PET/CT imaging of lungs in patients with cystic fibrosis. *Chest* **2009**, *136*, 1220–1228. [CrossRef]
105. Amin, R.; Charron, M.; Grinblat, L.; Shammas, A.; Grasemann, H.; Graniel, K.; Ciet, P.; Tiddens, H.; Ratjen, F. Cystic fibrosis: Detecting changes in airway inflammation with FDG PET/CT. *Radiology* **2012**, *264*, 868–875. [CrossRef]
106. Cremers, J.P.; Van Kroonenburgh, M.J.; Mostard, R.L.; Vöö, S.A.; Wijnen, P.A.; Koek, G.H.; Drent, M. Extent of disease activity assessed by 18F-FDG PET/CT in a Dutch sarcoidosis population. *Sarcoidosis Vasc. Diffus. Lung Dis.* **2014**, *31*, 37–45.
107. Dolovich, M.B.; Schuster, D.P. Positron emission tomography and computed tomography versus positron emission tomography computed tomography: tools for imaging the lung. *Proc. Am. Thorax Soc.* **2007**, *4*, 328–333. [CrossRef]
108. Groves, A.M.; Win, T.; Screaton, N.J.; Berovic, M.; Endozo, R.; Booth, H.; Kayani, I.; Menezes, L.J.; Dickson, J.C.; Ell, P.J. Idiopathic pulmonary fibrosis and diffuse parenchymal lung disease: implications from initial experience with 18F-FDG PET/CT. *J. Nucl. Med.* **2009**, *50*, 538–545. [CrossRef]
109. Chen, D.L.; Wang, X.; Yamamoto, S.; Carpenter, D.; Engle, J.T.; Li, W.; Lin, X.; Kreisel, D.; Krupnick, A.S.; Huang, H.J.; et al. Increased T cell glucose uptake reflects acute rejection in lung grafts. *Am. J. Transpl.* **2013**, *13*, 2540–2549. [CrossRef]
110. Kothekar, E.; Borja, A.J.; Gerke, O.; Werner, T.J.; Alavi, A.; Revheim, M.E. Assessing respiratory muscle activity with 18F-FDG-PET/CT in patients with COPD. *Am. J. Nucl. Med. Mol. Imaging.* **2019**, *9*, 309–315.
111. Braune, J.; Hofheinz, F.; Bluth, T.; Kiss, T.; Wittenstein, J.; Scharffenberg, M.; Kotzerke, J.; Gama de Abreu, M. Comparison of static 18F-FDG-PET/CT (SUV, SUR) and dynamic 18F-FDG-PET/CT (Ki) for quantification of pulmonary inflammation in acute lung injury. *J. Nucl. Med.* **2019**, *60*, 1629–1634. [CrossRef] [PubMed]
112. Verleden, S.E.; Gheysens, O.; Goffin, K.E.; Vanaudenaerde, B.M.; Verbeken, E.K.; Weynand, B.; Van Raemdonck, D.E.; Verleden, G.M.; Vos, R. Role of 18F-FDG PET/CT in restrictive allograft syndrome after lung transplantation. *Transplantation* **2019**, *103*, 823–831. [CrossRef]
113. Hara, T.; Kosaka, N.; Suzuki, T.; Kudo, K.; Niino, H. Uptake rates of 18F-fluorodeoxyglucose and 11C-choline in lung cancer and pulmonary tuberculosis: A positron tomography study. *Chest* **2003**, *124*, 893–901. [CrossRef] [PubMed]
114. Liu, Q.; Peng, Z.M.; Liu, Q.W.; Yao, S.Z.; Zhang, L.; Meng, L.; Chen, J.H. The role of 11C-choline positron emission tomography– computed tomography and videomediastinoscopy in the evaluation of diseases of middle mediastinum. *Chin. Med. J.* **2006**, *119*, 634–639. [CrossRef] [PubMed]
115. Hara, T.; Inagaki, K.; Kosaka, N.; Morita, T. Sensitive detection of mediastinal lymph node metastasis of lung cancer with 11C-choline PET. *J. Nucl. Med.* **2000**, *41*, 1507–1513.

116. Norikane, T.; Yamamoto, Y.; Maeda, Y.; Noma, T.; Dobashi, H.; Nishiyama, Y. Comparative evaluation of 18F-FLT and 18F-FDG for detecting cardiac and extra-cardiac thoracic involvement in patients with newly diagnosed sarcoidosis. *Ejnmmi Res.* **2017**, *7*, 69. [CrossRef]
117. Win, T.; Screaton, N.J.; Porter, J.; Endozo, R.; Wild, D.; Kayani, I.; Dickson, J.; Shortman, R.I.; Reubi, J.C.; Ell, P.J.; et al. Novel positron emission tomography/computed tomography of diffuse parenchymal lung disease combining a labeled somatostatin receptor analogue and 2-deoxy-2[18F]fluoro-D-glucose. *Mol. Imaging* **2012**, *11*, 91–98. [CrossRef]
118. Ordenez, A.A.; DeMarco, V.P.; Klunk, M.H.; Pokkali, S.; Jain, S.K. Imaging chronic tuberculosis lesions using sodium [18F] Fluoride positron emission tomography in mice. *Mol. Imaging. Biol.* **2015**, *17*, 609–614. [CrossRef]
119. Mirsadraee, S.; Marin, A.; Jenkins, W.; Connell, M.; Tavares, A.; Flecher, A.; Hirani, N.; van Beek, E.J. The identification of systemic integrin activation in idiopathic and systemic sclerosis pulmonary fibrosis using 18F-fluciclatide positron emission tomography. *Insights Imaging* **2016**, *7*, S424.
120. Knudsen, L.; Atochina-Vasserman, E.N.; Massa, C.B.; Birkelbach, B.; Guo, C.J.; Scott, P.; Haenni, B.; Beers, M.F.; Ochs, M.; Gow, A.J. The role of inducible nitric oxide synthase for interstitial remodeling of alveolar septa in surfactant protein D-deficient mice. *Am. J. Physiol. Lung Cell. Mol. Physiol.* **2015**, *309*, 959–969. [CrossRef]
121. Zhou, D.; Lee, H.; Rothfuss, J.M.; Chen, D.L.; Ponde, D.E.; Welch, M.J.; March, R.H. Design and synthesis of 2-amino-4-methylpyridine analogues as inhibitors for inducible nitric oxide synthase and in vivo evaluation of [18F]6-(2-fluoropropyl)-4-methyl-pyridin-2-amine as a potential PET tracer for inducible nitric oxide synthase. *J. Med. Chem.* **2009**, *52*, 2443–2453. [CrossRef] [PubMed]
122. Huang, H.L.; Isakow, W.; Byers, D.E.; Engle, J.T.; Griffin, E.A.; Kemp, D.; Brody, S.L.; Gropler, R.J.; Miller, J.P.; Chu, W.; et al. Imaging pulmonary inducible nitric oxide synthase expression with PET. *J. Nucl. Med.* **2015**, *56*, 76–81. [CrossRef] [PubMed]
123. Ebenhan., T.; Mokaleng, B.; Venter, J.; Kruger, H.; Zeevaart, J.; Sathekge, M. Preclinical assessment of a 68Ga-DOTA-functionalized depsipeptide as a radiodiagnostic infection imaging agent. *Molecules* **2017**, *22*, 1403. [CrossRef] [PubMed]
124. Mukherjee, A.; Bhatt, J.; Shinto, A.; Korde, A.; Kumar, M.; Kamaleshwaran, K.; Joseph, J.; Sarma, H.D.; Dash, A. 68Ga-NOTA-ubiquicidin fragment for PET imaging of infection: From bench to bedside. *J. Pharm. Biomed. Anal.* **2018**, *159*, 245–251. [CrossRef] [PubMed]
125. Ebenhan, T.; Zeevaart, J.R.; Venter, J.D.; Govender, T.; Kruger, G.H.; Jarvis, N.V.; Sathekge, M. Preclinical evaluation of 68Ga-labeled 1,4,7-Triazacyclononane-1,4,7-Triacetic acid-ubiquicidin as a radioligand for PET infection imaging. *J. Nucl. Med.* **2014**, *55*, 308–314. [CrossRef] [PubMed]
126. Kapur, S.; Bhalla, A.S.; Jana, M. Pediatric Chest MRI: A Review. *Indian J. Pediatr.* **2019**, *86*, 842–853. [CrossRef]
127. Richard, J.-C.; Chen, D.L.; Ferkol, T.; Schuster, D.P. Molecular imaging for pediatric lung diseases. *Pediatr. Pulmonol.* **2004**, *37*, 286–296. [CrossRef]
128. Syrjala, H.; Broas, M.; Ohtonen, P.; Jartti, A.; Pääkkö, E. Chest magnetic resonance imaging for pneumonia diagnosis in outpatients with lower respiratory tract infection. *Eur. Respir. J.* **2016**, *49*, 1601303. [CrossRef]
129. Hirsch, W.; Sorge, I.; Krohmer, S.; Weber, D.; Meier, K.; Till, H. MRI of the lungs in children. *Eur. J. Radiol.* **2008**, *68*, 278–288. [CrossRef]
130. Poelmans, J.; Hillen, A.; Vanherp, L.; Govaerts, K.; Maertens, J.; Dresselaers, T.; Himmelreich, U.; Lagrou, K.; Vande Velde, G. Longitudinal, in vivo assessment of invasive pulmonary aspergillosis in mice by computed tomography and magnetic resonance imaging. *Lab. Investig.* **2016**, *96*, 692–704. [CrossRef]
131. Tournebize, R.; Doan, B.-T.; Dillies, M.-A.; Maurin, S.; Beloeil, J.-C.; Sansonetti, P.J. Magnetic resonance imaging of Klebsiella pneumoniae-induced pneumonia in mice. *Cell. Microbiol.* **2006**, *8*, 33–43. [CrossRef] [PubMed]
132. Marzola, P.; Lanzoni, A.; Nicolato, E.; Di Modugno, V.; Cristofori, P.; Osculati, F.; Sbarbati, A. 1H MRI of pneumococcal pneumonia in a murine model. *J. Magn. Reson. Imaging* **2005**, *22*, 170–174. [CrossRef] [PubMed]
133. Hoerr, V.; Faber, C. Magnetic resonance imaging characterization of microbial infections. *J. Pharm. Biomed. Anal.* **2014**, *93*, 136–146. [CrossRef] [PubMed]
134. Asanuma, T.; Kawahara, T.; Inanami, O.; Nakao, M.; Nakaya, K.; Ito, A.; Takiguchi, M.; Hashimoto, A.; Kuwabara, M. Magnetic resonance imaging of alveolar echinococcosis experimentally induced in the rat lung. *J. Vet. Med. Sci.* **2006**, *68*, 15–20. [CrossRef]

135. Mc Fadden, R.G.; Carr, T.J.; Mackie, I.D. Thoracic magnetic resonance imaging in the evaluation of HIV-1/AIDS pneumonitis. *Chest* **1992**, *101*, 371–374. [CrossRef]
136. Kuhlman, J.E. Pneumocystic infections: the radiologist's perSPETive. *Radiology* **1996**, *198*, 623–635. [CrossRef]
137. Nishimura, A.; Yamaguchi, H.; Ito, Y.; Tokumoto, S.; Toyoshima, D.; Kasai, M.; Maruyama, A. Empyema necessitatis due to Pseudomonas aeruginosa in a child with cerebral palsy. *J. Infect. Public Health* **2019**, *13*, 140–142. [CrossRef]
138. Liszewski, M.C.; Görkem, S.; Sodhi, K.S.; Lee, E.Y. Lung magnetic resonance imaging for pneumonia in children. *Pediatr. Radiol.* **2017**, *47*, 1420–1430. [CrossRef]
139. Ekinci, A.; Yucel Ucarkus, T.; Okur, A.; Ozturk, M.; Dogan, S. MRI of pneumonia in immunocompromised patients: comparison with CT. *Diagn. Interv. Radiol.* **2017**, *23*, 22–28. [CrossRef]
140. Ozcan, H.N.; Gormez, A.; Ozsurekci, Y.; Karakaya, J.; Oguz, B.; Unal, S.; Haliloglu, M. Magnetic resonance imaging of pulmonary infection in immunocompromised children: Comparison with multidetector computed tomography. *Pediatric Radiol.* **2016**, *47*, 146–153. [CrossRef]
141. Yan, C.; Tan, X.; Wei, Q.; Feng, R.; Li, C.; Wu, Y.; Xu, Y. Lung MRI of invasive fungal infection at 3 Tesla: Evaluation of five different pulse sequences and comparison with multidetector computed tomography (MDCT). *Eur. Radiol.* **2014**, *25*, 550–557. [CrossRef] [PubMed]
142. Yan, C.; Xu, J.; Xiong, W.; Wei, Q.; Feng, R.; Wu, Y.; Xu, Y. Use of intravoxel incoherent motion diffusion-weighted MR imaging for assessment of treatment response to invasive fungal infection in the lung. *Eur. Radiol.* **2016**, *27*, 212–221. [CrossRef] [PubMed]
143. Ohno, Y.; Hatabu, H.; Takenaka, D.; Adachi, S.; Kono, M.; Sugimura, K. Solitary Pulmonary Nodules: Potential Role of Dynamic MR Imaging in Management—Initial Experience. *Radiology* **2002**, *224*, 503–511. [CrossRef] [PubMed]
144. Chung, M.H.; Lee, H.G.; Kwon, S.S.; Park, S.H. MR imaging of solitary pulmonary lesion: Emphasis on tuberculomas and comparison with tumors. *J. Magn. Reson. Imaging* **2000**, *11*, 629–637. [CrossRef]
145. Chung, J.H.; Huitt, G.; Yagihashi, K.; Hobbs, S.B.; Faino, A.V.; Bolster, B.D.; Lynch, D.A. Proton Magnetic Resonance Imaging for Initial Assessment of Isolated Mycobacterium avium Complex Pneumonia. *Ann. Am. Thorac. Soc.* **2016**, *13*, 49–57. [CrossRef]
146. Blum, U.; Windfuhr, M.; Buitrago-Tellez, C.; Sigmund, G.; Herbst, E.W.; Langer, M. Invasive Pulmonary Aspergillosis. *Chest* **1994**, *106*, 1156–1161. [CrossRef]
147. Sodhi, K.S.; Gupta, P.; Shrivastav, A.; Saxena, A.K.; Mathew, J.L.; Singh, M.; Agarwal, R. Evaluation of 3 T lung magnetic resonance imaging in children with allergic bronchopulmonary aspergillosis: Pilot study. *Eur. J. Radiol.* **2019**, *111*, 88–92. [CrossRef]
148. Moore, E.; Webb, W.; Muller, N.; Sollitto, R. MRI of pulmonary airspace disease: experimental model and preliminary clinical results. *Am. J. Roentgenol.* **1986**, *146*, 1123–1128. [CrossRef]
149. Cohen, M.D.; Scales, R.L.; Eigen, H.; Scott, P.; Tepper, R.; Cory, D.A.; Smith, J.A. Evaluation of pulmonary parenchymal disease by magnetic resonance imaging. *Br. J. Radiol.* **1987**, *60*, 223–230. [CrossRef]
150. Montella, S.; Maglione, M.; Bruzzese, D.; Mollica, C.; Pignata, C.; Aloj, G.; Santamaria, F. Magnetic resonance imaging is an accurate and reliable method to evaluate non-cystic fibrosis paediatric lung disease. *Respirology* **2011**, *17*, 87–91. [CrossRef]
151. Owrangi, A.M.; Parraga, G. Chest MRI in children: Why bother? *Respirology* **2011**, *17*, 3–4. [CrossRef] [PubMed]
152. Jacob, R.E.; Amidan, B.G.; Soelberg, J.; Minard, K.R. In vivo MRI of altered proton signal intensity and T2 relaxation in a bleomycin model of pulmonary inflammation and fibrosis. *J. Magn. Reson. Imaging* **2010**, *31*, 1091–1099. [CrossRef] [PubMed]
153. Yi, C.A.; Lee, K.S.; Han, J.; Chung, M.P.; Chung, M.J.; Shin, K.M. 3-T MRI for Differentiating Inflammation- and Fibrosis-Predominant Lesions of Usual and Nonspecific Interstitial Pneumonia: Comparison Study with Pathologic Correlation. *Am. J. Roentgenol.* **2008**, *190*, 878–885. [CrossRef] [PubMed]
154. Wallace, W.A.; Fitch, P.M.; Simpson, A.J.; Howie, S.E. Inflammation-associated remodelling and fibrosis in the lung – a process and an end point. *Int. J. Exp. Pathol.* **2007**, *88*, 103–110. [CrossRef] [PubMed]
155. Romei, C.; Turturici, L.; Tavanti, L.; Miedema, J.; Fiorini, S.; Marletta, M.; Ciet, P. The use of chest magnetic resonance imaging in interstitial lung disease: a systematic review. *Eur. Respir. Rev.* **2018**, *27*, 180062. [CrossRef]

156. Lutterbey, G.; Grohé, C.; Gieseke, J.; von Falkenhausen, M.; Morakkabati, N.; Wattjes, M.P.; Schild, H.H. Initial experience with lung-MRI at 3.0T: Comparison with CT and clinical data in the evaluation of interstitial lung disease activity. *Eur. J. Radiol.* **2007**, *61*, 256–261. [CrossRef]
157. Cutillo, A.G.; Morris, A.H.; Ailion, D.C.; Durney, C.H. Clinical Implications of Nuclear Magnetic Resonance Lung Research. *Chest* **1989**, *96*, 643–652. [CrossRef]
158. Buzan, M.T.A.; Eichinger, M.; Kreuter, M.; Kauczor, H.-U.; Herth, F.J.; Warth, A.; Dinkel, J. T2 mapping of CT remodelling patterns in interstitial lung disease. *Eur. Radiol.* **2015**, *25*, 3167–3174. [CrossRef]
159. Müller, C.d.S.; Warszawiak, D.; Paiva, E.d.S.; Escuissato, D.L. Pulmonary magnetic resonance imaging is similar to chest tomography in detecting inflammation in patients with systemic sclerosis. *Rev. Bras. Reumatol.* **2017**, *57*, 419–424. [CrossRef]
160. Buzan, M.T.A.; Wetscherek, A.; Heussel, C.P.; Kreuter, M.; Herth, F.J.; Warth, A.; Dinkel, J. Texture analysis using proton density and T2 relaxation in patients with histological usual interstitial pneumonia (UIP) or nonspecific interstitial pneumonia (NSIP). *PloS ONE* **2017**, *12*, e0177689. [CrossRef]
161. Gaeta, M.; Blandino, A.; Scribano, E.; Minutoli, F.; Barone, M.; Andò, F.; Pandolfo, I. Chronic Infiltrative Lung Diseases. *Chest* **2000**, *117*, 1173–1178. [CrossRef] [PubMed]
162. Bianchi, A.; Ozier, A.; Ousova, O.; Raffard, G.; Crémillieux, Y. Ultrashort-TE MRI longitudinal study and characterization of a chronic model of asthma in mice: Inflammation and bronchial remodeling assessment. *NMR Biomed.* **2013**, *26*, 1451–1459. [CrossRef] [PubMed]
163. Caravan, P.; Yang, Y.; Zachariah, R.; Schmitt, A.; Mino-Kenudson, M.; Chen, H.H.; Lanuti, M. Molecular Magnetic Resonance Imaging of Pulmonary Fibrosis in Mice. *Am. J. Respir. Cell Mol. Biol.* **2013**, *49*, 1120–1126. [CrossRef] [PubMed]
164. Vogel-Claussen, J.; Renne, J.; Hinrichs, J.; Schönfeld, C.; Gutberlet, M.; Schaumann, F.; Hohlfeld, J.M. Quantification of Pulmonary Inflammation after Segmental Allergen Challenge Using Turbo-Inversion Recovery-Magnitude Magnetic Resonance Imaging. *Am. J. Respir. Crit. Care Med.* **2014**, *189*, 650–657. [CrossRef]
165. Evans, R.L.; Changani, K.K.; Hotee, S.; Pindoria, K.; Campbell, S.; Nials, A.T.; Kidd, E.J. Pulmonary edema measured by MRI correlates with late-phase response to allergen challenge. *Exp. Lung Res.* **2015**, *41*, 189–198. [CrossRef]
166. Quintana, H.K.; Cannet, C.; Schaeublin, E.; Zurbruegg, S.; Sugar, R.; Mazzoni, L.; Beckmann, N. Identification with MRI of the pleura as a major site of the acute inflammatory effects induced by ovalbumin and endotoxin challenge in the airways of the rat. *Am. J. Physiol. Lung Cell. Mol. Physiol.* **2006**, *291*, L651–L657. [CrossRef]
167. Renne, J.; Hinrichs, J.; Schönfeld, C.; Gutberlet, M.; Winkler, C.; Faulenbach, C.; Vogel-Claussen, J. Noninvasive Quantification of Airway Inflammation Following Segmental Allergen Challenge with Functional MR Imaging: A Proof of Concept Study. *Radiology* **2015**, *274*, 267–275. [CrossRef]
168. Castro, M.; Fain, S.B.; Hoffman, E.A.; Gierada, D.S.; Erzurum, S.C.; Wenzel, S. Lung imaging in asthmatic patients: The picture is clearer. *J. Allergy Clin. Immunol.* **2011**, *128*, 467–478. [CrossRef]
169. Aysola, R.; de Lange, E.E.; Castro, M.; Altes, T.A. Demonstration of the heterogeneous distribution of asthma in the lungs using CT and hyperpolarized helium-3 MRI. *J. Magn. Reson. Imaging* **2010**, *32*, 1379–1387. [CrossRef]
170. Haczku, A.; Emami, K.; Fischer, M.C.; Kadlecek, S.; Ishii, M.; Panettieri, R.A.; Rizi, R.R. Hyperpolarized 3He MRI in Asthma. *Acad. Radiol.* **2005**, *12*, 1362–1370. [CrossRef]
171. Fiel, S.B.; Friedman, A.C.; Caroline, D.F.; Radecki, P.D.; Faerber, E.; Grumbach, K. Magnetic Resonance Imaging in Young Adults with Cystic Fibrosis. *Chest* **1987**, *91*, 181–184. [CrossRef] [PubMed]
172. Biederer, J.; Mirsadraee, S.; Beer, M.; Molinari, F.; Hintze, C.; Bauman, G.; Puderbach, M. MRI of the lung (3/3)—current applications and future perSPETives. *Insights Imaging* **2012**, *3*, 373–386. [CrossRef] [PubMed]
173. Wielpütz, M.O.; Heußel, C.P.; Herth, F.J.F.; Kauczor, H.-U. Radiological Diagnosis in Lung Disease. *Dtsch. Aerzteblatt Online* **2014**, *111*, 181–187. [CrossRef] [PubMed]
174. Ciet, P.; Serra, G.; Andrinopoulou, E.R.; Bertolo, S.; Ros, M.; Catalano, C.; Morana, G. Diffusion weighted imaging in cystic fibrosis disease: beyond morphological imaging. *Eur. Radiol.* **2016**, *26*, 3830–3839. [CrossRef] [PubMed]
175. Ciet, P.; Bertolo, S.; Ros, M.; Andrinopoulou, E.R.; Tavano, V.; Lucca, F.; Morana, G. Detection and monitoring of lung inflammation in cystic fibrosis during respiratory tract exacerbation using diffusion-weighted magnetic resonance imaging. *Eur. Respir. J.* **2017**, *50*, 1601437. [CrossRef]

176. Tiddens, H.A.W.M.; Stick, S.M.; Wild, J.M.; Ciet, P.; Parker, G.J.M.; Koch, A.; Vogel-Claussen, J. Respiratory tract exacerbations revisited: Ventilation, inflammation, perfusion, and structure (VIPS) monitoring to redefine treatment. *Pediatr. Pulmonol.* **2015**, *50*, S57–S65. [CrossRef]

177. Baues, M.; Dasgupta, A.; Ehling, J.; Prakash, J.; Boor, P.; Tacke, F.; Kiessling, F.; Lammers, T. Fibrosis imaging: Current concepts and future directions. *Adv. Drug. Deliv. Rev.* **2017**, *121*, 9–26. [CrossRef]

178. Toma, P.; Bertaina, A.; Castagnola, E.; Colafati, G.S.; D'Andrea, M.L.; Finocchi, A.; Granata, C. Fungal infections of the lung in children. *Pediatr. Radiol.* **2016**, *46*, 1856–1865. [CrossRef]

179. Sodhi, K.S.; Khandelwal, N.; Saxena, A.K.; Singh, M.; Agarwal, R.; Bhatia, A.; Lee, E.Y. Rapid lung MRI in children with pulmonary infections: Time to change our diagnostic algorithms. *J. Magn. Reson. Imaging* **2016**, *43*, 1196–1206. [CrossRef]

180. Bray, M.; Lawler, J.; Paragas, J.; Jahrling, P.B.; Mollura, D.J. Molecular Imaging of Influenza and Other Emerging Respiratory Viral Infections. *J. Infect. Dis.* **2011**, *203*, 1348–1359. [CrossRef]

181. Peltola, V.; Ruuskanen, O.; Svedström, E. Magnetic resonance imaging of lung infections in children. *Pediatr. Radiol.* **2008**, *38*, 1225–1231. [CrossRef] [PubMed]

182. Rieger, C.; Herzog, P.; Eibel, R.; Fiegl, M.; Ostermann, H. Pulmonary MRI—a new approach for the evaluation of febrile neutropenic patients with malignancies. *Support. Care Cancer* **2007**, *16*, 599–606. [CrossRef] [PubMed]

183. Sodhi, K.S.; Bhatia, A.; Khandelwal, N. Rapid lung magnetic resonance imaging in children with pulmonary infection. *Pediatr. Radiol.* **2017**, *47*, 764–765. [CrossRef] [PubMed]

184. Serra, G.; Milito, C.; Mitrevski, M.; Granata, G.; Martini, H.; Pesce, A.M.; Quinti, I. Lung MRI as a Possible Alternative to CT Scan for Patients With Primary Immune Deficiencies and Increased Radiosensitivity. *Chest* **2011**, *140*, 1581–1589. [CrossRef] [PubMed]

185. Heusch, P.; Köhler, J.; Wittsack, H.J.; Heusner, T.A.; Buchbender, C.; Poeppel, T.D.; Nensa, F.; Wetter, A.; Gauler, T.; Hartung, V.; et al. Hybrid [^{18}F]-FDG PET/MRI including non-Gaussian diffusion-weighted imaging (DWI): Preliminary results in non-small cell lung cancer (NSCLC). *Eur. J. Radiol.* **2013**, *82*, 2055–2060. [CrossRef]

186. Raad, R.A.; Friedman, K.P.; Heacock, L.; Ponzo, F.; Melsaether, A.; Chandarana, H. Outcome of small lung nodules missed on hybrid PET/MRI in patients with primary malignancy. *J. Magn. Reson. Imaging* **2016**, *43*, 504–511. [CrossRef]

187. Heusch, P.; Buchbender, C.; Köhler, J.; Nensa, F.; Gauler, T.; Gomez, B.; Reis, H.; Stamatis, G.; Kühl, H.; Hartung, V.; et al. Thoracic staging in lung cancer: prospective comparison of 18F-FDG PET/MR imaging and 18F-FDG PET/CT. *J. Nucl. Med.* **2014**, *55*, 373–378. [CrossRef]

188. Lee, S.M.; Goo, J.M.; Park, C.M.; Yoon, S.H.; Paeng, J.C.; Cheon, G.J.; Kim, Y.T.; Park, Y.S. Preoperative staging of non-small cell lung cancer: prospective comparison of PET/MR and PET/CT. *Eur. Radiol.* **2016**, *26*, 3850–3857. [CrossRef]

189. Ohno, Y.; Koyama, H.; Yoshikawa, T.; Takenaka, D.; Seki, S.; Yui, M.; Yamagata, H.; Aoyagi, K.; Matsumoto, S.; Sugimura, K. Three-way Comparison of Whole-Body MR, Coregistered Whole-Body FDG PET/MR, and Integrated Whole-Body FDG PET/CT Imaging: TNM and Stage Assessment Capability for Non-Small Cell Lung Cancer Patients. *Radiology* **2015**, *275*, 849–861. [CrossRef]

190. Schaarschmidt, B.M.; Buchbender, C.; Nensa, F.; Grueneisen, J.; Gomez, B.; Köhler, J.; Reis, H.; Ruhlmann, V.; Umutlu, L.; Heusch, P. Correlation of the apparent diffusion coefficient (ADC) with the standardized uptake value (SUV) in lymph node metastases of non-small cell lung cancer (NSCLC) patients using hybrid 18F-FDG PET/MRI. *PloS ONE* **2015**, *10*, e0120606. [CrossRef]

191. Thomas, B.A.; Molton, J.S.; Leek, F.; Pang, Y.; Totman, J.J.; Paton, N.I.; Townsend, D.W. A comparison of 18F-FDG PET/MR with PET/CT in pulmonary tuberculosis. *Nucl. Med. Commun.* **2017**, *38*, 971–978. [CrossRef] [PubMed]

192. Ebner, B.; Behm, P.; Jacoby, C.; Burghoff, S.; French, B.A.; Schrader, J.; Flogel, U. Early Assessment of Pulmonary Inflammation by 19F MRI In Vivo. *Circ. Cardiovasc. Imaging* **2010**, *3*, 202–210. [CrossRef] [PubMed]

193. Stoll, G.; Basse-Lüsebrink, T.; Weise, G.; Jakob, P. Visualization of inflammation using 19F-magnetic resonance imaging and perfluorocarbons. *Wiley Interdiscip. Rev. Nanomed. Nanobiotechnol.* **2012**, *4*, 438–447. [CrossRef] [PubMed]

194. Schuster, D.P.; Kovacs, A.; Garbow, J.; Piwnica-Worms, D. Recent Advances in Imaging the Lungs of Intact Small Animals. *Am. J. Respir. Cell Mol. Biol.* **2004**, *30*, 129–138. [CrossRef] [PubMed]
195. Kashefi, A.; Kuo, J.; Shelton, D.K. Molecular Imaging in Pulmonary Diseases. *Am. J. Roentgenol.* **2011**, *197*, 295–307. [CrossRef] [PubMed]

2

Diagnostic Performance of ^{18}F-FDG PET/CT in Native Valve Endocarditis

Christel H. Kamani [1], Gilles Allenbach [1], Mario Jreige [1], Anna G. Pavon [2], Marie Meyer [1], Nathalie Testart [1], Maria Firsova [1], Victor Fernandes Vieira [1], Sarah Boughdad [1], Marie Nicod Lalonde [1], Niklaus Schaefer [1,3], Benoit Guery [3,4], Pierre Monney [2,3], John O. Prior [1,3,†] and Giorgio Treglia [1,3,5,6,*,†]

1 Department of Nuclear Medicine and Molecular Imaging, Lausanne University Hospital, CH-1011 Lausanne, Switzerland; Christel-Hermann.Kamani@chuv.ch (C.H.K.); Gilles.Allenbach@chuv.ch (G.A.); Mario.Jreige@chuv.ch (M.J.); Marie-Madeleine.Meyer@chuv.ch (M.M.); Nathalie.Testart@chuv.ch (N.T.); Maria.Firsova@chuv.ch (M.F.); Victor.Fernandes-Vieira@chuv.ch (V.F.V.); Sarah.Boughdad@chuv.ch (S.B.); Marie.Nicod-Lalonde@chuv.ch (M.N.L.); Niklaus.Schaefer@chuv.ch (N.S.); John.Prior@chuv.ch (J.O.P.)

2 Department of Cardiology, Lausanne University Hospital, CH-1011 Lausanne, Switzerland; Anna-Giulia.Pavon@chuv.ch (A.G.P.); Pierre.Monney@chuv.ch (P.M.)

3 University of Lausanne, CH-1011 Lausanne, Switzerland; Benoit.Guery@chuv.ch

4 Department of Infectious Diseases, Lausanne University Hospital, CH-1011 Lausanne, Switzerland

5 Clinic of Nuclear Medicine and Molecular Imaging, Imaging Institute of Southern Switzerland, Ente Ospedaliero Cantonale, CH-6500 Bellinzona, Switzerland

6 Health Technology Assessment Unit, Academic Education, Research and Innovation Area, Ente Ospedaliero Cantonale, CH-6500 Bellinzona, Switzerland

* Correspondence: Giorgio.Treglia@eoc.ch

† These authors contributed equally to this work and they share the last authorship.

Abstract: Background: Infectious endocarditis is a life-threatening disease, requiring prompt and accurate diagnosis. The aim of this article is to perform a systematic review and meta-analysis of the literature to estimate the performance of fluorine-18 fluorodeoxyglucose positron emission tomography/computed tomography (^{18}F-FDG PET/CT) for the diagnosis of native valve endocarditis (NVE). Methods: Selected articles evaluating the diagnostic accuracy of ^{18}F-FDG PET/CT in patients with suspected NVE, resulting from a comprehensive literature search through the PubMed/MEDLINE and Cochrane library databases until April 2020, were included for the systematic review and meta-analysis. Results: Seven studies (351 episodes of suspected NVE) were included. ^{18}F-FDG PET/CT yielded a pooled sensitivity of 36.3% and a pooled specificity of 99.1% for the diagnosis of NVE. The pooled positive likelihood ratio, negative likelihood ratio, and diagnostic odds ratio were 8.3, 0.6, and 15.3, respectively. The sensitivity increased using contemporary PET/CT device with state-of-the-art patient preparation as well as innovative image acquisitions or adding the results of ^{18}F-FDG PET/CT in a multimodality strategy. Conclusions: In our systematic review and meta-analysis, ^{18}F-FDG PET/CT yielded a poor pooled sensitivity with an otherwise excellent pooled specificity for the diagnosis of NVE, however, several factors may increase the sensitivity without affecting the specificity and these factors should be better evaluated in future studies.

Keywords: diagnostic performance; ^{18}F-FDG; PET/CT; positron emission tomography; native valve endocarditis; infectious endocarditis; infectious diseases; meta-analysis; systematic review

1. Introduction

Infective endocarditis (IE) is a multisystem infectious disease affecting the damaged endocardial surface of the heart valve as well as the surface of an indwelling cardiac device [1]. It was first described as a pathological infectious process in 1885 by Sir William Osler [2]. It is a relatively rare disease, with a prevalence ranging from 1.5 to 11.6 cases per 100,000 person-years [3]. IE occurs in more than half of cases in the native valve [4] and it remains a life-threatening disease despite the improvement in diagnosis and therapy, with contemporary mortality rates up to 25% [5]. The diagnosis of native valve endocarditis (NVE) is based on the presence of positive blood cultures and evidence of endocardial involvement in echocardiography as major criteria [6]. However, using the Duke criteria (DC) alone leads to about 24% misclassification of patients with proven IE to possible IE, especially by negative blood culture endocarditis [7]. This is of clinical importance, since delay in the diagnosis and thus initiation of an appropriate treatment results in poorer clinical outcome [8]. Therefore, further strategies for prompt and accurate diagnosis are still needed.

In recent years, promising studies on the role of fluorine-18 fluorodeoxyglucose positron emission tomography/computed tomography (^{18}F-FDG PET/CT) in the diagnosis of active inflammatory and infectious processes in patients with fever of unknown origin, with endovascular prosthesis and implantable pacemaker/defibrillators have been published [9]. Moreover, the potential of this technique to diagnose prosthetic valve endocarditis (PVE) [10] has also been investigated. This investigation tool relies on the increase glycolytic activity of inflammatory cells following pathogen invasion, allowing their visualization by ^{18}F-FDG PET/CT [11]. Based on accumulating evidence, ^{18}F-FDG PET/CT has been included as a new major criterion for PVE in the modified Duke criteria (mDC) endorsed by the European Society of Cardiology in 2015 [6]. However, the evidence is not in favor of the use of this technique for the diagnosis of NVE due to its limited sensitivity [6].

New evidence on the value of ^{18}F-FDG PET/CT in IE has been published in over the last few years. Some of these studies were pooled in three systematic reviews and/or meta-analyses with mixed population of IE patients [12–14]. We perform this systematic review and meta-analysis to investigate the current value of ^{18}F-FDG PET/CT in the detection of NVE only.

2. Materials and Methods

The authors performed a systematic review and meta-analysis according to the "Preferred Reporting Items for a Systematic Review and Meta-Analysis of Diagnostic Test Accuracy Studies" (PRISMA-DTA statement), a guideline which describes the items required for reporting in systematic reviews and meta-analyses of diagnostic accuracy studies [15].

2.1. Search Strategy

We performed a comprehensive computer literature search through PubMed/MEDLINE and Cochrane library databases for published studies evaluating the diagnostic accuracy of ^{18}F-FDG PET/CT in patients with suspected NVE until April 27, 2020. For this purpose, a search algorithm based on a combination of terms was created and used: (A) "PET" OR "positron" OR "FDG" AND (B) "endocarditis". There were no date limit nor language restrictions applied to the database search. Moreover, in order to achieve a more comprehensive search, we also manually screened the references of the selected articles.

2.2. Study Selection

Titles and abstracts of the records obtained by using our search strategy were independently screened by two reviewers (C.K. and G.T.) based on predefined inclusion and exclusion criteria. Inclusion criteria were original articles reporting information on the diagnostic performance of ^{18}F-FDG PET/CT in NVE. Exclusion criteria were: (a) reviews, editorials, comments related to the review question; (b) case reports related to the review question; (c) articles outside the field of interest of this review (including those focused on the role of ^{18}F-FDG PET/CT in detecting PVE or extra-cardiac foci of IE). The full text of letters and original articles which were related to the review question was independently screened to assess for their inclusion for both the systematic review and the meta-analysis. From these selected articles, those who did not provide sufficient data to reassess the sensitivity and specificity of ^{18}F-FDG PET/CT in NVE were excluded from the meta-analysis. In the case of data overlap, all the selected articles were included in the systematic review, whereas only the article with the most complete information was included in the meta-analysis. Disagreements were solved through a consensus meeting between both reviewers.

2.3. Data Extraction

For each included study, data were extracted by two reviewers (C.K. and G.T.), including general information on study characteristics (authors name, year of publication, country, study design), patient characteristics (age, sex ratio, type and number of patients evaluated, clinical and biological findings), technical details (patient preparation protocol, ^{18}F-FDG injected activity, time interval between radiotracer injection and image acquisition, acquisition of delayed images, and protocol for the image analysis). Moreover, data on the diagnostic accuracy of ^{18}F-FDG PET/CT on a per patient-based analysis (including true positive and true negative findings, false positive and false negative findings, sensitivity, specificity, positive and negative predictive values, diagnostic accuracy), name of the most common microbiological pathogen involved in NVE and information about the extent of the infection were also collected. For some articles, extraction of data from available figures, followed by mathematic calculations, was needed to calculate the diagnostic value of ^{18}F-FDG PET/CT.

2.4. Quality Assessment

The quality of the included studies was assessed according to the revised "Quality Assessment of Diagnostic Accuracy Studies" tool (QUADAS-2) by 2 independent investigators (C.K. and G.T.). Of note, QUADAS-2 includes four domains: patient selection, index test, reference standard, and flow and timing. Each domain was assessed in terms of risk of bias, and also in terms of concerns regarding applicability (except the flow and timing domain for this latest) [16]. Any discrepancies in the quality assessment were solved by consensus.

2.5. Statistical Analysis

On a per patient-based analysis, accuracy data (true positive, false positive, true negative, and false negative) were extracted from each study to assess the pooled sensitivity and specificity, using a bivariate random-effects model for statistical pooling of data, which takes into account any possible correlation between sensitivity and specificity. Further diagnostic measures were calculated, including positive and negative likelihood ratios (LR+ and LR–) as well as diagnostic odds ratio (DOR). A random-effects model was also used for statistical pooling of LR+, LR–, as well as DOR. Pooled data were given with 95% confidence intervals (95% CI) and displayed using forest plots. Heterogeneity was assessed using the I-square index (I^2). Statistical analyses were performed using OpenMeta [Analyst]® software (version 0.1503) funded by the Agency for Healthcare Research and Quality (AHRQ) (Rockville, Maryland, United States).

3. Results

3.1. Literature Search

A total of 340 records were identified through the comprehensive electronic database search of PubMed/MEDLINE and Cochrane library databases. Overall, 327 records were excluded: 254 as not in the field of interest, 46 as reviews, editorials, or letters, and 27 as case reports. Thus, 13 articles were eligible for full-text screening. No pertinent studies were added after screening the references of these articles. After full-text screening, six articles were excluded from the systematic review as well as from the meta-analysis, because of missing information to assess both sensitivity and specificity of ^{18}F-FDG PET/CT. Therefore, seven articles with a total of 351 episodes of suspected NVE were included in the qualitative (systematic review) as well as in the quantitative analysis (meta-analysis) [17–23]. Figure 1 summarizes the literature search results.

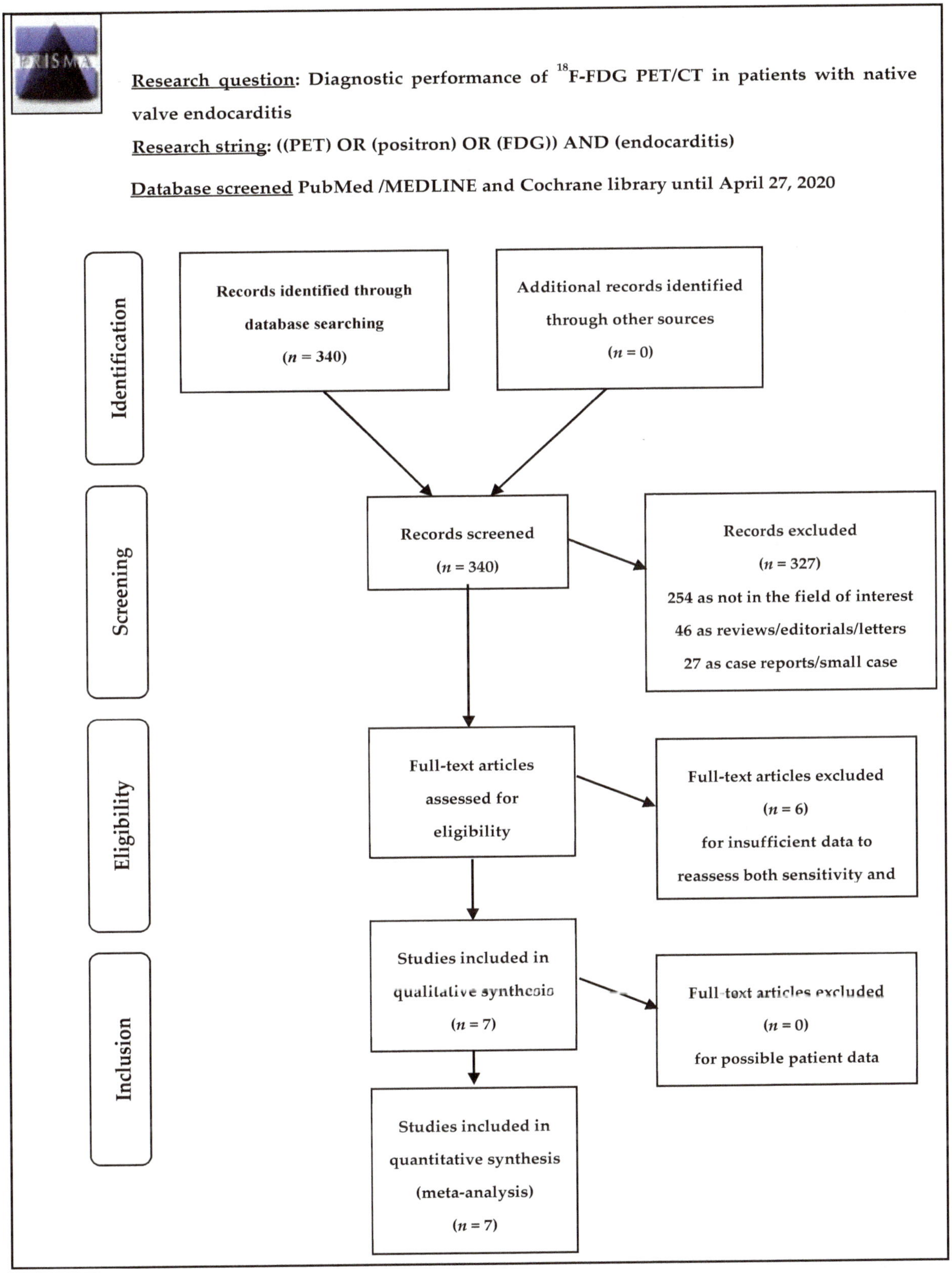

Figure 1. Flowchart of study selection and search results.

3.2. *Qualitative Analysis (Systematic Review)*

3.2.1. Basic Study and Patient Characteristics

Table 1a,b summarize the main characteristics of the included studies. Of note, the selected studies were mostly performed in Europe, except for two which were performed in North America [17] and South America [19]. There were all monocentric and mostly prospective, except for two retrospective studies [17,22]. The articles were published between 2016 and 2020. Five studies included a total of 722 episodes with clinical suspicion of IE, with a subgroup of 209 episodes with suspected NVE [18–21,23]. Two studies were exclusively dedicated to assess the accuracy of ^{18}F-FDG PET/CT in 142 patients with clinical suspected NVE [17,22]. In six studies, the mean age of the patients ranged from 58 to 71 years with a proportion of 68.1% of males, whereas corresponding data could not be assessed in one study [23]. Two studies reported the percentage of positive echocardiographic findings, ranging from 19% to 42% [20,22]. These two studies reported a rate of positive blood culture of 52% and 100% of the study population, partly because only blood culture positive patients were included in the second study by Kouijzer et al. [22]. A third study reported a 74% rate of positive blood culture [19]. Two studies reported the presence of fever in about 70% of their study population [17,19], with a C-reactive protein (CRP) mean value of 78.5 mg/L in one of these studies [17], similar to the CRP mean value of another study [18]. Most patients were treated with antibiotics prior to ^{18}F-FDG PET/CT, with a mean duration of treatment ranging from 7 to 30 days [17,19–21].

Table 1. (**a**) Basic study and patient characteristics; (**b**) Basic study and patient characteristics.

(a)					
Authors	**Year**	**Country**	**Study Design**	**Type of Patients Evaluated**	**No. of Episodes with Suspicion of IE (NVE) Undergoing ^{18}F-FDG PET/CT**
Abikhzer et al. [17]	2020	Canada	Retrospective monocentric	Patients with clinical suspicion of NVE	54 (54)
Abou Jokh Casas et al. [18]	2019	Spain	Prospective monocentric	Patients with clinical suspicion of IE, including a subgroup of patients with suspicion of NVE	43 (12)
de Camargo et al. [19]	2020	Brazil	Prospective monocentric	Patients with clinical suspicion of IE, including a subgroup of patients with suspicion of NVE	303 (115)
Gomes et al. [20]	2018	Netherlands	Prospective monocentric	Patients with clinical suspicion of IE, including a subgroup of patients with suspicion of NVE	176 (27)
Granados et al. [21]	2016	Spain	Prospective monocentric	Patients with clinical suspicion of IE, including a subgroup of patients with suspicion of NVE	80 (21)
Kouijzer et al. [22]	2018	Netherlands	Retrospective monocentric	Patients with clinical suspicion of NVE	88 (88)
Sánchez-Enrique et al. [23]	2018	Spain	Prospective monocentric	Patients with clinical suspicion of IE, including a subgroup of patients with suspicion of NVE	120 (34)

Table 1. *Cont.*

(b)							
Authors	**Age (Years)**	**%Male**	**Vegetation in TTE/TEE**	**Positive Blood Cultures**	**Presence of Fever**	**Value of CRP**	**Antibiotic Treatment Prior to the Exam (days)**
Abikhzer et al. [17]	Mean: 63 ± 15 Range: 33–93	64.8%	NR	NR	37/54 (68.5%)	78.5 ± 43.2 (0.2–193)	Median duration: 7 (range 1–61 days).
Abou Jokh Casas et al. [18]	Median: 71 Range: 25–88	88.4%	NR	NR	NR	76 ± 75 (0–349)	NR
de Camargo et al. [19]	Mean: 58 ± 17	58%	NR	40/54 (74%)	82/115 (71%)	NR	6 ± 8 (1–62)
Gomes et al. [20]	Mean: 64 Range: 18–95	60%	5/27 (19%)	14/27 (51.8%)	NR	NR	Yes, length not specified
Granados et al. [21]	Mean: 68 ± 13	81%	NR	NR	NR	NR	Definite IE: 20 (12–30) Possible IE: 13 (8–25)
Kouijzer et al. [22]	Mean: 61 Range: 17–90	56.8%	37/88 (42%)	88/88 (100%)	NR	NR	NR
Sánchez-Enrique et al. [23]	NR	NR	NR	NR	NR	NR	NR

Legend: ^{18}F-FDG = Fluorine-18 Fluorodeoxyglucose; IE = infective endocarditis; NVE = native valve endocarditis; PET/CT = positron emission tomography/computed tomography. CRP = C-reactive protein; IE = infective endocarditis; TTE = transthoracic echocardiography; TEE = transesophageal echocardiography; NR = not reported.

3.2.2. Technical Aspects

Table 2a,b summarize the technical aspects of ^{18}F-FDG PET/CT in the included studies. In all studies, the physiological myocardial ^{18}F-FDG uptake suppression was obtained through high-fat low-carbohydrate (HFLC) diet for 12 to 24 h and at least 6 to 8 h prolonged fasting prior administration of ^{18}F-FDG. Moreover, a bolus of unfractionated heparin (50 IU/kg) was injected, when not contraindicated [17,18,21]. No indication about heparin administration was given in four studies [19,20,22,23]. The images were acquired 60 min after administration of ^{18}F-FDG in the vast majority of studies, except for one, where the images were performed earlier at 45 min [18]. Four studies used a Biograph mCT hybrid PET/CT (Siemens) [17,20–22] with different technical performance, and one used a Gemini-TF hybrid PET/CT (Philips) [19]. No information about the type of hybrid device was given in two studies [18,23]. The mean injected activity ranged from 3 to 5 MBq/kg in four studies [19–22]. A fixed dose of 370 MBq was administered in two studies [17,18]. The images were visually assessed in all studies by two experienced physicians, all blinded to the patient clinical information. In two studies, involvement of a third experienced physician was required in case of disagreement [18,21]. For the vast majority of studies, a focal or heterogeneous ^{18}F-FDG uptake greater than the surrounding tissue, after exclusion of potential residual physiological myocardial activity, was used as positive criterion [17,19–21,23]. Two studies considered any increased ^{18}F-FDG uptake in the native heart valve as a positive criterion [18,22]. In addition, visual assessment was standardized using a scoring system in two studies [20,21]. Three studies used in addition to the visual analysis a semi-quantitative assessment of the ^{18}F-FDG uptake, i.e., through the calculation of the maximal standardized uptake values (SUVmax) [18,19,21].

Table 2. (**a**) Technical aspects of fluorine-18 fluorodeoxyglucose positron emission tomography/computed tomography (^{18}F-FDG PET/CT) in the included studies; (**b**)Technical aspects of 18F-FDG PET/CT in the included studies.

(a)

Authors	Hybrid Imaging Modality Name of the Device	Myocardial Suppression of ^{18}F-FDG Uptake	Protocol for Myocardial Suppression of ^{18}F-FDG Uptake	Injection of Heparin (50 UI/Kg) 15 min Prior Injection of ^{18}F-FDG	Mean Injected Activity
Abikhzer et al. [17]	PET/CT (with low-dose CT) Biograph mCT Flow 40 with TrueV, Siemens	Yes	Prolonged fasting (at least 12 h), HFLC diet in the 24 h prior injection of ^{18}F-FDG	Yes, when not CI (10 patients excluded)	370 MBq
Abou Jokh Casas et al. [18]	PET/CT (with low-dose CT) NR	Yes	Prolonged fasting (at least 6 h), HFLC diet at in the 12 h prior injection of ^{18}F-FDG	Yes, when not CI	370 MBq
de Camargo et al. [19]	PET/CT (with low-dose CT) Gemini-TF 64-Slice, Philips Medical Systems	Yes	Prolonged fasting (at least 8 h), HFLC diet in the 24 h prior injection of ^{18}F-FDG	NR	5 MBq/kg
Gomes et al. [20]	PET/CT (with low-dose CT) Biograph mCT 64-Slice, Siemens	Yes	Prolonged fasting (at least 6 h), HFLC diet in the 24 h prior injection of ^{18}F-FDG	NR	244 MBq (3 MBq/Kg)
Granados et al. [21]	PET/CT (with low-dose CT) Biograph mCT 64-Slice, Siemems	Yes	Prolonged fasting (at least 12 h)	Yes, when not CI	4 MBq/kg
Kouijzer et al. [22]	PET/CT (with low-dose CT) Biograph mCT 40, Siemens	Yes	Prolonged fasting (at least 6 h), HFLC diet in the 24 h prior injection of ^{18}F-FDG	NR	3.3 MBq/kg
Sánchez-Enrique et al. [23]	PET/CT (with low-dose CT) NR	NR	NR	NR	NR

Table 2. *Cont.*

(b)					
Authors	**Time Interval between Radiotracer Injection and Image Acquisition**	**Delayed PET/CT Imaging**	**Image Interpretation**	**Visual Criteria for Positive ^{18}F-FDG PET/CT**	**Semi-Quantitative Analysis**
Abikhzer et al. [17]	60 min	in selected cases	2 experienced physicians, blinded to the patient clinical information	Presence of focally increased ^{18}F-FDG uptake in and around the native heart valve, excluding the papillary muscle	No
Abou Jokh Casas et al. [18]	45 min	NR	2 experienced physicians, with involvement of a third physician by disagreement	Presence of any increased ^{18}F-FDG uptake in the native heart valve,	SUV_{max}
de Camargo et al. [19]	60 min	NR	2 experienced physicians, blinded to the patient clinical information	Presence of focal or heterogeneous ^{18}F-FDG uptake that persisted in the non-corrected images	SUV_{max}
Gomes et al. [20]	60 min	NR	2 experienced physicians, blinded to the patient clinical information	Focal/heterogeneous ^{18}F-FDG uptake, at least greater than uptake in mediastinum	No
Granados et al. [21]	60 min	NR	2 experienced physicians, with involvement of a third physician by disagreement	Presence of focal or heterogeneous ^{18}F-FDG uptake that persisted in the non-corrected images	SUV_{max}
Kouijzer et al. [22]	60 min	NR	2 experienced physicians, blinded to the patient clinical information	Presence of any increased ^{18}F-FDG uptake in and around the native heart valve, distinguishable from normal heart uptake	No
Sánchez-Enrique et al. [23]	NR	NR	NR	Presence of focal or heterogeneous ^{18}F-FDG uptake that persisted in the non-corrected images	No

Legend: ^{18}F-FDG = Fluorine-18 Fluorodeoxyglucose; CI = contra-indicated; CT = computed tomography; HFLC = high-fat low-carbohydrate; MBq/kg = Mega Becquerel per kilogram; NR = not reported; PET/CT = positron emission tomography/computed tomography; min = minutes; mDC = modified Duke criteria; NR = not reported; PET/CT = positron emission tomography/computed tomography; SUVmax = maximal standardized uptake value.

3.2.3. Main Findings

Table 3a,b summarize the diagnostic performance of ^{18}F-FDG PET/CT in patients suspected of NVE in the included studies, whereas Figure 2 illustrates the overall quality assessment of these studies. No adverse effects were reported in any of the patients after ^{18}F-FDG administration. In most of the included studies, we observed a poor sensitivity of ^{18}F-FDG PET/CT in patients with suspected NVE, except for one recent study with improved sensitivity by 67.7% [17]. In contrast, the specificity of ^{18}F-FDG PET/CT was excellent in all included studies, reaching 100% in four studies. The diagnostic accuracy ranged from 61.8% to 85.2%.

The most common microbiological pathogens found in blood cultures were Gram-positive bacteria from the Staphylococcus species, followed by Streptococcus species and Enterococcus species. Due to the acquisition from the base of the skull to at least the mid-tights in all the studies, it was possible to assess for the presence of metastatic foci. These were reported in the majority of studies in patients with confirmed NVE, in up to 54.5% of the patients [22]. Alternative diagnoses, such as systemic inflammatory diseases or neoplastic diseases, were reported in the majority of studies in patients with rejected diagnosis of NVE, in up to 45% of the patients [21]. These studies, except one [23], also reported alternative foci of infections. It should be mentioned that the exact percentage of metastatic foci and alternative diagnosis in patients with confirmed or rejected diagnosis of NVE could not be extracted for all the included studies, since these data were given for the mixed population of PVE and NVE rather than specifically for the NVE population. All studies used, as gold standard for the diagnosis of IE, the decision of a multidisciplinary endocarditis team (MET), applying the mDC while integrating clinical, imaging, and microbiological findings. Three studies used, additionally in the final decision, the histological analyses of the valve tissue obtained after surgery [17,19,23]. Three studies excluded the ^{18}F-FDG PET/CT findings from the final decision [17–19], whereas four studies integrated them in the final decision [20–23].

Two from seven studies [22,23] reported false positive cases. False negative cases were reported in all studies, ranging from 32% to even 100%; this latest in a study with limited number of patients [21]. One study reported incomplete ^{18}F-FDG myocardial suppression as a potential cause of the false negative findings [17]. Two studies did not report any significant difference in the performance of ^{18}F-FDG PET/CT between different groups based on the duration of antibiotic treatment [19,20], whereas one study reported the administration of antibiotics in the vast majority of patients with false negative results [17].

Echocardiography performed globally better than ^{18}F-FDG PET/CT in the majority of studies [18,21,23]. Two studies reported a better performance of ^{18}F-FDG PET/CT compared to the mDC [17,22]. However, in one study, only transthoracic echocardiography (TTE) and not transesophageal echocardiography (TEE) was performed in the majority of patients with the diagnosis of possible or rejected NVE [22]. Two studies reported a greater size of the vegetation in patients with positive ^{18}F-FDG PET/CT findings [17,23]. When adding ^{18}F-FDG PET/CT as major and minor criterion in the mDC, we observed a significant improvement of the mDC sensitivity up to 78% (95%CI 66–90%), without excellent specificity by up to 91% (95%CI 85–98), as reported in two studies [17,19].

Table 3. (**a**): Diagnostic performance of ^{18}F-FDG PET/CT in patients with suspected native valve endocarditis; (**b**) Diagnostic performance of 18F-FDG PET/CT in patients with suspected native valve endocarditis.

(a)							
Authors.	**Reference Standard for Diagnostic Performance Assessment**	**True Positive**	**False Positive**	**True Negative**	**False Negative**	**Sensitivity**	**Specificity**
Abikhzer et al. [17]	histological analysis of valve tissue or mDC and decision of MET taking into account clinical, imaging, and microbiological findings. ^{18}F-FDG PET/CT excluded from the final decision	21	0	23	10	67.7%	100%
Abou Jokh Casas et al. [18]	mDC determined by MET. ^{18}F-FDG PET/CT excluded from the final decision	2	0	6	4	33.3%	100%
de Camargo et al. [19]	microbiological and histological analysis of valve tissue or modified Duke criteria determined by MET. ^{18}F-FDG PET/CT excluded from the final decision	10	0	69	36	22%	100%
Gomes et al. [20]	mDC and decision of MET taking into account clinical, imaging, and microbiological findings. ^{18}F-FDG PET/CT included in the final decision	2	0	20	5	28.6%	100%
Granados et al. [21]	mDC and decision of MET taking into account clinical, imaging, and microbiological findings. ^{18}F-FDG PET/CT included in the final decision	0	0	15	6	0%	100%
Kouijzer et al. [22]	mDC and decision of MET taking into account clinical, imaging, and microbiological findings. ^{18}F-FDG PET/CT included in the final decision	9	2	66	11	45%	97.1%
Sánchez-Enrique et al. [23]	histological analysis of valve tissue or mDC and decision of MET taking into account clinical, imaging, and microbiological findings. ^{18}F-FDG PET/CT included in the final decision	10	2	11	11	47.6%	84.6%

Table 3. *Cont.*

(b)

Authors	PPV	NPV	Diagnostic Accuracy	Metastatic Foci	Alternative Diagnosis/ Foci for Infection	Most Common Microbiological Findings
Abikhzer et al. [17]	100%	69.7%	81.5%	45.1%	5 (21.7%)	NR
Abou Jokh Casas et al. [18]	100%	60%	66.7%	NR	NR	1. Staph. epidermidis/ 2. Staph. aureus / 3. Strepto. bovis
de Camargo et al. [19]	100%	66%	68.7%	Identified in 47 patients with final diagnosis, but not specifically reported for NVE cases	Identified in 29 patients with excluded IE, but not specifically reported for NVE cases	1. Strepto. sp. / 2. Staph. aureus / 3. Entero. sp.
Gomes et al. [20]	100%	80%	81.5%	Identified in 6 patients with final diagnosis, but not specifically reported for NVE cases	Identified in 94% of patients with excluded IE, but not specifically reported for NVE cases	1. Staph. aureus / 2. Staph. others groups / 3. T. Whippeli
Granados et al. [21]	NR	71.4%	71.4%	Identified in 8 patients with final diagnosis, but not specifically reported for NVE cases	7 (45%)	Staph. aureus
Kouijzer et al. [22]	81.8%	85.7%	85.2%	Identified in 54.5% of patients with final diagnosis	NR	1. Staph. aureus / 2. Strepto. sp. / 3. Entero. sp.
Sánchez-Enrique et al. [23]	83.3%	50%	61.8%	NR	NR	NR

Legend: ^{18}F-FDG PET/CT = fluorine-18 fluorodeoxyglucose positron emission tomography/computed tomography; mDC = modified Duke criteria; MET = multidisciplinary endocarditis team; Entero = Enterococcus; IE = infectious endocarditis; NPV = negative predictive value; NR = not reported; NVE = native valve endocarditis; PPV = positive predictive value; sp. = species; Staph = Staphylococcus; Strepto= Streptococcus; T = Tropheryma.

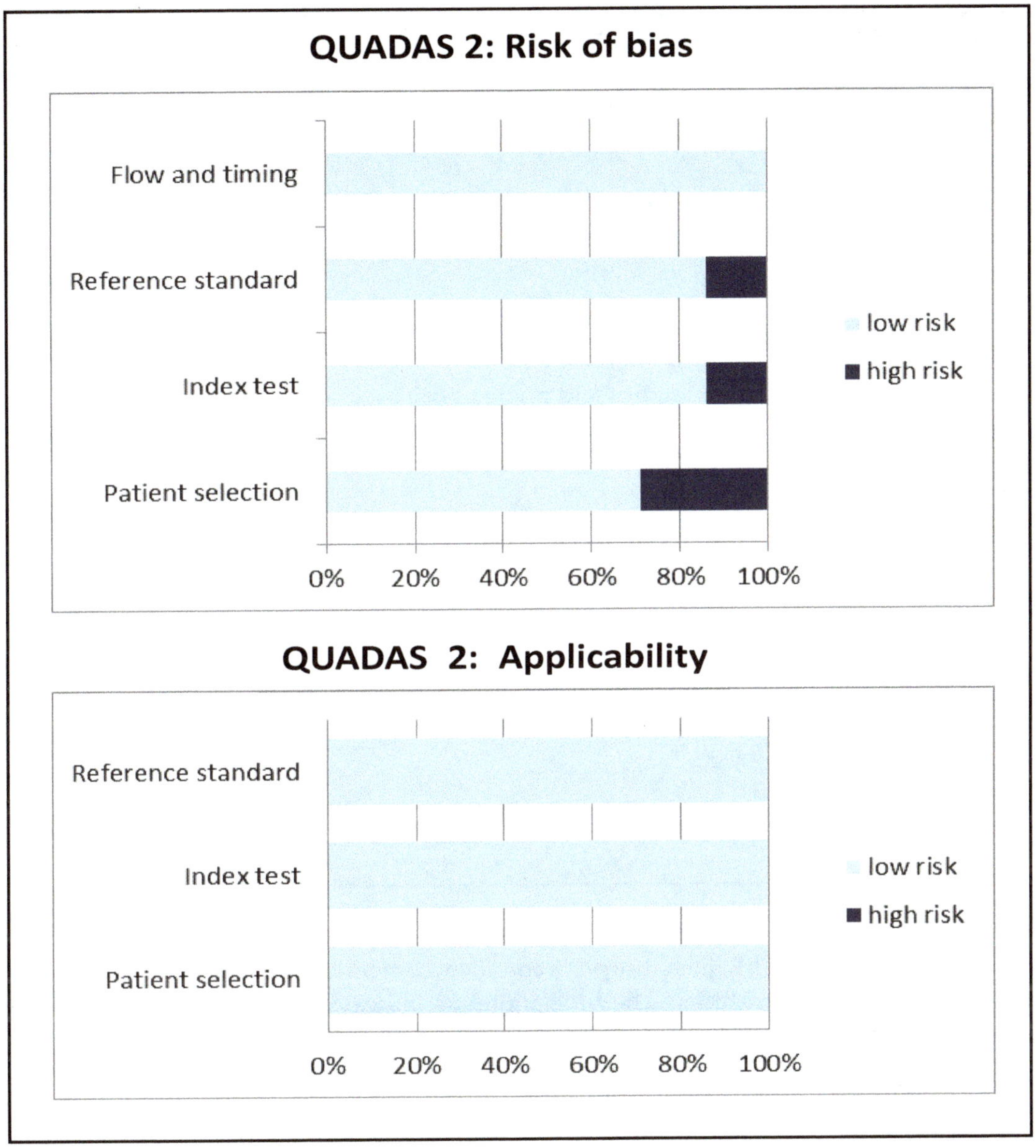

Figure 2. Overall quality assessment of the studies included in the systematic review according to Quality Assessment of Diagnostic Accuracy Studies (QUADAS-2) tool.

3.3. *Quantitative Analysis (Meta-Analysis)*

Seven studies with 351 episodes of suspected NVE were included for the bivariate meta-analysis [17–23]. Results of the meta-analysis are presented in Figure 3, Figure 4, and Figure 5. The sensitivity of ^{18}F-FDG PET/CT in patients with suspected NVE ranged from 22% to 67.7%, with a pooled estimate of 36.3% (95%CI: 21.8–53.9%). The specificity of ^{18}F-FDG PET/CT in patients with suspected NVE ranged from 84.6% to 100% with a pooled estimate of 99.1% (95%CI: 88.6–99.9%). The pooled LR+, LR−, and DOR were 8.3 (95%CI: 3.7–18.3), 0.6 (95%CI: 0.27–1.33), and 15.3 (95%CI: 6.14–38.38), respectively. No significant statistical heterogeneity among the studies was found for all the metrics evaluated (I^2 = 0%).

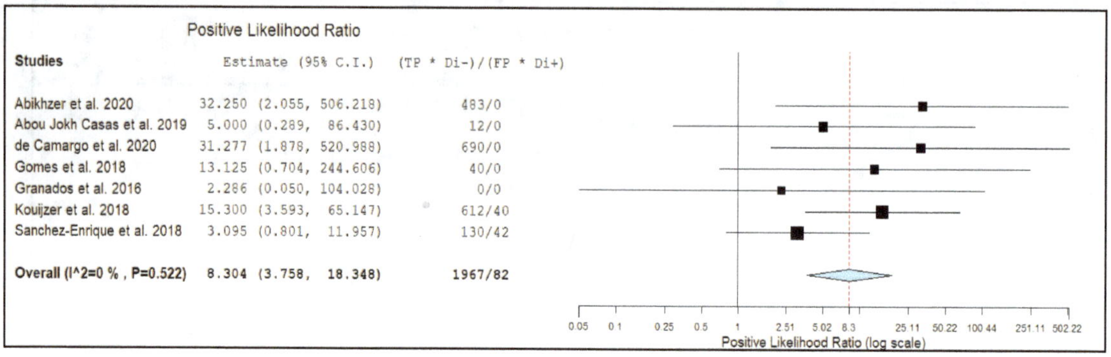

Figure 3. Forest plot of individual studies and pooled positive likelihood ratio of ^{18}F-FDG PET/CT in patients with suspicious native valve endocarditis (NVE), including 95% confidence interval (95% CI). The size of the squares indicates the weight of each study. The blue rhombus indicates the pooled estimate with 95% confidence intervals.

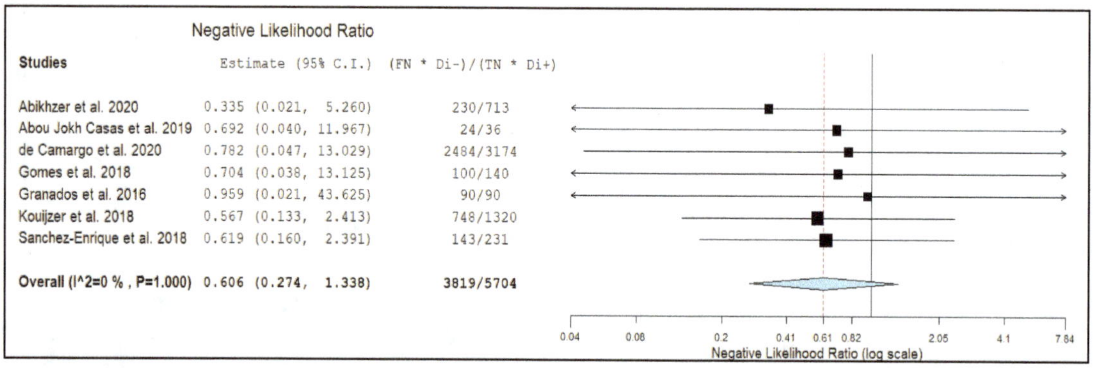

Figure 4. Forest plot of individual studies and pooled negative likelihood ratio of ^{18}F-FDG PET/CT in patients with suspicious NVE, including 95% confidence interval (95%CI). The size of the squares indicates the weight of each study. The blue rhombus indicates the pooled estimate with 95% confidence intervals.

Bivariate summary

Pooled sensitivity: 36.3% (95%CI: 21.8-53.9%)

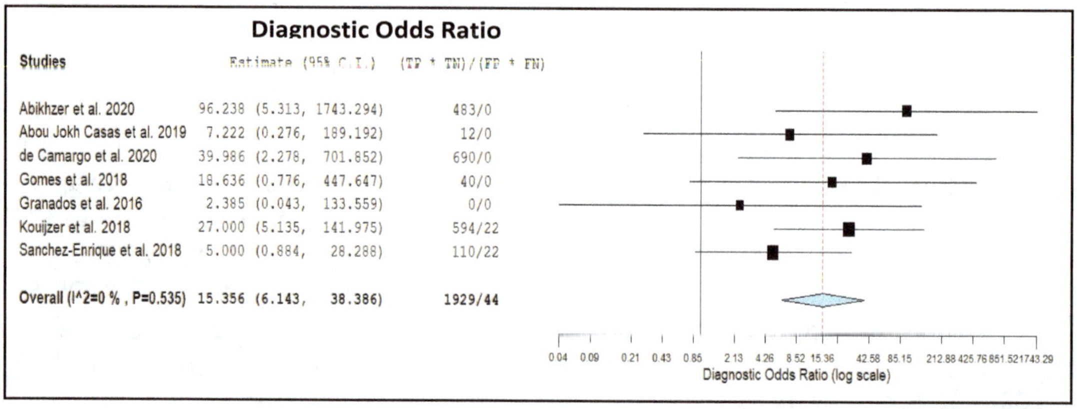

Figure 5. Forest plot of individual studies and pooled diagnostic odds ratio of ^{18}F-FDG PET/CT in patients with suspicious NVE, including 95% confidence interval (95%CI). The size of the squares indicates the weight of each study. The blue rhombus indicates the pooled estimate with 95% confidence intervals.

4. Discussion

Three recent systematic reviews and/or meta-analyses have questioned the performance of ^{18}F-FDG PET/CT in the diagnosis of IE [12–14]. In recent years, several articles assessing the diagnostic performance of ^{18}F-FDG PET/CT in NVE became available. To better understand the potential role of ^{18}F-FDG PET/CT in the diagnosis of NVE, we pooled the results from several studies to increase the statistical power.

In this meta-analysis of seven mostly prospective studies including 351 episodes with suspected NVE, ^{18}F-FDG PET/CT showed a poor pooled sensitivity (36.3%) but an excellent pooled specificity (99.1%) for the diagnosis of NVE. Moreover, whole body ^{18}F-FDG PET/CT was able to assess the extent of the infection, being the first modality to diagnose extra-cardiac foci in up to 79% of cases [22]. ^{18}F-FDG PET/CT was also able to provide alternative infectious foci by rejected NVE diagnosis as well as noninfectious relevant diagnosis, such as neoplastic or inflammatory disease [17–22].

In four studies, ^{18}F-FDG PET/CT findings were included in the final decision of the MET [20–23]. This could have led to an underestimation of the false positive cases, and thus contribute to the excellent specificity. However, three others studies [17–19] excluded the ^{18}F-FDG PET/CT results from the final decision, always with an excellent specificity by 100%. Moreover, two of these studies had an external validation using histopathological findings, whenever available. These observations confirm the excellent specificity of ^{18}F-FDG PET/CT for this indication. This specificity is clearly superior in this indication in comparison to PVE [12,13]. The reason for this superiority is the absence of prosthetic material that can cause reactive post-operative ^{18}F-FDG uptake.

Heterogeneity in patient preparation has contributed to the poor sensitivity of ^{18}F-FDG PET/CT in the diagnosis of NVE. Due to the physiological myocardial glucose uptake, a metabolic shift of the myocardium exclusively towards fatty acid metabolism is required before administration of ^{18}F-FDG, an analog of glucose. This can be achieved using different techniques, including dietary manipulation, as well as administration of some drugs such as heparin, known to increase the lipolysis [24]. The only study not including a HFLC diet in the patient preparation reported a relatively low rate of complete myocardial glucose uptake suppression (61% of patients with suspected PVE and NVE) and the poorest sensitivity (0%) of the included articles [21]. Some studies decided to exclude patients with inadequate ^{18}F-FDG myocardial suppression [19,22], introducing a selection bias in their results. This inadequate patient preparation is likely the reason for the false positive cases reported in two studies, since no physiological valvular or paravalvular ^{18}F-FDG uptake is expected, except from the surrounding myocardium [22,23]. Abikhzer et al. [17] reported incomplete ^{18}F-FDG myocardial suppression in 60% of the false negative studies. Interestingly, after excluding these patients, the ^{18}F-FDG PET/CT sensitivity significantly increased from 67.7% to 80%, without altering the excellent specificity. This sensitivity remains lower than the reported high sensitivity of TEE for NVE, in the range of 95%–100% [25]. However, based on its higher specificity, ^{18}F-FDG PET/CT could be considered in patients with possible NVE after doubtful or negative TTE or with a contra-indication for TEE [17,22]. Since the scans results have major implications on patient management, it is of the utmost importance to implement standardized preparation protocols with higher rate of adequate ^{18}F-FDG myocardial suppression [26].

Inflammatory cells, especially monocytes, are constituents of the inflammatory response following adhesion and invasion of the valvular site by pathogens, with a marked increase of their glycolytic activity, allowing their visualization by ^{18}F-FDG PET/CT [11]. In 54 patients with NVE, De Carmargo et al. [19] compared the ^{18}F-FDG uptake pattern with histopathological analysis, including the presence of fibrin, inflammatory infiltrate, and fibrosis. They demonstrated a significantly lower accumulation of fibrin, inflammatory cells, especially polymorphonuclear cells, and a significant higher content of fibrosis in NVE samples in comparison to PVE samples. These authors associated the reduced accumulation of inflammatory cells in NVE with the fact that vegetations are avascular and mostly of small size (less than 10 mm). The direct consequence is the reduced ^{18}F-FDG uptake by NVE, insufficient to be clearly differentiated from the background activity, and thus to be visualized by ^{18}F-FDG PET/CT. Moreover, the constant movement of the valve makes the situation worse since the already low ^{18}F-FDG signal is being blurred by this valve's motion [6]. In one study, the use of innovative acquisition sequence, such as delayed acquisitions (134 ± 42 min post injection of ^{18}F-FDG, compared to the standard acquisition performed 45-60 min post injection of ^{18}F-FDG) was shown to contribute to a significant increase the ^{18}F-FDG PET/CT performance to diagnose NVE [17]. Indeed, the authors demonstrated an increase of the target to background ratio (TBR) on delayed images in comparison to standard images, allowing the identification of a large number of positive findings. Moreover, in this study, acquisitions of simultaneous electrocardiogram- and respiratory-gated cardiac images with motion correction provided a better contrast resolution (more counts per pixel), a better spatial resolution (larger matrix and smaller pixel size), as well as less scattering, leading to an improved sensitivity to detect lower metabolic activity, as well as better metabolic and anatomic image fusion [17]. This evidence points out the technical differences of the PET/CT systems, and explains the superiority in the detection rate of NVE in the one recent study using a contemporary PET/CT device [17].

Since the diagnosis of NVE is challenging, this meta-analysis emphasizes the need for a MET to include as much clinical and imaging information as possible in the final diagnosis. Four studies reported the performance of mDC in the detection of NVE as compared to ^{18}F-FDG PET/CT. In two of them, ^{18}F-FDG PET/CT was superior to mDC: in one of these studies [22], mostly TTE rather than TEE was performed in patients with possible or rejected diagnosis of NVE, whereas in the other one [17], use of delayed PET/CT acquisitions as well as a contemporary PET/CT device allowed for the diagnosis of most of the positive cases. In the two other studies, mDC was superior to ^{18}F-FDG PET/CT [19,21]. Thus, compared individually to mDC, ^{18}F-FDG PET/CT showed variable performance. Two studies [17,19] proposed new criteria of the mDC based on the ^{18}F-FDG PET/CT findings and assessed their additive value on the overall performance of mDC. The major criterion was defined as a focal valvular or paravalvular ^{18}F-FDG uptake. The minor criterion was defined as the presence of septic emboli. Indeed, ^{18}F-FDG PET/CT as whole-body imaging method can detect septic emboli (except for the brain due to the increased cerebral glycolytic activity [11]), allowing the diagnosis of peripheral infectious complications. When integrating these new criteria in the mDC, its sensitivity increased up to 78%, without significantly affecting its specificity, which was up to 91% [17,19]. This led to a reclassification for up to 44% of patients from possible to definite NVE [17,19]. In the absence of an external gold standard, this performance could have been bias. Indeed, in this specific subgroup of patients with persistent suspicion of NVE and normal or doubtful echocardiography, no histological correlation between ^{18}F-FDG uptake and the presence of infection can be made, since these patients usually had no indication for valve surgery. De Carmago et al. [19] made a histological correlation between ^{18}F-FDG uptake and the histological confirmation of NVE in patients with confirmed NVE which undergone valve surgery. Thus, this evidence could be translated in this specific subgroup of patients, since no physiological ^{18}F-FDG uptake is expected in the valvular area. However, the present data did not report on the number of patients with NVE with negative echocardiography, but positive valvular ^{18}F-FDG uptake. This information would have allowed a better assessment of the valvular ^{18}F-FDG uptake performance, since the value of septic emboli is still established in this specific group of patients [6]. Nevertheless, based on these promising results, in patients with doubtful echocardiography findings, the use of ^{18}F-FDG PET/CT may be helpful in the final diagnosis of NVE [17,19]. Furthermore, ^{18}F-FDG PET/CT in some cases revealed the presence of malignant lesions, alternative infectious foci, or other inflammatory diseases, such as cardiac sarcoidosis, with the possibility of an early curative management [17–22]. Gomes et al. [20] pointed out the additive value of the use of flowchart integrating multimodality imaging to increase the detection performance of NVE. Integrating the findings of ^{18}F-FDG PET/CT with cardiac computed tomography angiography (CTA) and echocardiography (TTE and TEE) following a specific flowchart was feasible in clinical practice, providing complementary information on the anatomical cardiac structures and the extension of the infection. This led to significant increase in sensitivity for the diagnosis of NVE up to 86%, as compared to the sensitivity of each individual imaging modality. Finally, the specific patient referral through an MET increased the prevalence of the IE in the population referred for imaging investigation, leading to increased performance of the imaging tool. All this evidence could be discussed by the update of the next guidelines on the diagnosis of IE.

The suspicion of NVE requires the administration of large spectral antibiotics [6]. Since cardiac ^{18}F-FDG PET/CT requires a dietary preparation, it is mostly performed a few days after introduction of an antibiotic treatment. Three studies reported on the impact of antibiotic treatment duration in the performance of ^{18}F-FDG PET/CT [17,19,20]. In one study, the vast majority of patients with false negative results (9/10) were under antibiotic treatment [17]. Even if no information about the length of the treatment prior to PET/CT was provided, it can be suggested that antibiotics treatment could have led to false negative ^{18}F-FDG PET/CT. This would be in line with observations in PVE. Indeed, a prolonged antibiotic therapy could bring the pathogens in a quiescent status, leading to less accumulation of the inflammatory cells at the site of infection and therefore less or absent ^{18}F-FDG accumulation [27,28]. However, two other studies showed no significant difference on the performance of ^{18}F-FDG PET/CT depending on the duration of the antibiotic treatment [19,20]. Of note, in these two studies, the sensitivity was much lower compared to the first study [17]. This controversy has to be further investigated in future studies.

The most common microbiological pathogens found as causes of NVE were Staphylococcus aureus (SA), followed by Streptococcus species (SS). The included studies did not perform cost-effectiveness analysis about the role of ^{18}F-FDG PET/CT in NVE. Interestingly, a previous study performed a cost-effectiveness analysis of the use of ^{18}F-FDG PET/CT in SA and SS bacteremia. This study demonstrated a decrease in morbidity and mortality when ^{18}F-FDG PET/CT was included in the diagnostic algorithm to search for metastatic foci in patients with suspected endocarditis, with mean incremental costs within the range considered to be efficient by Dutch guidelines [29]. In this study, specific criteria to stratify the patient embolic risk were defined, such as persistent fever more than 72 h after administration of appropriate treatment, persistent positive blood culture over 48 h after administration of appropriate treatment, signs of infection 48 h prior administration of appropriate treatment, and community acquisition. The authors concluded that in patients with one or more of these risk features, there was a clinical, cost-effective benefit when ^{18}F-FDG PET/CT was performed for the search of embolic foci.

Finally, no studies evaluating the accuracy of SUVmax could demonstrate any utility compared to the visual assessment. Therefore, this semi-quantitative score value is not recommended for the diagnosis of NVE in the clinical routine. This can be explained by the fact that many external factors (i.e., time interval between injection of ^{18}F-FDG and image acquisition, plasma glucose, PET/CT scanner performances, etc.) can influence the SUVmax, resulting in wide variation among patients [18]. Thus, establishing a threshold to detect infection can be challenging.

In this meta-analysis, we focused on the diagnostic performance of ^{18}F-FDG PET/CT for the detection of NVE. However, the diagnostic performance of an imaging test is not the only component of a successful clinical management. Other factors influence the clinical management of patients with suspected NVE, such as availability, local expertise in images interpretation, radiation dose, safety, examination time, organization, and cost-effectiveness.

In this meta-analysis, ^{18}F-FDG PET/CT demonstrated poor pooled sensitivity and excellent specificity. However, many limiting factors were identified, which can be considered in future larger prospective and multicenter studies. Specifically, the use of standardized preparation protocol for ^{18}F-FDG myocardial suppression with higher success rates should be implemented in further studies. Moreover, the value of semi-quantitative analysis of PET/CT images should be further assessed. Additional studies are also needed to evaluate the simultaneous acquisition of ^{18}F-FDG PET/CT with cardiac CTA as well as the diagnostic accuracy of new PET/CT generation with higher timing and spatial resolution.

Some limitations and biases of our meta-analysis should be mentioned. First of all, a limited number of studies were available. Due to this limited number of studies, no significant biases among the included studies were identified. Heterogeneity among the studies (i.e., due to different characteristics among the included patients, difference in methodological aspects, and difference in gold standard) could also represent a potential source of bias in our meta-analysis [30]. On the other hand, we did not find a significant statistical heterogeneity among the studies included in our pooled analysis. The absence of a true independent gold standard could have introduced a certain bias in the evaluation of the ^{18}F-FDG PET/CT performance to detect NVE. More, in the specific subgroup of patients with possible NVE, but normal or doubtful echocardiography, the added value of valvular ^{18}F-FDG uptake needs to be better assessed.

5. Conclusions

In this meta-analysis specifically designed to assess the performance of ^{18}F-FDG PET/CT in the diagnosis of NVE, we demonstrated the poor pooled sensitivity and excellent pooled specificity of ^{18}F-FDG PET/CT in this setting. However, when using contemporary PET/CT device with innovative image acquisitions, the sensitivity increased, with still excellent specificity. Moreover, including ^{18}F-FDG PET/CT findings in the mDC further increased the mDC sensitivity for the detection of NVE without affecting its specificity. Finally, when adding the results of ^{18}F-FDG PET/CT in a multimodality strategy, the overall sensitivity for the detection of NVE can be improved. However, these findings need to be confirmed in larger prospective multicenter studies.

Author Contributions: Conceptualization, C.H.K. and J.O.P.; methodology, G.T.; software, G.T. and C.H.K.; validation, J.O.P.; A.G.P.; B.G. and P.M.; formal analysis, C.H.K.; G.A.; M.M.; N.T.; M.F.; V.F.V.; S.B.; writing—original draft preparation, C.H.K.; G.T.; J.O.P.; G.A.; M.J.; M.M.; N.T.; M.F.; V.F.V.; S.B.; M.N.L., N.S.; writing—review and editing, C.H.K.; G.T.; J.O.P.; A.G.P.; B.G. and P.M. All authors have read and agreed to the published version of the manuscript.

References

1. Holland, T.L.; Baddour, L.M.; Bayer, A.S.; Hoen, B.; Miro, J.M.; Fowler, V.G., Jr. Infective endocarditis. *Nat. Rev. Dis. Primers* **2016**, *2*, 16059. [CrossRef] [PubMed]
2. Osler, W. The Gulstonian Lectures, on Malignant Endocarditis. *Br. Med. J.* **1885**, *1*, 5775–5779. [CrossRef] [PubMed]
3. Bin Abdulhak, A.A.; Baddour, L.M.; Erwin, P.J.; Hoen, B.; Chu, V.H.; Mensah, G.A.; Tleyjeh, I.M. Global and regional burden of infective endocarditis, 19902–010: A systematic review of the literature. *Glob. Heart* **2014**, *9*, 1311–1343.
4. Habib, G.; Erba, P.A.; Iung, B.; Donal, E.; Cosyns, B.; Laroche, C.; Popescu, B.A.; Prendergast, B.; Tornos, P.; Sadeghpour, A.; et al. Clinical presentation, aetiology and outcome of infective endocarditis. Results of the ESC-EORP EURO-ENDO (European infective endocarditis) registry: A prospective cohort study. *Eur. Heart J.* **2019**, *40*, 32223–32232. [CrossRef] [PubMed]
5. Murdoch, D.R.; Corey, G.R.; Hoen, B.; Miro, J.M.; Fowler, V.G., Jr.; Bayer, A.S.; Karchmer, A.W.; Olaison, L.; Pappas, P.A.; Moreillon, P.; et al. Clinical presentation, etiology, and outcome of infective endocarditis in the 21st century: The International Collaboration on Endocarditis-Prospective Cohort Study. *Arch. Intern. Med.* **2009**, *169*, 4634–4673. [CrossRef]
6. Habib, G.; Lancellotti, P.; Antunes, M.J.; Bongiorni, M.G.; Casalta, J.P.; Del Zotti, F.; Dulgheru, R.; El Khoury, G.; Erba, P.A.; Iung, B.; et al. 2015 ESC Guidelines for the management of infective endocarditis: The Task Force for the Management of Infective Endocarditis of the European Society of Cardiology (ESC). Endorsed by: European Association for Cardio-Thoracic Surgery (EACTS), the European Association of Nuclear Medicine (EANM). *Eur. Heart J.* **2015**, *36*, 3075–3128.
7. Habib, G.; Derumeaux, G.; Avierinos, J.F.; Casalta, J.P.; Jamal, F.; Volot, F.; Garcia, M.; Lefevre, J.; Biou, F.; Maximovitch-Rodaminoff, A.; et al. Value and limitations of the Duke criteria for the diagnosis of infective endocarditis. *J. Am. Coll. Cardiol.* **1999**, *33*, 2023–2029. [CrossRef]
8. Fukuchi, T.; Iwata, K.; Ohji, G. Failure of early diagnosis of infective endocarditis in Japan—A retrospective descriptive analysis. *Medicine (Baltimore)* **2014**, *93*, e237. [CrossRef]

9. Treglia, G. Diagnostic Performance of (18)F-FDG PET/CT in Infectious and Inflammatory Diseases according to Published Meta-Analyses. *Contrast Media Mol. Imaging* **2019**, *2019*, 3018349. [CrossRef]
10. Saby, L.; Laas, O.; Habib, G.; Cammilleri, S.; Mancini, J.; Tessonnier, L.; Casalta, J.P.; Gouriet, F.; Riberi, A.; Avierinos, J.F.; et al. Positron emission tomography/computed tomography for diagnosis of prosthetic valve endocarditis: Increased valvular 18F-fluorodeoxyglucose uptake as a novel major criterion. *J. Am. Coll. Cardiol.* **2013**, *61*, 2374–2382. [CrossRef]
11. Vaidyanathan, S.; Patel, C.N.; Scarsbrook, A.F.; Chowdhury, F.U. FDG PET/CT in infection and inflammation–current and emerging clinical applications. *Clin. Radiol.* **2015**, *70*, 787–800. [CrossRef]
12. Mahmood, M.; Kendi, A.T.; Ajmal, S.; Farid, S.; O'Horo, J.C.; Chareonthaitawee, P.; Baddour, L.M.; Sohail, M.R. Meta-analysis of 18F-FDG PET/CT in the diagnosis of infective endocarditis. *J. Nucl. Cardiol.* **2019**, *26*, 9229–9235. [CrossRef] [PubMed]
13. Wang, T.K.M.; Sanchez-Nadales, A.; Igbinomwanhia, E.; Cremer, P.; Griffin, B.; Xu, B. Diagnosis of Infective Endocarditis by Subtype Using (18)F-Fluorodeoxyglucose Positron Emission Tomography/Computed Tomography: A Contemporary Meta-Analysis. *Circ. Cardiovasc. Imaging* **2020**, *13*, e010600. [CrossRef]
14. Gomes, A.; Glaudemans, A.W.J.M.; Touw, D.J.; van Melle, J.P.; Willems, T.P.; Maass, A.H.; Natour, E.; Prakken, N.H.J.; Borra, R.J.H.; van Geel, P.P.; et al. Diagnostic value of imaging in infective endocarditis: A systematic review. *Lancet Infect. Dis.* **2017**, *17*, e1–e14. [CrossRef]
15. McInnes, M.D.F.; Moher, D.; Thombs, B.D.; McGrath, T.A.; Bossuyt, P.M.; Clifford, T.; Cohen, J.F.; Deeks, J.J.; Gatsonis, C.; the PRISMA-DTA Group; et al. Preferred Reporting Items for a Systematic Review and Meta-analysis of Diagnostic Test Accuracy Studies: The PRISMA-DTA Statement. *JAMA* **2018**, *319*, 3883–3896. [CrossRef]
16. Whiting, P.F.; Rutjes, A.W.; Westwood, M.E.; Mallett, S.; Deeks, J.J.; Reitsma, J.B.; Leeflang, M.M.; Sterne, J.A.; Bossuyt, P.M. Group Q-. QUADAS-2: A revised tool for the quality assessment of diagnostic accuracy studies. *Ann. Intern. Med.* **2011**, *155*, 529–536. [CrossRef]
17. Abikhzer, G.; Martineau, P.; Gregoire, J.; Finnerty, V.; Harel, F.; Pelletier-Galarneau, M. [(18)F]FDG-PET CT for the evaluation of native valve endocarditis. *J. Nucl. Cardiol.* **2020**. [CrossRef]
18. Abou Jokh Casas, E.; Pubul Nunez, V.; Pombo Pasin, M.D.C.; Garrido Pumar, M.; Martinez, M.A.; Abou Jokh Casas, C.; Martinez de Alegria, A.; Dominguez, M.J.; Ruibal Morell, A. Advantages and limitations of 18-fluoro-2-deoxy-d-glucose positron emission tomography/computed tomography in the diagnosis of infective endocarditis. *Rev. Port. Cardiol.* **2019**, *38*, 5735–5780. [CrossRef]
19. de Camargo, R.A.; Sommer Bitencourt, M.; Meneghetti, J.C.; Soares, J.; Goncalves, L.F.T.; Buchpiguel, C.A.; Paixao, M.R.; Felicio, M.F.; de Matos Soeiro, A.; Varejao Strabelli, T.M.; et al. The Role of 18F-Fluorodeoxyglucose Positron Emission Tomography/Computed Tomography in the Diagnosis of Left-sided Endocarditis: Native vs Prosthetic Valves Endocarditis. *Clin. Infect. Dis.* **2020**, *70*, 5835–5894. [CrossRef] [PubMed]
20. Gomes, A.; van Geel, P.P.; Santing, M.; Prakken, N.H.J.; Ruis, M.L.; van Assen, S.; Slart, R.; Sinha, B.; Glaudemans, A. Imaging infective endocarditis: Adherence to a diagnostic flowchart and direct comparison of imaging techniques. *J. Nucl. Cardiol.* **2020**, *27*, 592–608. [CrossRef] [PubMed]
21. Granados, U.; Fuster, D.; Pericas, J.M.; Llopis, J.L.; Ninot, S.; Quintana, E.; Almela, M.; Pare, C.; Tolosana, J.M.; Falces, C.; et al. Diagnostic Accuracy of 18F-FDG PET/CT in Infective Endocarditis and Implantable Cardiac Electronic Device Infection: A Cross-Sectional Study. *J. Nucl. Med.* **2016**, *57*, 17261–17732. [CrossRef] [PubMed]
22. Kouijzer, I.J.E.; Berrevoets, M.A.H.; Aarntzen, E.; de Vries, J.; van Dijk, A.P.J.; Oyen, W.J.G.; de Geus-Oei, L.F.; Bleeker-Rovers, C.P. 18F-fluorodeoxyglucose positron-emission tomography combined with computed tomography as a diagnostic tool in native valve endocarditis. *Nucl. Med. Commun.* **2018**, *39*, 747–752. [CrossRef] [PubMed]
23. Sanchez-Enrique, C.; Olmos, C.; Jimenez-Ballve, A.; Fernandez-Perez, C.; Ferrera, C.; Perez-Castejon, M.J.; Ortega Candil, A.; Delgado-Bolton, R.; Carnero, M.; Maroto, L.; et al. Usefulness of (18)F Fluorodeoxyglucose Positron Emission Tomography/Computed Tomography in Infective Endocarditis in Daily Practice: Individualized Analysis of Each Potential Focus of Infection: A Prospective Cohort Study. *JACC Cardiovasc. Imaging* **2018**, *11*, 19201–19922. [CrossRef] [PubMed]
24. Osborne, M.T.; Hulten, E.A.; Murthy, V.L.; Skali, H.; Taqueti, V.R.; Dorbala, S.; DiCarli, M.F.; Blankstein, R. Patient preparation for cardiac fluorine-18 fluorodeoxyglucose positron emission tomography imaging of inflammation. *J. Nucl. Cardiol.* **2017**, *24*, 86–99. [CrossRef]

25. De Castro, S.; d'Amati, G.; Cartoni, D.; Venditti, M.; Magni, G.; Gallo, P.; Beni, S.; Fiorelli, M.; Fedele, F.; Pandian, N.G. Valvular perforation in left-sided infective endocarditis: A prospective echocardiographic evaluation and clinical outcome. *Am. Heart J.* **1997**, *134*, 656–664. [CrossRef]
26. Larson, S.R.; Pieper, J.A.; Hulten, E.A.; Ficaro, E.P.; Corbett, J.R.; Murthy, V.L.; Weinberg, R.L. Characterization of a highly effective preparation for suppression of myocardial glucose utilization. *J. Nucl. Cardiol.* **2020**, *27*, 849–861. [CrossRef]
27. Scholtens, A.M.; Swart, L.E.; Verberne, H.J.; Tanis, W.; Lam, M.G.; Budde, R.P. Confounders in FDG-PET/CT Imaging of Suspected Prosthetic Valve Endocarditis. *JACC Cardiovasc Imaging* **2016**, *9*, 1462–1465. [CrossRef]
28. Scholtens, A.M.; van Aarnhem, E.E.; Budde, R.P. Effect of antibiotics on FDG-PET/CT imaging of prosthetic heart valve endocarditis. *Eur. Heart J. Cardiovasc. Imaging* **2015**, *16*, 1223. [CrossRef]
29. Vos, F.J.; Bleeker-Rovers, C.P.; Kullberg, B.J.; Adang, E.M.; Oyen, W.J. Cost-effectiveness of routine (18)F-FDG PET/CT in high-risk patients with gram-positive bacteremia. *J. Nucl. Med.* **2011**, *52*, 1673–1678. [CrossRef]
30. Sadeghi, R.; Treglia, G. Systematic reviews and meta-analyses of diagnostic studies: A practical guideline. *Clin. Transl. Imaging* **2017**, *5*, 83–87. [CrossRef]

3

^{64}Cu-DOTATATE Positron Emission Tomography (PET) of *Borrelia Burgdorferi* Infection: In Vivo Imaging of Macrophages in Experimental Model of Lyme Arthritis

Anne Skovsbo Clausen [1,2], Mathilde Ørbæk [3], Regitze Renee Pedersen [4], Peter Oestrup Jensen [4,5,6], Anne-Mette Lebech [3,7] and Andreas Kjaer [1,2,*]

1. Department of Clinical Physiology, Nuclear Medicine & PET, Rigshospitalet, DK-2100 Copenhagen, Denmark; anne.clausen@sund.ku.dk
2. Cluster for Molecular Imaging, Department of Biomedical Sciences, University of Copenhagen, DK-2200 Copenhagen, Denmark
3. Department of Infectious Diseases, Copenhagen University Hospital, Rigshospitalet, DK-2100 Copenhagen, Denmark; mathilde.daniele.oerbaek.thalund@regionh.dk (M.Ø.); anne-mette.lebech@regionh.dk (A.-M.L.)
4. Costerton Biofilm Center, Department of Immunology and Microbiology, University of Copenhagen, DK-2200 Copenhagen, Denmark; regitze.pedersen@sund.ku.dk (R.R.P.); pojensen@sund.ku.dk (P.O.J.)
5. Department of Clinical Microbiology, Copenhagen University Hospital, Rigshospitalet, DK-2100 Copenhagen, Denmark
6. Center for Rheumatology and Spine Diseases, Institute for Inflammation Research, Copenhagen University Hospital, Rigshospitalet, DK-2100, Copenhagen, Denmark
7. Institute of Clinical Medicine, University of Copenhagen, DK-2100 Copenhagen, Denmark

* Correspondence: akjaer@sund.ku.dk

Abstract: Macrophages play a key role in the inflammatory response in Lyme arthritis (LA) and could be a target for diagnosing and monitoring active *Borrelia burgdorferi* sensu lato (*Bb*) infection. Therefore, we evaluated the potential of macrophage imaging using ^{64}Cu-DOTATATE PET/CT for detection of *Bb* activity in a murine model of LA. LA was established in C3H/HeNRj mice infected with *Bb* B31 strain ML23 pBBE22*luc*. Bioluminescence imaging was performed to detect migration of spirochetes and inflammatory phagocytes to the joints. Three weeks post-infection ^{64}Cu-DOTATATE PET/CT imaging was performed at an early (3 h) and late (48 h) time point. Plasma levels of a systemic macrophage marker in plasma CD163 were measured. ^{64}Cu-DOTATATE uptake in infected joints was increased at the early ($p < 0.0001$) and late time points ($p = 0.0005$) compared with uptake in non-infected controls. No significant difference in plasma levels of CD163 was measured. ^{64}Cu-DOTATATE PET allows for in vivo detection and quantification of LA locally in the joints through non-invasive visualization of macrophages. In contrast, measurement of a systemic macrophage marker in plasma, CD163, did not allow to detect disease. We suggest that ^{64}Cu-DOTATATE PET could become a valuable diagnostic tool for in situ detection of *Bb* infection-related inflammation.

Keywords: lyme borreliosis; *borrelia burgdorferi* sensu lato complex; animal model; macrophage; positron emission tomography (PET); ^{64}Cu-DOTATATE PET

---

1. Introduction

Lyme borreliosis (LB) caused by the *Borrelia burgdorferi* sensu lato (*Bb* s.l.) complex is the most prevalent vector-borne infection in Europe and the US with estimates of annual incidence ranging from

10–80 per 100,000 inhabitants. *Bb* s.l. can cause a variety of clinical manifestations including erythema migrans, Lyme neuroborreliosis and Lyme arthritis. The heterogeneity in the clinical expression of human LB is in part explained by different organotropism of the more than 20 species in the *Bb* s.l. complex. *B. burgdorferi* sensu stricto (*Bb* sensu stricto) is especially arthritogenic and causes Lyme arthritis, whereas *B. garinii* and *B. afzelii* cause Lyme neuroborreliosis and dermatoborreliosis, respectively [1–3].

A diagnosis of disseminated LB is based on possible exposure to tick bites, compatible clinical symptoms and objective signs in combination with antibody detection [4]. However, seropositivity alone is insufficient to make a diagnosis of active LB, as antibodies may first be detectable after weeks of infection and may persist for years after the infection has been treated. Additionally, direct detection of *Bb* s.l. by culture or molecular methods have a variable and suboptimal sensitivity. Likewise, *Borrelia* DNA can persist for months in the skin or in synovial fluid even after successful treatment, which renders the difficulty for direct detection of *Borrelia* DNA to unequivocally verify an active infection [5–7]. Therefore, new methods to monitor disease activity in patients with LB would be of paramount interest to practice precision medicine in these patients and to promote a shift from empirical treatment to personalized medicine with expected improvement in patient outcome.

During *Bb* s.l. infection, the early immune response is characterized by activation of monocytes/macrophages, which is sustained as long as active infection is present [2,8]. Furthermore, increased recruitment and number of macrophages with high phagocytic activity have been found in the joints of *Bb*-infected mice [9] as well as in studies of LB in rhesus macaques [10,11]. Thus, macrophages play a key role in the inflammatory response in Lyme arthritis and could be a potential target for diagnosing, localizing and monitor active inflammation caused by *Bb* infection [12,13].

We previously developed the positron emission tomography (PET) tracer ^{64}Cu-DOTATATE targeting somatostatin receptor subtype-2 (sstr2), which is known to be overexpressed on activated macrophages both in mice and humans [14,15]. Therefore, ^{64}Cu-DOTATATE could potentially serve as non-invasive imaging agent for detection and monitoring of LB. In addition, the long half-life of ^{64}Cu of 12.7 h and the high spatial resolution on PET using this isotope make it attractive for clinical routine use. However, macrophages also have significant impact on the inflammatory response in other diseases including rheumatoid arthritis (RA). The collagen-induced arthritis (CIA) mouse model that mimics human autoimmune arthritis is a widely studied animal model of human RA and was in the present study used to confirm tracer uptake in inflamed joints [16]. Moreover, in vivo bioluminescence imaging using lucigenin, which is activated by phagocyte NADPH oxidase in macrophages, was performed [17].

Furthermore, cluster of differentiation (CD) 163, a biomarker of macrophages gene expression, is known to correlate with ^{64}Cu-DOTATATE uptake, indicating that ^{64}Cu-DOTATATE PET is detecting activated macrophages [18,19]. Moreover, the development of arthritis in CIA mice is dependent on the macrophage biomarker: CD163 [20].

The aim of the present study was to evaluate the potential of macrophage imaging using ^{64}Cu-DOTATATE positron emission tomography/computed tomography (PET/CT) for non-invasive in vivo detection and quantification of *Bb* activity in a murine model of Lyme arthritis. In addition, we wanted to test if plasma levels of CD163 could be used to detect *Bb* infection.

2. Materials and Methods

2.1. Mice

Six-week-old, female C3H/HeNRj and DBA/1 mice were purchased (Janvier, Le Genest-Saint-Isle, France) and housed in groups of 4–8 mice in individually ventilated cages under standardized lighting conditions and fed pathogen-free food and water ad libitum. All animal experiments had been approved by The Danish Working Environment Authority and by The Animal Experiments Inspectorate in Denmark under the license number 2016-15-0201-00920, approved on 5 July 2016.

2.2. Induction of Bb Infection

Bb B31 strain ML23 was made competent and transformed with the bioluminescent plasmid pBBE22*luc*, and the transformants were selected for resistance to kanamycin. *Bb* B31 strain ML23 pBBE22*luc* was kindly provided by Dr. Jon T. Skare. Cultures were grown in Barbour–Stoenner–Kelly medium (BSK-H) supplemented with 6% rabbit serum (Merck KGaA, Darmstadt, Germany) under conventional microaerobic conditions (1–5% CO_2, 33 °C) created in Oxoid^{TM} Compact Plastic Pouches (Thermo Fisher Scientific, Waltham, MA, USA) with a OxoidTM Campygen^{TM} Compact sachet (Thermo Fisher Scientific), sealed airtight with a sealing clip [21]. Medium was filter-sterilized with 0.2 μm filter and incubated with kanamycin (300 μg/mL) [22]. After incubation, the cultures were checked with fluorescence microscopy (Axio Imager.Z2, LSM880 CLSM; Zeiss, Jena, Germany) using Syto9 (Molecular Probes, Eugene, OR, USA) emitting a green fluorescent signal to ensure the morphologies of the spirochete before being used for infection. Prior to infection, confocal fluorescence microscopy confirmed the helical shaped morphology of spirochetes. Images were processed using IMARIS 9.2 software (Bitplane, Zurich, Switzerland). Total cell counting of the bacterial culture was performed in duplicate by flow cytometry using a FacsCanto II (BD Biosciences, La Jolla, CA, USA). A volume of 10 μL bacterial solution in 1 mL Dulbecco's Phosphate Buffered Saline (PBS) (Biowest, Nuaillé, France) was stained with 5 μM Syto9 and added to a TruCount tube (BD Bioscience). Bacteria were discriminated according to their light scatter and Syto9 fluorescence. The counting beads were identified according to their fluorescens at 485-535 nm and above 610 nm. Propidium iodide (Merck KGaA, Darmstadt, Germany) was used for bacterial viability staining as it only enters cells with compromised membranes, binds to DNA and RNA and emits red fluorescence [23]. The bacterial culture was adjusted with PBS to a concentration of 20×10^6 cells/mL. Two setups of C3H/HeNRj mice were anaesthetized (2–3% isoflurane in O_2) and inoculated intradermally in the lower back with 10^6 ML23 pBBE22*luc* (50 μL) ($n = 2 \times 16$) or with PBS (50 μL) ($n = 2 \times 6$). Blood samples (50–100 μL of blood) were collected from *Bb*-infected and PBS control mice by submandibular bleeding using single-use lancet without the use of anesthesia [24]. Blood was centrifuged (1800× *g*, 10 min, 4 °C), and plasma was stored at −80 °C until analysis.

2.3. Collagen-Induced Arthritis

DBA/1 mice were immunized with chicken type II collagen (Chondrex, Redmond, WA, USA) emulsified in complete Freund's adjuvant (Sigma-Aldrich, St. Louis, MO, USA) by subcutaneous injection in the tail (100 μL). After three weeks, mice received a booster immunization with type II collagen emulsified in incomplete Freund's adjuvant (Sigma-Aldrich) (100 μL) [25]. Mice were anesthetized in 3–4% sevoflurane in 65% N_2 and 35% O_2 during both immunizations. Four weeks after initial immunization, signs of arthritis in the paws developed. Each paw was scored three times a week on a scale from 0 to 4. The following criteria were used: 0, normal paw; 1, one toe inflamed and swollen; 2, more than one toe, but not entire paw, inflamed and swollen or mild swelling of entire paw; 3, entire paw inflamed and swollen and 4, very inflamed and swollen paw or ankylosed paw. A mean score of 2.5 for all paws was considered maximum per animal.

2.4. In Vivo Bb Bioluminescence Imaging

Mice were intraperitoneally (ip.) injected with 5 mg D-luciferin (30 mg/mL in PBS) 10 min before bioluminescence imaging using an IVIS Lumina XR imaging system (Caliper Life Sciences, Hopkinton, MA, USA). Luciferase bioluminescence intensities were measured using 120–180 s exposure on the mice in ventral/sternal recumbency followed by 120–180 s exposure in dorsal recumbency (f/stop = 1, emission filter = open and binning = 8). Imaging was performed the 1st day after inoculation and subsequently 1, 2, 3, 4, 5, 6 and 8 weeks after inoculation with *Bb*. Control mice were measured for bioluminescence after injection of D-luciferin 1, 2, 3, 4, 5 and 6 weeks after PBS injection. Additionally, inflammatory bioluminescence activities were detected using lucigenin (bis-N-methylacridinium nitrate, 1.25 mg/mL in isotonic saline solution). Mice were ip. injected with lucigenin (12.5 mg/kg) and imaging was performed 10 min after injection. Lucigenin bioluminescence imaging was performed 3 weeks after inoculation with *Bb*. All images were analyzed using Living Image Software version 4.2 (Caliper Life Sciences, Hopkinton, MA, USA). ROIs were drawn for quantitative measurement of the luminescence (total flux) in photons/second (p/s) using equal ROI size for carpal joints as well as for tarsal joints for all mice, infected and negative controls. The geometrical mean of each carpal or tarsal joint was calculated from both ventral and dorsal ROI quantification.

2.5. *Synthesis and Radiolabeling of [^{64}Cu]Cu-DOTATATE*

The ligand [1,4,7,10-tetraazacyclododecane-*N,N′,N′′,N′′′*-tetraacetic acid]-*d*-Phe1,Tyr3-octreotate (DOTATATE) was labeled with the long-lived PET isotope ^{64}Cu. [^{64}Cu]Cu-DOTATATE was produced at DTU Nutech Hevesy Lab, Risør, Denmark, as previously described and approved under good manufacturing practice [26].

2.6. *PET/CT Imaging Acquisition and Analysis*

PET/CT imaging (Inveon, Siemens Medical Systems, Malvern, PA, USA) was performed as a double-bed (two mice at a time), 3 weeks after inoculation with *Bb* ($n = 16$) or PBS for control mice ($n = 6$). Mice were injected intravenously with [^{64}Cu]Cu-DOTATATE in a radioactive dose of 10.0 ± 0.2 MBq (mean ± SD). After injection, mice were returned to cages to rest before PET/CT scan. Animals were anesthetized (3–5% sevoflurane in 35% O_2/65% N_2) and PET imaging was performed 3 h (termed early scan, 300 s PET acquisition) and 48 h (termed late scan, 900 s PET acquisition) after [^{64}Cu]Cu-DOTATATE injection. CT was performed for anatomical reference and for attenuation correction. Emission data were corrected for dead time and decay. PET scans were reconstructed with the maximum a posterior reconstruction algorithm. Inveon Research Workstation software (Siemens Medical Systems, PA, USA) was used for quantitative analysis. ROIs were manually drawn on the carpal and tarsal joints of each mouse, using CT as an anatomical guide. The uptake of [^{64}Cu]Cu-DOTATATE was quantified as maximal percentage of injected dose per gram tissue (%Max ID/g)

2.7. *CD163 Enzyme-Linked Immunosorbent Assay*

Murine CD163 concentrations were measured in 200-fold diluted plasma by CD163 ELISA Kit (antibodies-online GmbH, Aachen, Germany) according to the manufacturer's instructions. The absorbance was measured at 450 nm with a FLUOstar Omega plate reader (BMG Labtech, Ortenberg, Germany) and subtracted with a reference value measured at 650 nm. The concentration of CD163 was calculated using a standard curve and the measured absorbance. Values above the standard curve was reported as 100 ng/mL.

2.8. *Statistical Analysis*

Unpaired t-test was used for comparisons of lucigenin total flux between *Bb*-infected and control mice, ^{64}Cu-DOTATATE uptake between early (3 h) and late scan (48 h) and CD163 plasma levels between *Bb*-infected and control mice at weeks 2, 3, 4 and 5 post-infection. A p value of less than 0.05 was considered statistically significant. Values are reported as mean ± SEM unless otherwise stated. Prism version 7.00 (GraphPad, San Diego, CA, USA) was used for all statistical analyses.

3. Results

3.1. *Bb Infection and Migration of Spirochetes to the Joints*

All *Bb* injected mice became successfully infected. Bioluminescence imaging detected *Bb*-infected mice, which showed focal bioluminescent signal centrally on the lower back at the initial imaging time point (day 1) post-infection at the site of injection. This local infection induced by injection of ML23 pBBE22*luc* strain of *Bb* B31 expanded in the mouse presumably due to dissemination throughout the skin, which was observed one week post-infection as an intensive signal from the dorsal surface of the mice. Two weeks post-infection, the emitted signal spread in the mice, and the bioluminescent signal appeared at the extremities (Figure 1a). All mice were imaged in ventral and dorsal recumbency at each time point. Based on these values, the geometrical mean of the total flux in each joint was calculated as a measure for total amount of bacteria per joint. A peak in the bioluminescence emission from each carpal and tarsal joint was observed 3 weeks post-infection compared with the control mice. Starting three weeks after inoculation, the signal started to diminish but remained visible until the last day of imaging (Figure 1b). Eight weeks after infection, the bioluminescent signal from the joints reached low geometrical means representing disappearance of *Bb*. Bioluminescence signals from the joints were $1.1 \times 10^4 \pm 2.5 \times 10^3$, $1.4 \times 10^5 \pm 9.5 \times 10^3$, $2.2 \times 10^5 \pm 1.4 \times 10^4$, $1.1 \times 10^5 \pm 8.7 \times 10^3$, $1.2 \times 10^5 \pm 1.1 \times 10^4$, $7.5 \times 10^4 \pm 8.6 \times 10^3$, $3.7 \times 10^4 \pm 2.8 \times 10^3$ p/s for the 1, 2, 3, 4, 5, 6 and 8 week time points, respectively. Quantitative data on lucigenin bioluminescence imaging 3 weeks post-infection are depicted in Figure 1c, and the average geometrical mean of the total flux was $2.0 \times 10^4 \pm 6.3 \times 10^2$ and $1.4 \times 10^4 \pm 7.0 \times 10^2$ for *Bb*-infected and control mice, respectively. Total flux (p/s) was significantly increased in *Bb*-infected mice 3 weeks post-infection compared with control mice ($p < 0.0001$).

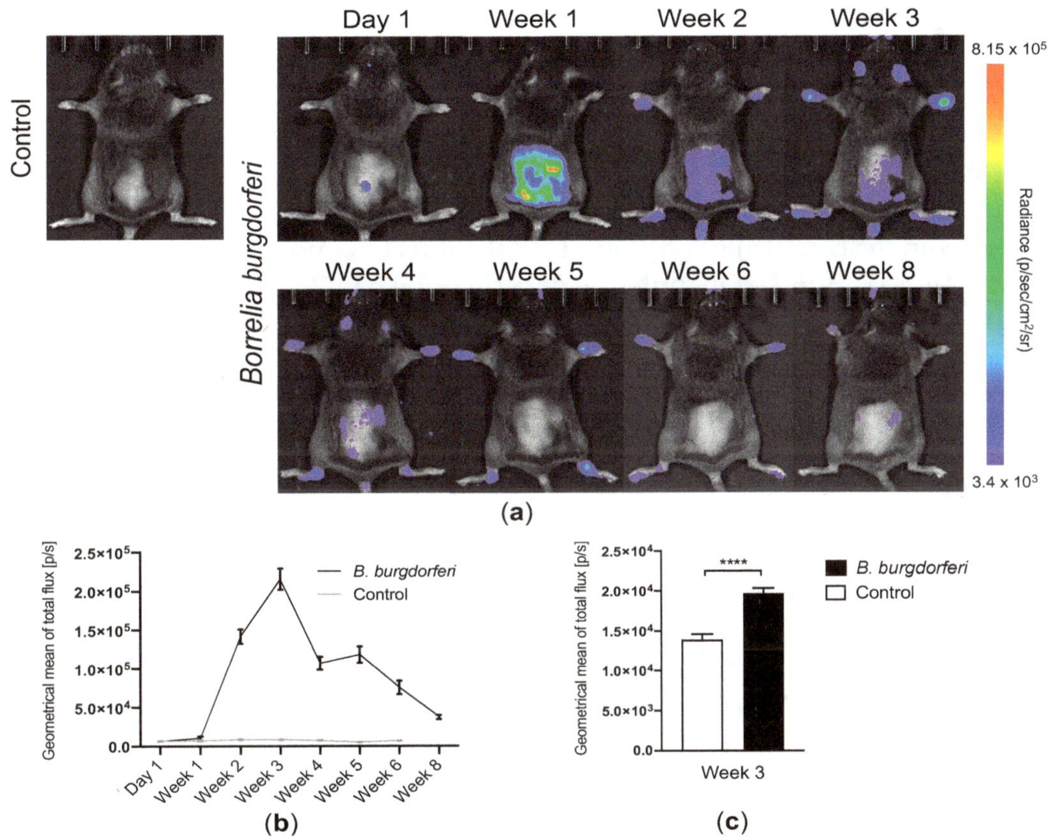

Figure 1. In vivo bioluminescence imaging of *B. burgdorferi* infection and inflammatory phagocytes: (**a**) Representative images of a control mouse and *Bb*-infected mice at day 1 followed by 1, 2, 3, 4, 5, 6 and 8 weeks after intradermal inoculation with *B. burgdorferi* strain ML23 pBBE22*luc*. Images were acquired following ip. injection of D-luciferin. (**b**) Geometrical mean of total flux (p/s) of mice after ip. injection of D-luciferin. In vivo imaging was performed on *Bb*-infected (n = 6–26/group) and control (n = 4–10/group) mice at day 1 followed by week 1, 2, 3, 4, 5, 6 and 8 after intradermal inoculation. All values are derived from ROI analysis of carpal and tarsal joints. Data are presented as mean ± SEM. (**c**) Quantitative representation of lucigenin bioluminescence from the ROI analysis of the carpal and tarsal joints after ip. injection of lucigenin (12.5 mg/kg) in *Bb*-infected (n = 18) and control (n = 6) mice on week 3 after inoculation. Data are presented as mean ± SEM. All images were acquired with a delay of 10 min post-injection (p.i.) of substrate before imaging was completed. The significance level is indicated by asterisks (*). $p < 0.0001$ (****).

3.2. [^{64}Cu]Cu-DOTATATE PET/CT Imaging of Macrophages in CIA and Lyme Arthritis

In addition to PET imaging of Lyme arthritis in *Bb* mice, ^{64}Cu-DOTATATE was tested in the inflammatory CIA mouse model. Quantitative data on the uptake in joints are depicted in Figure 2. The maximum ^{64}Cu-DOTATATE uptake in joints with high CIA arthritis score (score 3) was 4.70% ± 0.38% 3 h p.i. Maximum tracer uptake was significantly increased in these joints compared with control mice ($p = 0.0032$). Maximum uptake in control mice was 2.85% ± 0.26% 3 h p.i.

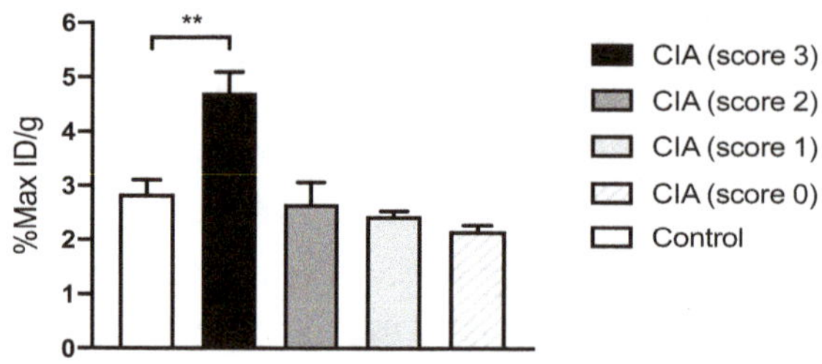

Figure 2. In vivo quantification of ^{64}Cu-DOTATATE uptake in collagen-induced arthritis (CIA) mice ($n = 7$) and controls ($n = 4$). Data are presented as maximal percentage of injected dose per gram tissue (%Max ID/g) in each joint acquired 3 h p.i. Data are presented as mean ± SEM. The significance level is indicated by asterisks (*). $p = 0.0032$ (**).

In vivo PET/CT imaging of *Bb*-induced Lyme arthritis 3 weeks post-infection in mice showed an increased, intense focal accumulation of ^{64}Cu-DOTATATE in the joints at the late scan (48 h p.i. of PET tracer) compared with uninfected control mice. Images acquired 3 h p.i. of tracer displayed a more diffuse uptake within the carpal and tarsal joints of the infected mice. Control mice showed little to no uptake in the joints (Figure 3). Quantitative data on uptake in *Bb*-infected joints are illustrated in Figure 4, and the maximum ^{64}Cu-DOTATATE uptake in infected joints (%Max ID/g) was 2.89% ± 0.06% 3 h p.i. (early scan) and 2.47% ± 0.31% 48 h p.i. (late scan). Maximum tracer uptake was significantly increased in the infected joints at the early ($p < 0.0001$) and late scan time point ($p = 0.0005$) compared with the uptake in control mice. Maximum uptake in control mice was 2.44% ± 0.07% 3 h p.i. (early scan) and 0.47% ± 0.20% 48 h p.i. (late scan) (Figure 4).

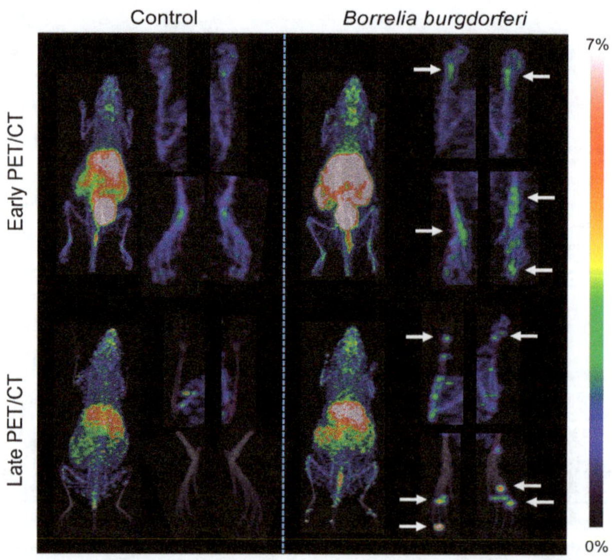

Figure 3. ^{64}Cu-DOTATATE coronal PET/CT imaging of *Bb*-infected and control mice. Representative images of mice inoculated intradermally with *B. burgdorferi* ($n = 18$) or PBS ($n = 6$). Images were acquired 3 weeks after inoculation at 3 h (early PET/CT) and 48 h (late PET/CT) p.i. Images of the ROIs drawn around the carpal and tarsal joints are shown next to the whole-body images. Arrows designate high tracer uptake in the carpal and tarsal joints.

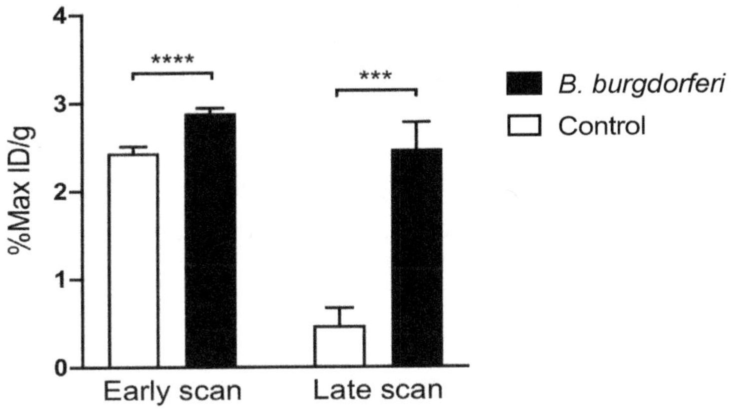

Figure 4. In vivo quantification of accumulated ^{64}Cu-DOTATATE in mice inoculated with *B. burgdorferi* ($n = 18$) or PBS ($n = 6$). Data are presented as maximal percentage of injected dose per gram tissue (%Max ID/g) in each joint and acquired 3 h (early scan) and 48 h (late scan) p.i. 3 weeks post-infection. Data are presented as mean ± SEM. The significance level is indicated by asterisks (*). $p = 0.0005$ (***) and $p < 0.0001$ (****).

3.3. CD163 as a Circulating Marker for Macrophages

Plasma levels of CD163 in infected mice were 56.4 ± 13.3, 58.3 ± 13.1, 25.3 ± 4.1 and 45.0 ± 9.1 ng/mL for the 2-, 3-, 4- and 5-week time points, respectively. No significant differences between *Bb*-infected and control mice were observed at any of the time points (Figure 5). In addition, samples from individual mice showed heterogeneous levels of CD163. Variations at each time point for both *Bb*-infected and control mice appeared, and 23.6% of all samples were higher than 100 ng/mL.

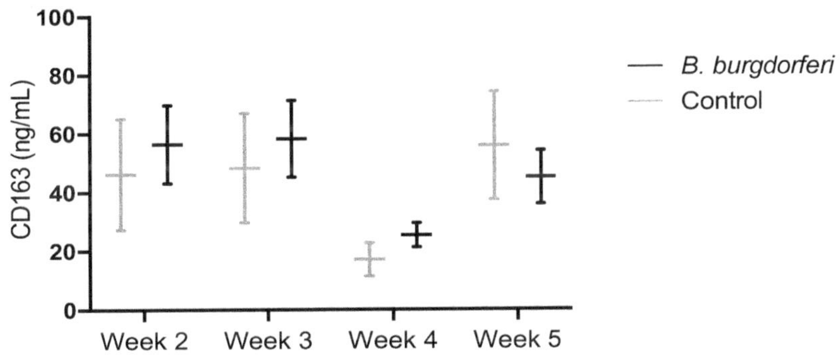

Figure 5. CD163 plasma levels (ng/mL) in a murine model of Lyme arthritis. Mice were infected with 10^6 *B. burgdorferi* intradermally in the lower back, and cheek blood was collected at week 2, 3, 4 ($n = 8$) and 5 ($n = 15$) post-infection. Data are presented as mean ± SEM.

4. Discussion

The major finding in the present study was that PET/CT imaging using ^{64}Cu-DOTATATE, a PET tracer demonstrating macrophages, could detect and monitor Lyme arthritis activity non-invasively, whereas levels of CD163, a marker of macrophages in the plasma during bacterial infection, could not be used for this purpose.

Using bioluminescence, we showed that ML23 pBBE22*luc* strain of *Bb* B31 administered intradermally migrated to the joints in the mice, and a peak of bacterial burden in the joints was observed 3 weeks after inoculation of the spirochetes representing direct evidence of pathogens within the joints. The stage of the joint invasion by *Bb* in this model represents the early phase of Lyme arthritis. Bioluminescence imaging also confirmed the presence of macrophages in Lyme arthritis lesions in the infected mice.

This is the first study to present data on somatostatin receptor imaging of infectious lesions in LB. ^{64}Cu-DOTATATE is mainly being used in the clinical setting for neuroendocrine tumors (NETs) [18,26,27] but has also been tested for detection of atherosclerotic inflammation [19]. In NETs, the basis for imaging is overexpression of somatostatin receptors on the tumors cells [28] whereas the basis for use in atherosclerosis is the macrophages in the atherosclerotic lesions [19,29]. Since *Bb* infection in the joints is likely to be characterized by macrophage invasion [12], we hypothesized that ^{64}Cu-DOTATATE could be a useful tool for diagnosis and monitoring of Lyme arthritis by imaging of macrophages.

Before testing our hypothesis, we showed that ^{64}Cu-DOTATATE can be used in another inflammatory model as the tracer significantly accumulates in the joints of CIA mice with high clinical score at an early time point. Data from this study confirmed that the tracer can be used to target a local inflammatory response and allowed us to continue the work with ^{64}Cu-DOTATATE on our *Bb*-infection model.

^{64}Cu has a half-life of 12.7 h giving the possibility for delayed imaging, and therefore, we tested two different time points for PET scanning, an early (3 h) and a late (48 h) after tracer injection. Our results indicate that PET imaging using ^{64}Cu-DOTATATE of Lyme arthritis in mice should be performed after 48 h to enable clearance of background activity. We showed a significantly increased uptake of tracer (%Max ID/g) in infected mice imaged at the late time point (48 h).

Currently, the most commonly used tracer in PET imaging for infection and inflammation is fluorine-18-fluorodeoxyglucose (^{18}F-FDG), a radiolabeled glucose analogue [30–32]. However, ^{18}F-FDG has major limitations including being non-specific for infection. FDG is taken up by cells via glucose transporters in the membrane, and many different cells are involved including leukocytes, macrophages, monocytes, lymphocytes and giant cells [33]. Due to these limitations, there is an unmet need for other, more specific, targeted radiotracers to improve imaging of infectious diseases and the adjacent inflammatory response. Only few other PET tracers have previously been tested to visualize the inflammatory response caused by *Bb*. Pietikäinen et al. tested ^{18}F-FDG [31] and showed increased uptake in affected joints. However, ^{18}F-FDG has limitations as previously described. Siitonen et al. tested ^{68}Ga-DOTA-Siglec-9 a PET tracer targeting vascular adhesion protein-1 (VAP-1) and showed uptake in infected joints. Both tracers where only tested in tibiotarsal joints in a Lyme arthritis murine model.

In our model, we utilized direct intradermal inoculation of bacteria that allowed bacteria to enter the bloodstream mimicking the pathogenesis in human Lyme arthritis although not transmitted by a vector. The C3H/HeN mouse is the most frequently used animal strain to investigate the immune mechanisms of Lyme arthritis. The model has the advantages of mimicking the early innate immune response that occurs when the bacteria enter the host when transmitted by a vector [34], and using C3H/HeN mice is a promising model for studying the inflammation of subacute Lyme arthritis as a response to spirochetes localized in the joint tissue [35]. This allow us to test our ^{64}Cu-DOTATATE PET tracer as an early marker for the bacterial infection. However, using bioluminescence, we showed that C3H/HeN mice cleared the *Bb* infection in the joints 3 to 6 weeks after inoculation, which is not consistent with human Lyme arthritis, and the model does not mimic the immunological events that result in severe arthritis. We know that our model displays mild and not sustained symptoms of arthritis indicating that the inflammatory response is mild, which makes it more difficult to show increased accumulation of ^{64}Cu-DOTATATE. Having this in mind, our findings on increased accumulation of the tracer within the joints of *Bb*-infected mice seem promising as an early marker for Lyme arthritis in the patients and have great potential in the clinic. In addition, previous studies have described that macrophages play a direct effector role in the induction of severe destructive Lyme arthritis [36], substantiating the clinical use of ^{64}Cu-DOTATATE as a biomarker for macrophages in the joints. Potentially, the severity of Lyme arthritis in regard to immune infiltration could be used in the clinic for initial treatment regimens. However, when using the tracer, it should be kept in mind that it is not specific for Lyme arthritis, and other inflammatory joint conditions may appear similar.

We previously showed that ^{64}Cu-DOTATATE is significantly associated with biomarkers of CD163 positive macrophage activation when studied in atherosclerotic patients [19]. This clearly demonstrates the systemic nature of atherosclerosis with inflammation in the vasculature. In contrast, the present study was not able to show any increased level of CD163 in the plasma during infection with *Bb* in mice. This might not be surprising as Lyme arthritis has a localized nature. Therefore, it seems CD163 cannot be used as a circulatory biomarker for Lyme arthritis as these results show no systemic upregulation of CD163$^+$ macrophages. Based on these results, we must assume that Lyme arthritis results in a localized macrophage response within the joint and not a systemically induced response in the blood of C3H/HeN mice. These results highlight the necessity and benefit of non-invasive in vivo imaging; local detection of the inflammatory response as seen in Lyme arthritis may be demonstrated. The reason for testing circulating CD163 was that this would constitute an easy method in the clinics. However, it did not turn out to be of value in our study.

In conclusion, ^{64}Cu-DOTATATE PET allows for detection of LB infection locally in the joints through non-invasive visualization of macrophages. In contrast, measurement of a systemic macrophage marker in plasma, CD163, did not allow to detect disease. We suggest, that ^{64}Cu-DOTATATE PET could become a valuable diagnostic tool for in situ detection of *Bb* infection-related inflammation.

Author Contributions: Conceptualization, A.K., A.-M.L. and A.S.C.; methodology, A.S.C.; validation, A.S.C., M.Ø. and A.K.; formal analysis, A.S.C. and M.Ø.; investigation, A.S.C., M.Ø., R.R.P. and P.O.J.; resources, A.K. and A.-M.L.; data curation, A.S.C. and A.K.; writing—original draft preparation, A.S.C.; writing—review and editing, A.S.C., M.Ø., R.R.P., P.O.J., A.-M.L. and A.K.; visualization, A.S.C.; supervision, A.K. and A.-M.L.; project administration, A.K., A.-M.L. and A.S.C.; funding acquisition, A.K. All authors have read and agreed to the published version of the manuscript.

References

1. Stanek, G.; Strle, F. Lyme borreliosis-from tick bite to diagnosis and treatment. *FEMS Microbiol. Rev.* **2018**, *42*, 233–258. [CrossRef] [PubMed]
2. Steere, A.C.; Strle, F.; Wormser, G.P.; Hu, L.T.; Branda, J.A.; Hovius, J.W.; Li, X.; Mead, P.S. Lyme borreliosis. *Nat. Rev. Dis. Primers* **2016**, *2*, 16090. [CrossRef] [PubMed]
3. Steere, A.C.; Glickstein, L. Elucidation of Lyme arthritis. *Nat. Rev. Immunol.* **2004**, *4*, 143–152. [CrossRef] [PubMed]
4. Dessau, R.B.; van Dam, A.P.; Fingerle, V.; Gray, J.; Hovius, J.W.; Hunfeld, K.P.; Jaulhac, B.; Kahl, O.; Kristoferitsch, W.; Lindgren, P.E.; et al. To test or not to test? Laboratory support for the diagnosis of Lyme borreliosis: A position paper of ESGBOR, the ESCMID study group for Lyme borreliosis. *Clin. Microbiol. Infect.* **2018**, *24*, 118–124. [CrossRef]
5. Obel, N.; Dessau, R.B.; Krogfelt, K.A.; Bodilsen, J.; Andersen, N.S.; Moller, J.K.; Roed, C.; Omland, L.H.; Christiansen, C.B.; Ellermann-Eriksen, S.; et al. Long term survival, health, social functioning, and education in patients with European Lyme neuroborreliosis: Nationwide population based cohort study. *BMJ* **2018**, *361*. [CrossRef]
6. Raffetin, A.; Saunier, A.; Bouiller, K.; Caraux-Paz, P.; Eldin, C.; Gallien, S.; Jouenne, R.; Belkacem, A.; Salomon, J.; Patey, O.; et al. Unconventional diagnostic tests for Lyme borreliosis: A systematic review. *Clin. Microbiol. Infect.* **2020**, *26*, 51–59. [CrossRef]
7. Shapiro, E.D.; Wormser, G.P. Lyme Disease in 2018: What Is New (and What Is Not). *JAMA* **2018**, *320*, 635–636. [CrossRef]
8. Strle, K.; Drouin, E.E.; Shen, S.; El Khoury, J.; McHugh, G.; Ruzic-Sabljic, E.; Strle, F.; Steere, A.C. Borrelia burgdorferi stimulates macrophages to secrete higher levels of cytokines and chemokines than Borrelia afzelii or Borrelia garinii. *J. Infect. Dis.* **2009**, *200*, 1936–1943. [CrossRef]
9. Lasky, C.E.; Olson, R.M.; Brown, C.R. Macrophage Polarization during Murine Lyme Borreliosis. *Infect Immun.* **2015**, *83*, 2627–2635. [CrossRef]

10. Ramesh, G.; Didier, P.J.; England, J.D.; Santana-Gould, L.; Doyle-Meyers, L.A.; Martin, D.S.; Jacobs, M.B.; Philipp, M.T. Inflammation in the pathogenesis of lyme neuroborreliosis. *Am. J. Pathol.* **2015**, *185*, 1344–1360. [CrossRef]
11. Eiffert, H.; Karsten, A.; Schlott, T.; Ohlenbusch, A.; Laskawi, R.; Hoppert, M.; Christen, H.J. Acute peripheral facial palsy in Lyme disease—A distal neuritis at the infection site. *Neuropediatrics* **2004**, *35*, 267–273. [CrossRef] [PubMed]
12. Wooten, R.M.; Weis, J.J. Host-pathogen interactions promoting inflammatory Lyme arthritis: Use of mouse models for dissection of disease processes. *Curr. Opin. Microbiol.* **2001**, *4*, 274–279. [CrossRef]
13. Xu, Q.; Seemanapalli, S.V.; Reif, K.E.; Brown, C.R.; Liang, F.T. Increasing the recruitment of neutrophils to the site of infection dramatically attenuates Borrelia burgdorferi infectivity. *J. Immunol.* **2007**, *178*, 5109–5115. [CrossRef] [PubMed]
14. Dalm, V.A.; van Hagen, P.M.; van Koetsveld, P.M.; Achilefu, S.; Houtsmuller, A.B.; Pols, D.H.; van der Lely, A.J.; Lamberts, S.W.; Hofland, L.J. Expression of somatostatin, cortistatin, and somatostatin receptors in human monocytes, macrophages, and dendritic cells. *Am. J. Physiol. Endocrinol. Metab.* **2003**, *285*, E344–E353. [CrossRef] [PubMed]
15. Perez, J.; Viollet, C.; Doublier, S.; Videau, C.; Epelbaum, J.; Baud, L. Somatostatin binds to murine macrophages through two distinct subsets of receptors. *J. Neuroimmunol.* **2003**, *138*, 38–44. [CrossRef]
16. Courtenay, J.S.; Dallman, M.J.; Dayan, A.D.; Martin, A.; Mosedale, B. Immunisation against heterologous type II collagen induces arthritis in mice. *Nature* **1980**, *283*, 666–668. [CrossRef] [PubMed]
17. Tseng, J.C.; Kung, A.L. In vivo imaging method to distinguish acute and chronic inflammation. *J. Vis. Exp.* **2013**, e50690. [CrossRef]
18. Johnbeck, C.B.; Knigge, U.; Loft, A.; Berthelsen, A.K.; Mortensen, J.; Oturai, P.; Langer, S.W.; Elema, D.R.; Kjaer, A. Head-to-Head Comparison of (64)Cu-DOTATATE and (68)Ga-DOTATOC PET/CT: A Prospective Study of 59 Patients with Neuroendocrine Tumors. *J. Nucl. Med.* **2017**, *58*, 451–457. [CrossRef]
19. Pedersen, S.F.; Sandholt, B.V.; Keller, S.H.; Hansen, A.E.; Clemmensen, A.E.; Sillesen, H.; Hojgaard, L.; Ripa, R.S.; Kjaer, A. 64Cu-DOTATATE PET/MRI for Detection of Activated Macrophages in Carotid Atherosclerotic Plaques: Studies in Patients Undergoing Endarterectomy. *Arter. Thromb. Vasc. Boil.* **2015**, *35*, 1696–1703. [CrossRef]
20. Svendsen, P.; Etzerodt, A.; Deleuran, B.W.; Moestrup, S.K. Mouse CD163 deficiency strongly enhances experimental collagen-induced arthritis. *Sci. Rep.* **2020**, *10*, 12447. [CrossRef]
21. Hubalek, Z.; Halouzka, J.; Heroldova, M. Growth temperature ranges of Borrelia burgdorferi sensu lato strains. *J. Med. Microbiol.* **1998**, *47*, 929–932. [CrossRef] [PubMed]
22. Hyde, J.A.; Weening, E.H.; Chang, M.; Trzeciakowski, J.P.; Hook, M.; Cirillo, J.D.; Skare, J.T. Bioluminescent imaging of Borrelia burgdorferi in vivo demonstrates that the fibronectin-binding protein BBK32 is required for optimal infectivity. *Mol. Microbiol.* **2011**, *82*, 99–113. [CrossRef] [PubMed]
23. Rosenberg, M.; Azevedo, N.F.; Ivask, A. Propidium iodide staining underestimates viability of adherent bacterial cells. *Sci. Rep.* **2019**, *9*, 6483. [CrossRef] [PubMed]
24. Golde, W.T.; Gollobin, P.; Rodriguez, L.L. A rapid, simple, and humane method for submandibular bleeding of mice using a lancet. *Lab. Anim. (NY)* **2005**, *34*, 39–43. [CrossRef] [PubMed]
25. Pietrosimone, K.M.; Jin, M.; Poston, B.; Liu, P. Collagen-Induced Arthritis: A model for Murine Autoimmune Arthritis. *Bio-Protocol* **2015**, *5*. [CrossRef]
26. Pfeifer, A.; Knigge, U.; Mortensen, J.; Oturai, P.; Berthelsen, A.K.; Loft, A.; Binderup, T.; Rasmussen, P.; Elema, D.; Klausen, T.L.; et al. Clinical PET of neuroendocrine tumors using 64Cu-DOTATATE: First-in-humans study. *J. Nucl. Med.* **2012**, *53*, 1207–1215. [CrossRef]
27. Kjaer, A.; Binderup, T.; Johnbeck, C.; Carlsen, E.; Langer, S.; Federspiel, B.; Knigge, U. Cu-64-DOTATATE somatostatin receptor Imaging in neuroendocrine tumors: Experience from 500 patients at Copenhagen ENETS Center of Excellence. *J. Nucl. Med.* **2019**, *60* (Suppl. 1), 504.
28. Binderup, T.; Knigge, U.; Loft, A.; Mortensen, J.; Pfeifer, A.; Federspiel, B.; Hansen, C.P.; Hojgaard, L.; Kjaer, A. Functional imaging of neuroendocrine tumors: A head-to-head comparison of somatostatin receptor scintigraphy, 123I-MIBG scintigraphy, and 18F-FDG PET. *J. Nucl. Med.* **2010**, *51*, 704–712. [CrossRef]
29. Pedersen, S.F.; Graebe, M.; Hag, A.M.; Hojgaard, L.; Sillesen, H.; Kjaer, A. (18)F-FDG imaging of human

atherosclerotic carotid plaques reflects gene expression of the key hypoxia marker HIF-1alpha. *Am. J. Nucl. Med. Mol. Imaging* **2013**, *3*, 384–392.

30. Jamar, F.; Buscombe, J.; Chiti, A.; Christian, P.E.; Delbeke, D.; Donohoe, K.J.; Israel, O.; Martin-Comin, J.; Signore, A. EANM/SNMMI guideline for 18F-FDG use in inflammation and infection. *J. Nucl. Med.* **2013**, *54*, 647–658. [CrossRef]
31. Pietikainen, A.; Siitonen, R.; Liljenback, H.; Eskola, O.; Soderstrom, M.; Roivainen, A.; Hytonen, J. In vivo imaging of Lyme arthritis in mice by [(18)F]fluorodeoxyglucose positron emission tomography/computed tomography. *Scand. J. Rheumatol.* **2018**, *47*, 37–47. [CrossRef] [PubMed]
32. Vaidyanathan, S.; Patel, C.N.; Scarsbrook, A.F.; Chowdhury, F.U. FDG PET/CT in infection and inflammation–current and emerging clinical applications. *Clin. Radiol.* **2015**, *70*, 787–800. [CrossRef] [PubMed]
33. Glaudemans, A.W.; Slart, R.H.; van Dijl, J.M.; van Oosten, M.; van Dam, G.M. Molecular imaging of infectious and inflammatory diseases: A terra incognita. *J. Nucl. Med.* **2015**, *56*, 659–661. [CrossRef] [PubMed]
34. Munson, E.; Nardelli, D.T.; Du Chateau, B.K.; Callister, S.M.; Schell, R.F. Hamster and murine models of severe destructive Lyme arthritis. *Clin. Dev. Immunol.* **2012**, *2012*, 504215. [CrossRef]
35. Barthold, S.W.; Beck, D.S.; Hansen, G.M.; Terwilliger, G.A.; Moody, K.D. Lyme borreliosis in selected strains and ages of laboratory mice. *J. Infect. Dis.* **1990**, *162*, 133–138. [CrossRef]
36. Du Chateau, B.K.; England, D.M.; Callister, S.M.; Lim, L.C.; Lovrich, S.D.; Schell, R.F. Macrophages exposed to Borrelia burgdorferi induce Lyme arthritis in hamsters. *Infect. Immun.* **1996**, *64*, 2540–2547. [CrossRef]

4

Relationship between ^{18}F-FDG Uptake in the Oral Cavity, Recent Dental Treatments and Oral Inflammation or Infection: A Retrospective Study of Patients with Suspected Endocarditis

Geertruida W. Dijkstra [1], Andor W. J. M. Glaudemans [2,*], Paola A. Erba [2,3], Marjan Wouthuyzen-Bakker [4], Bhanu Sinha [4], David Vállez García [2], Luc W. M. van der Sluis [1] and Riemer H. J. A. Slart [2,5]

1 Center for Dentistry and Oral Hygiene, University Medical Center Groningen, University of Groningen, PO 9700 RB Groningen, The Netherlands; g.w.dijkstra@umcg.nl (G.W.D.); l.w.m.van.der.sluis@umcg.nl (L.W.M.v.d.S.)
2 Department of Nuclear Medicine and Molecular Imaging, University Medical Center Groningen, University of Groningen, PO 9700 RB Groningen, The Netherlands; paola.erba@unipi.it (P.A.E.); d.vallez-garcia@umcg.nl (D.V.G.); r.h.j.a.slart@umcg.nl (R.H.J.A.S.)
3 Department of Nuclear Medicine, Department of Translational Research and New Technology in Medicine, University of Pisa, 56128 Pisa, Italy
4 Department of Medical Microbiology and Infection Prevention, University Medical Center Groningen, University of Groningen, PO 9700 RB Groningen, The Netherlands; m.wouthuyzen-bakker@umcg.nl (M.W.-B.); b.sinha@umcg.nl (B.S.)
5 Department of Biomedical Photonic Imaging, University of Twente, 7522 NB Enschede, The Netherlands
* Correspondence: a.w.j.m.glaudemans@umcg.nl

Abstract: [^{18}F]-fluorodeoxyglucose positron emission tomography ([^{18}F]FDG PET/CT) has proven to be a useful diagnostic tool in patients with suspected infective endocarditis (IE), but is conflicting in relation to dental procedures. Questions: Is there a correlation between [^{18}F]FDG PET/CT findings, recent dental treatment, and an affected oral cavity? (2) Is there a correlation between infective endocarditis (IE), oral health status, and (extra)cardiac findings on [^{18}F]FDG PET/CT? Methods: This retrospective study included 52 patients. All [^{18}F]FDG PET/CT scans were examined visually by pattern recognition using a three-point scale and semi-quantified within the volume of interest (VOI) using SUV_{max}. Results: 19 patients were diagnosed with IE (group 1), 14 with possible IE (group 2), and 19 without IE based on the modified Duke criteria (group 3). No correlation was found between visual PET and SUV_{max} and sites of oral inflammation and infection. The visual PET scores and SUV_{max} were not significantly different between all groups. A significant difference in the SUV_{max} of the valve between all groups was observed. Conclusions: This study suggests that no correlation exists between the PET findings in the oral cavity and dental treatments or inflammation/infection. No correlation between IE, actual oral health status, and extra-cardiac findings was demonstrated. Additional research is needed to conclude whether [^{18}F]FDG PET/CT imaging is a reliable diagnostic modality for oral inflammation and infection sites.

Keywords: infective endocarditis; oral health; FDG PET/CT

---

1. Introduction

The oral cavity is a natural habitat for more than 500 species of microorganisms [1,2]. These microorganisms can form biofilms on dental surfaces. In the case of an unbalance among the microbial species in the biofilm, oral diseases can emerge, such as caries and periodontitis, the most prevalent microbial diseases in humans [2]. Indeed, any disruption of the natural integrity between the biofilm and the subgingival epithelium, which is at most about 10 cell layers thick, could lead to a bacteremic state. Oral microorganisms can also enter the circulation and cause bacteremia during and after routine oral activities (e.g., chewing and tooth brushing) or dental procedures (e.g., dental extractions, scaling, and root planing) [3,4]. The presence of gingivitis, periodontitis, or other odontogenic infections (following dental procedures—e.g., extractions, dental scaling) increases the incidence of bacteremia, since the periodontal vasculature proliferates and dilates, providing an even greater surface area to allow the entry of microorganisms into the bloodstream [5]. This may lead to the seeding of organisms in different target organs, resulting in subclinical, acute, or chronic infections. Infective endocarditis (IE), a microbial infection of a native or prosthetic heart valve, the endocardial surface, other organs, or an indwelling cardiac device [6], is a well-known complication of odontogenic bacteremia [7]. IE is a serious condition with a 30% incidence of mortality [3,8,9].

The bacteria that cause IE are in 85% of cases of Gram-positive cocci (streptococci, staphylococci, and enterococci) that can be considered as commensals with *Staphylococcus aureus* (*S. aureus*), associated with the most severe form of IE [10]. The most prevalent species of the streptococci group causing IE is *Streptococcus viridans* (*S. viridans*) [10–12]. The blood-circulating bacteria responsible for IE enter the bloodstream via the mouth (29%, of which 59% have an oral or dental infectious focus, and 12% are due to recent dental procedures), the skin (40%), and the gastrointestinal and urinary tracts (23%) [13]. A higher microbial load would facilitate such dissemination, as it is known that individuals with poor oral hygiene are at higher risk of developing bacteremias during oral manipulative procedures [14].

In case of infection, [^{18}F]-fluorodeoxyglucose positron emission tomography ([^{18}F]FDG PET/CT) is used to provide diagnostic information based on increased glucose metabolism by inflammatory cells recruited at the site of infection [15–17]. In addition, Heuker et al. (2017) [17] observed that the clinical isolates of many major Gram-positive and Gram-negative bacterial pathogens can actively take up [^{18}F]FDG. Since both types of bacteria are present in the oral cavity, [^{18}F]FDG PET/CT can be used to detect periodontal disease and apical periodontitis [18–20]. Furthermore, a correlation was described between peri-implant hypermetabolism and peri-implantitis diagnosed in [^{18}F]FDG PET/CT scans [21].

Whole-body [^{18}F]FDG PET/CT has been demonstrated to successfully identify cardiac and extra-cardiac infection, providing information on possible portals of infection (POEs)—e.g., in the case of IE, the oral cavity [22,23]. According to the recently published guidelines of the European Society of Cardiology, [^{18}F]FDG PET/CT should be a routine part of the diagnostic algorithm of patients with suspected IE [24]. However, no systematic analysis has examined the role of [^{18}F]FDG PET/CT in detecting infection in the oral cavity in patients with IE. Therefore, this study aims (1) to explore the correlation of [^{18}F]FDG uptake in patients with recent dental treatments and/or inflammation and infection in the oral cavity; (2) the correlation between IE, oral health status, and (extra)cardiac findings on [^{18}F]FDG PET/CT.

2. Materials and Methods

2.1. Study Design and Patients

Between 2011 and 2018, 60 patients (39 men, 21 women; median age 60 years; IQR (48–69) years) with suspected IE underwent [^{18}F]FDG PET/CT imaging at the University Medical Center Groningen (UMCG), the Netherlands. Status praesens and dental records were requested from the dental offices of the included patients. Exclusion criteria were patients who did not visit a dentist during the two years preceding the [^{18}F]FDG PET/CT scan, and edentate patients without dental implants. All the patients were divided into three groups based on their final diagnosis: group 1—patients diagnosed with IE; group 2—patients diagnosed with possible IE; and group 3—patients without IE based on the modified Duke criteria [24]. The final diagnosis of IE was established through expert consensus based on all available clinical and diagnostic data, and with at least one year of follow-up. [^{18}F]FDG PET/CT scans, transoesophageal echocardiograms, transthoracic echocardiograms, and blood cultures were analyzed for all the patients. The local institutional review board approved this retrospective study and waived the requirement for written informed consent (2015/033 (date: March 2016)).

2.2. *Status Praesens, Oral Health, and Dental Records*

Patient characteristics and dental records were reviewed for the relevant clinical data at the time of the [^{18}F]FDG PET/CT scan, including age; sex; clinical risk factors; acute dental infection; decayed, missing, and filled teeth (DMFT index); and the status praesens of the oral cavity (number and sites of dental procedures). All the dental treatments such as dental restorations, extractions, implants, root canal treatments, non-surgical procedures (scaling and root planing), and surgical periodontal treatment within two years before the [^{18}F]FDG PET/CT scan were assessed to verify whether a dental treatment could have caused the infection. The treatments were registered in six sextants (upper and lower jaw, incisor/canine region, left and right premolar/molar region) (Figure 1).

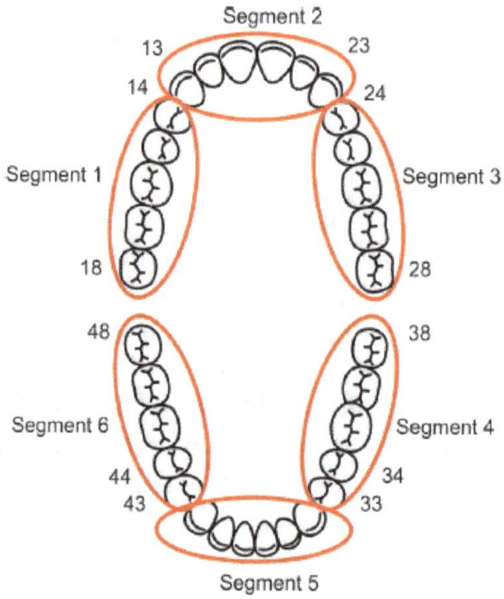

Figure 1. Oral cavity divided into six sextants. Sextant/segment 1: upper right premolar/molar region (18–14); Sextant/segment 2: upper jaw incisor/canine region (13–23); Sextant 3: upper left premolar/molar region (24–28); Sextant 4: lower left premolar/molar region (38–34); Sextant 5: lower jaw incisor/canine region (33–43); Sextant 6: lower right premolar/molar region (44–48).

2.3. *[^{18}F]FDG PET/CT Acquisition and Interpretation*

[^{18}F]FDG PET/CT imaging was performed on a BioGraph 40- or 64-slice mCT (Siemens Healthcare, Knoxville, TN, USA), and reconstructions were performed according to the EANM-SNMMI guidelines and IE recommendations [24,25]. For all scans, the patients followed a 24 h low-carbohydrate/fat-allowed diet and fasted for a minimum of 6 h. All the patients were scanned from the skull base to mid-thigh. The [^{18}F]FDG activity of 3 MBq/kg of body weight was injected intravenously 60 min before the PET data acquisition, according to existing guidelines [26]. All the scans were accompanied by low-dose CT scanning for attenuation correction and anatomical positioning and were performed early in the diagnostic process, within four days and no later than seven days after the start of antimicrobial therapy. All the scans were separately analyzed in consensus by two experienced readers (AWJMG, RHJAS), blinded for all clinical information. Image analysis was performed using Siemens Syngo.via (Client version 3.0; Siemens, Erlangen, Germany).

2.4. *[^{18}F]FDG PET/CT Scan Analyses of the Oral Cavity and Extra-Cardiac Areas*

All the [^{18}F]FDG PET/CT scans (with and without attenuation correction) were examined visually using a three-point scale per sextant: 0 = no [^{18}F]FDG uptake visible; 1 = mildly increased uptake (equal to muscle background); 2 = moderately increased uptake (higher than muscle activity, lower than [^{18}F]FDG brain activity); or 3 = highly increased uptake (equal or higher than brain activity). Uptake scores of 2 and 3 were defined as positive.

The [^{18}F]FDG uptake was further evaluated qualitatively by pattern recognition (homogeneous or focal/heterogeneous). The [^{18}F]FDG accumulation uptake was also semi-quantified by drawing a volume of interest (VOI) in all six sextants and calculating the SUV_{max} (Figure 1). Furthermore, the SUV_{max} was determined in the valve region. The valve culture was determined in patients who underwent a surgical valve replacement.

Extra-cardiac findings (lungs, mediastinum, sternum, CIED, liver, pancreas, gastrointestinal, lymphatic system, oropharynx, thyroid, musculoskeletal, abdominal, vascular, cutaneous, atrial, and sinuses) were measured as negative (0: no [^{18}F]FDG uptake visible) or positive (1: [^{18}F]FDG uptake visible).

2.5. Statistical Analyses

For continuous variables (age, SUV_{max}, and the number of dental treatments), the normality of the distribution was visually explored using Q-Q-plots, histograms, and box-plots. Fisher's exact probability test was used to analyze the visual [^{18}F]FDG uptake scores for the oral cavity and dental treatments performed in 312 sextants in the two years before the [^{18}F]FDG PET/CT scan. Furthermore, Pearson's correlation was used to determine the relationship between the SUV_{max} values and the number of dental treatments.

[^{18}F]FDG PET/CT was considered to be true-positive for oral findings when the SUV_{max} and visual scores per sextant matched with the dental treatments and true-negative when no [^{18}F]FDG uptake was visually identified and no dental treatments were performed or disease was reported in the same sextant. [^{18}F]FDG PET/CT was considered false-positive when positive findings were not related to any dental procedure or disease and false-negative in the case of negative PET/CT findings in patients with dental disease and if there were recent dental treatments.

To analyze a possible difference in the prevalence of dental treatments (0: no dental treatments performed; 1: dental treatments performed), Fisher's exact probability test was conducted. The Kruskal–Wallis H test was used to compare the ordinal variable DMFT index within groups 1, 2, and 3, as well as the differences between PET/CT scores. A one-way ANOVA was conducted to compare the SUV_{max} measured in the oral cavity.

Furthermore, to analyze the difference between the SUV_{max} valve scores in groups 1, 2, and 3, a one-way ANOVA and Tukey's post-hoc test were used. Pearson's correlations were used to determine whether the oral visual [^{18}F]FDG uptake scores were correlated with the presence of a visual uptake of [^{18}F]FDG in a heart valve. Fisher's exact probability test was used to analyze a possible difference in the prevalence of extra-cardiac [^{18}F]FDG PET/CT findings between groups 1, 2, and 3.

P values < 0.05 were considered statistically significant. Statistical analyses were performed using the IBM Statistical Package for Social Sciences (SPSS), version 25 (IBM SPSS).

3. Results

Between 2011 and 2018, 60 consecutive [^{18}F]FDG PET/CT scans were performed in patients with suspected IE. After the exclusion of six edentate patients and two patients who did not visit a dental professional in the two years before the PET/CT, 52 patients (32 men, 20 women; median age, 58 years; IQR (44–66) years) were included. Clinical parameters, including the echocardiography findings and blood cultures at the time of imaging, are summarized in Table 1. Of the 52 patients, 19 had a final diagnosis of IE (group 1: 12 men, 7 women; median age, 57 years; IQR (40–66) years), 14 had a final diagnosis of possible IE (group 2: 7 men, 7 women; median age, 60 years; IQR (37–65) years), and the remaining 19 patients were diagnosed as not having IE based on the modified Duke criteria (group 3: 13 men, 6 women; median age, 60 years; IQR (51–70) years).

Table 1. Patient characteristics and clinical data at the time of [^{18}F]FDG PET/CT imaging.

	Group 1 (*n* = 19)	Group 2 (*n* = 14)	Group 3 (*n* = 19)
Demographics			
Age (median (IQR), years)	57 (42–66)	60 (37–65)	60 (51–70)
Male sex, *n* (%)	12 (63%)	7 (50%)	13 (68%)
BMI (mean ±SD, kg/m^2)	25.1 ± 7.9	24.7 ± 2.7	25.5 ± 5.5
Diabetes, n (%)	3 (16%)	3 (21%)	4 (21%)
Previous IE, *n* (%)	5 (26%)	1 (7%)	4 (21%)
CIED, n (%)	2 (11%)	2 (14%)	3 (16%)
Previous PHV ○, *n* (%)	**16 (84%)**	**7 (50%)**	**6 (32%)**
Aortic	10 (63%)	6 (86%)	5 (83%)
Mitral	1 (6%)	1 (14%)	1 (17%)
Pulmonary	4 (25%)	0	0
Tricuspid	1 (6%)	0	0
Echocardiography data available ○, *n* (%)	**18 (95%)**	**14 (100%)**	**11 (58%)**
Vegetation ○○	12 (67%)	1 (7%)	0
Aortic	6 (50%)	0	0
Mitral	3 (25%)	0	0
Pulmonary	1 (8%)	1 (7%)	0
Tricuspid	2 (17%)	0	0
Abscess	2 (11%)	1 (7%)	0
Fistula	0	0	0
Prosthetic valve dehiscence	1 (6%)	0	0
Paravalvular leakage	6 (33%)	1 (7%)	0
CIED infection	1 (6%)	0	1 (10%)
Microbiology data available ○○○, *n* (%)	**19 (100%)**	**13 (93%)**	**13 (68%)**
Positive blood cultures ○	12 (63%)	8 (62%)	6 (46%)
Staphylococcus aureus	4 (33%)	6 (75%)	4 (67%)
Staphylococcus lugdunesis	0	0	1 (17%)
HACCEK ++	2 (17%)	0	0
Streptococcus mitis	3 (25%)	0	0
Streptococcus bovis	1 (8%)	0	0
Streptococcus gallolyticus	1 (8%)	1 (13%)	0
Streptococcus angiosus	0	0	1 (17%)
Other ##	1 (8%)	1 (13%)	0
PCR and/or serology positive ○, n (%)	**5 (26%)**	**0**	**0**
Haemophilus parainfluenzae	1 (5%)	0	0
Tropheryma whipplei	1 (5%)	0	0
Enterobacter cloacae	1 (5%)	0	0
Escherichia coli	1 (5%)	0	0
Proprionibacterium acnes	1 (5%)	0	0
Valve culture, n (%)	**10 (53%)**	**0**	**1 (5%)**
Staphylococcus aureus	2 (20%)	0	0
Haemophilus parainfluenzae	1 (10%)	0	0
Streptococcus mitis	1 (10%)	0	0
Proprionibacterium acnes	1 (10%)	0	1 (100%)
No bacteria and yeast on the valve	5 (50%)	0	0
Lab test, n (%)			
CRP (median (IQR), mg/L)	7.4 (2.8–46)	89 (36.3–148.5)	51 (19–145)
Leucocytes (median (IQR), ×109/L	8.2 (5.8–9.9)	10.1 (7–13.8)	9.6 (6.5-12)
Treatment, n (%)			
Antibiotic therapy	19 (100%)	6 (43%)	5 (26%)
Days of antibiotic therapy (median (IQR)) ^^	14 (8–38)	6 (6–9)	6 (2–8)
Valve surgery replacement	13 (68%)	0	2 (11%)

AV, aortic valve; BMI, body mass index; CIED, cardiovascular implantable electronic device; CRP, C-reactive protein; CT, computed tomography; [^{18}F]FDG, 18F-fluorodeoxyglucose; IQR, interquartile range; MV, mitral valve; PCR, polymerase chain; PET, positron-emission tomography; PHV, prosthetic heart valve; PV, pulmonary valve; and TV, tricuspid valve. ○ Percentages of PHV, abnormal echocardiographic findings, positive blood cultures, and PCR/positive serology are relative to the number of available PHV, echocardiograms, and positive blood findings, and a positive PCR/serology. ○○ One patient had vegetation on both AV and TV. Another patient had vegetation on both AV and TV. ○○○ For blood cultures, PCR, and serology, even if they were no longer positive at the time of [^{18}F]FDG PET/CT imaging, they were classified as positive if they had been positive during the clinical episode prior to the [^{18}F]FDG PET/CT scan. ++ HACCEK: Haemophilus spp., Aggregatibacter- (Actinobacillus) actinomycetemcomitans (A. actinomycetemcomitans), Capnocytophaga spp., Cardiobacterium hominis, Eikenella corrodens, and Kingella bacteria. ## S. epidermidis, Gram-negative staph bacteria. ^^ For 8 patients, data about the days of antibiotic therapy before the [^{18}F]FDG PET/CT scan could not be retrieved from the patient's electronic files.

3.1. Dental Procedures Prior to [^{18}F]FDG PET/CT Imaging

In the two years before the [^{18}F]FDG PET/CT scans, a total of 97 dental restorations, 43 extractions, 0 implants, and 5 root canal treatments were performed by 48 different dentists. The prevalence of patients who received dental restorations in groups 1, 2, and 3 was 47%, 86%, and 53%, respectively. The prevalence of patients who underwent extractions in groups 1, 2, and 3 was 21%, 7%, and 21%, respectively. For root canal treatments, the figures for groups 1, 2, and 3 were 16%, 7%, and 5%, respectively. No significant differences between groups were observed for the prevalence of dental restorations (p = 0.061), extractions (p = 0.590), or root canal treatments (p = 0.615).

Furthermore, all 52 patients routinely visited a dentist once or twice per year, which is the standard in the Netherlands. The removal of supragingival calculus by scaling was performed regularly in 17 patients (90%) in group 1, 11 patients (79%) in group 2, and 9 (47%) patients in group 3. The removal of subgingival calculus by scaling and root planing was performed in 1 patient (5%) in group 1, 0 patients in group 2, and 4 patients (21%) in group 3. None of the 52 patients had been subjected to periodontal surgery.

3.2. Oral Status Praesens at Time of [^{18}F]FDG PET/CT Imaging

Fifty status praesens and DMFT indices (median 12; IQR [7.3–16.5]) were determined by the information obtained from dental records. A Kruskal–Wallis H test revealed no difference (H(2) = 4.724, p = 0.094) between the mean DMFT scores of the three groups. The DMFT score in group 1 (median 10.5; IQR [5–14]) was not significantly different than the DMFT score in group 3 (median 12.5; IQR [10.3–23.8]). Based on the dental records, the periodontal health was good in all patients. Only one patient had acute dental problems at the time of the scan (Figure 2).

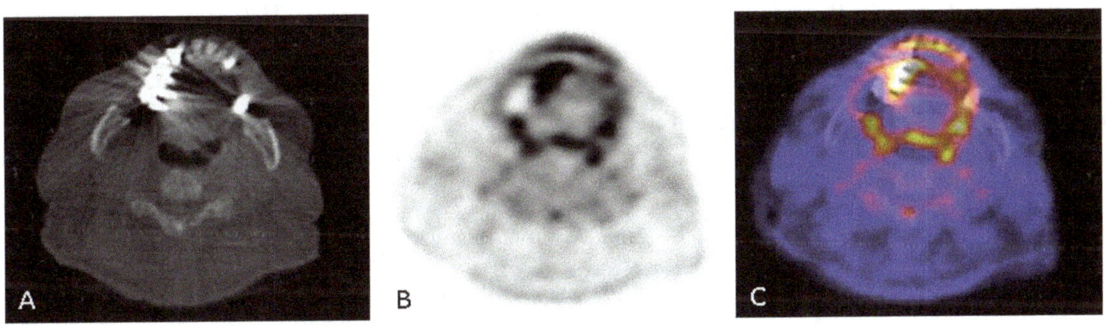

Figure 2. (**A**) a low dose CT on dental level acquired in combination with the PET. Seventy-eight-year-old male suspected of IE with a dental history of periapical inflammation related to tooth 16. Sextant 1 (**B**,**C**) shows a markedly increased [^{18}F]FDG uptake (score 2, SUVmax 4.0), possibly due to the extraction of tooth 16. Sextant 3 (**B**,**C**) shows a markedly increased [^{18}F]FDG uptake (score 3, SUVmax 7.7), possibly due to the extraction of tooth 25. Furthermore, periapical inflammation related to tooth 13 and tooth 27 was detected in panoramic radiographs but not in the PET scan. The patient had positive blood cultures for Streptococcus mitis.

3.3. Visual [^{18}F]FDG Uptake Scores and SUV_{max} Compared with Dental Treatments

In 54 sextants (17.3%) the positive visual scores were between 2 and 3 (median 2.0) (Table 2). Dental restorations were performed in 69 sextants, of which only 13 had a positive visual score. Furthermore, extractions were performed in 16 sextants, of which only 2 had a positive visual score. All the root canal treatments were performed in sextants with a visual [^{18}F]FDG uptake score of 0. Regarding the true-positive findings of [^{18}F]FDG PET/CT scans, the number of dental treatments did not correlate with the visual [^{18}F]FDG uptake scores (dental restorations, $p = 0.546$; extractions, $p = 0.985$; and root canal treatments, $p = 1.000$).

The SUV_{max} was measured in all sextants, and was above zero in 72 sextants (23%) (3.56 ± 1.67). The number of dental treatments also did not correlate with the SUV_{max} (dental restorations, $p = 0.209$; extractions, $p = 0.933$; root canal treatments, $p = 0.593$).

The visual [^{18}F]FDG uptake scores in groups 1, 2, and 3 were not significantly different ($H(2) = 4.359$, $p = 0.113$). There was also no significant difference in the SUV_{max} for the three groups ($F(2, 69) = 0.27$, $p = 0.798$).

3.4. Cardiac and Extra-Cardiac [^{18}F]FDG PET/CT Findings

There was a significant difference in the SUV_{max} of the valve for the three groups ($F(2, 309) = 28.06$, $p < 0.001$). A Tukey post-hoc test revealed that the SUV_{max} of the valve was significantly lower for group 2 (3.04 ± 1.39, $p < 0.001$) and group 3 (2.83 ± 0.55, $p < 0.001$) compared to group 1 (4.11 ± 1.85, $p < 0.001$). No significant correlation was demonstrated between the presence of the pathological visual uptake of [^{18}F]FDG in a heart valve and the visual uptake of [^{18}F]FDG in the oral cavity ($p = 0.160$) for the three groups.

In group 1, 13 patients underwent surgical valve replacement. The bacterial species on the valve was determined by culture after surgical valve replacement for 10 patients. The valve culture was positive for oral flora (*Streptococcus mitis, Heamophilus parainfluenzae*) in only two patients diagnosed with IEs. In group 3, two patients underwent surgical valve replacement. The valve culture was not positive for the oral flora in group 3 (Table 1).

Furthermore, in all three groups, the extra-cardiac visual [^{18}F]FDG PET/CT findings were mainly noticed in the lymph nodes, mediastinum, and lungs. The prevalence of patients who had extra-cardiac findings in groups 1, 2, and 3 was 95%, 86%, and 90%, respectively. No significant difference between groups was observed for the extra-cardiac findings ($p = 0.842$).

For groups 1, 2, and 3, the visual [^{18}F]FDG uptake scores, oral SUV_{max}, extra-cardiac [^{18}F]FDG PET/CT findings, and valve SUV_{max} are summarized in Table 3.

Table 2. Visual [18F]FDG uptake score and dental treatments.

	Visual [^{18}F]FDG Uptake Score ○				
	0	**1**	**2**	**3**	***Total***
Dental Restorations					
0	185	17	30	11	243
1	33	6	6	3	48
2	14	0	2	1	17
3	0	0	1	0	1
4	3	0	0	0	3
Total	235	23	39	15	312
Root Canal Treatment					
0	230	23	39	15	307
1	5	0	0	0	5
Total	235	23	39	15	312

Table 2. *Cont.*

	Visual [18F]FDG Uptake Score ○				
	0	1	2	3	*Total*
Extractions					
0	219	23	37	15	294
1	7	0	2	0	9
2	3	0	0	0	3
4	4	0	0	0	4
6	2	0	0	0	2
Total	235	23	39	15	312

○ Visual [18F]FDG uptake score, 0; no [18F]FDG uptake is visible, (1); mildly increased uptake (=muscle background), (2); moderately increased uptake (>muscle activity, <[18F]FDG brain activity), (3); ≥brain activity.

Table 3. [18F]FDG PET/CT scan in oral cavity and valve, and extra-cardiac findings.

	Visual Score [18F]FDG Uptake (Mean ± SD) ○	Oral SUV_{max} (Mean ± SD)	Extra-Cardiac Findings (MEAN ± SD) ○○	Valve SUV_{max} (mean ± SD) ○○○
Group 1	**0.51 ± 0.85**	**3.64 ± 2.18**		
Sextant 1	0.53 ± 0.84	3.24 ± 0.59		
Sextant 2	0.47 ± 0.84	3.80 ± 2.09		
Sextant 3	0.89 ± 1.05	4.17 ± 4.01	1.95 ± 1.43	4.11 ± 1.84
Sextant 4	0.32 ± 0.75	2.98 ± 1.29		
Sextant 5	0.53 ± 0.77	3.97 ± 1.46		
Sextant 6	0.32 ± 0.82	3.17 ± 1.77		
Group 2	**0.57 ± 1.01**	**3.65 ± 1.19**		
Sextant 1	0.43 ± 0.85	3.13 ± 0.70		
Sextant 2	1.21 ± 1.31	4.50 ± 1.25		
Sextant 3	0.50 ± 1.02	3.77 ± 0.51	2.00 ± 1.47	3.04 ± 1.38
Sextant 4	0.43 ± 0.85	3.05 ± 0.76		
Sextant 5	0.50 ± 0.94	2.80 ± 1.74		
Sextant 6	0.36 ± 0.93	4.70 ± 0.00		
Group 3	**0.35 ± 0.82**	**3.35 ± 1.08**		
Sextant 1	0.42 ± 0.90	3.40 ± 0.94		
Sextant 2	0.32 ± 0.82	3.97 ± 1.21		
Sextant 3	0.32 ± 0.82	2.80 ± 1.21	2.84 ± 1.61	2.83 ± 0.54
Sextant 4	0.74 ± 1.15	3.52 ± 1.38		
Sextant 5	0.21 ± 0.54	3.28 ± 0.26		
Sextant 6	0.11 ± 0.46	2.10 ± 0.00		

[18F]FDG, 18F-fluorodeoxyglucose; SD, standard deviation; Sextant 1, upper right premolar/molar region; Sextant 2, upper jaw incisor/canine region; Sextant 3, upper left premolar/molar region; Sextant 4, lower left premolar/molar region; Sextant 5, lower jaw incisor/canine region; Sextant 6, lower right premolar/molar region; SUVmax, maximum standardized uptake value. ○ Visual [18F]FDG uptake score, 0; no 18F-FDG uptake visible, 1; mildly increased uptake (=muscle background), 2; moderately increased uptake (>muscle activity, <[18F]FDG brain activity), 3; =>brain activity. ○○ Extra-cardiac findings: lungs, mediastinum, sternum, CIED, liver, pancreas, gastro-intestinal, lymphatic system, oropharynx, thyroid, musculoskeletal, abdominal, vascular, cutaneous, atrial, and sinuses. ○○○ Valve: aortic valve, mitral valve, tricuspid valve, and pulmonic valve.

4. Discussion

In this retrospective study, no significant correlation was found between the visual [18F]FDG uptake scores or SUV_{max}, the possible locations of oral inflammation and infection, and recent dental treatments.

Two previous studies found a correlation between the visual [18F]FDG uptake and oral inflammation/infection, periodontitis, and apical periodontitis [27,28]. In the Kito et al. (2012) study [28], periodontitis was scored by panoramic radiograph, which is not a reliable way to measure the severity and extension of this typical disease. Shimamoto et al. (2008) [27] used clinical measurements of periodontitis, resulting in a more reliable severity score. These measurements were performed by calibrated dentists, in contrast to our study in which dental records were used as a reference. This may have resulted in an underestimation of periodontal disease in our study. Furthermore, for both studies, it must be mentioned that it is technically impossible to accurately measure the severity and extension of apical periodontitis. Therefore, the reliability of the data related to apical periodontitis is questionable [29]. Panoramic radiographs were acquired to measure the severity of dental caries, periodontitis, and apical periodontitis [27,28]. However, intraoral bitewing radiography or a solo radiograph is superior to panoramic radiography in diagnosing the severity and extension of periodontitis and apical periodontitis [29].

The positive correlation between the visual [^{18}F]FDG uptake scores and oral inflammation and infection in the previously mentioned studies could also be explained by the extension and severity of periodontitis in that particular study population, which could be more pronounced than our included patients who regularly visited a dentist [27,28].

In this study, we compared the visual [^{18}F]FDG uptake scores and SUV_{max} to dental restorations performed within two years before [^{18}F]FDG PET/CT imaging, and found no significant correlation. In contrast to our study, Kao et al. (2003) [29] reported incidental findings on the [^{18}F]FDG uptake in patients with dental caries. A dental restoration is a filling of the mineral tooth loss due to caries and an indication of caries in the past. This may indicate possible inflammation of the tooth pulp. In our study, no dental caries were found, probably because the patients were regularly checked by dental professionals. The dental treatments performed in sextants with true-positive findings were 90% dental restorations. A possible explanation is that dental restorations are, for the most part, performed by dentists.

The normal physiologic uptake in the oral cavity could be an explanation for the false-positive results. In addition to the teeth, the oral cavity and oropharynx also consist of structures such as mucosal surfaces, salivary glands, muscle, lymphoid tissue, and brown fat, which is responsible for higher glucose uptake [30].

Regarding oral health status and IE, no difference in the dental health or amount or type of dental treatments before the diagnosis of IE was found between the groups diagnosed with IE and those not diagnosed with IE. Tubiania et al. (2017) [31] observed that, in her study of dental treatments, antibiotic prophylaxes, and IE in patients with prosthetic heart valves, invasive dental treatments may be associated with oral streptococcal IE. The prosthetic heart valve is recognized as a risk factor for IE [31]. Interestingly, 84% of group 1 had previously had a prosthetic heart valve, compared to only 32% of group 3. These data are in line with the literature, wherein for around 20% of patients diagnosed with IE oral microorganisms (commensals) are found on infected valves [4,5]. Bacteremia with oral microorganisms is a normal condition, and the number of microorganisms is higher when the infection and inflammation are more severe [32]. Therefore, one could logically assume that only acute dental problems are a preventable risk for IE.

The nature, duration, and incidence of bacteremia caused by routine oral behavior such as eating, tooth brushing, and dental procedures question the importance of and emphasis on endocarditis antibiotic prophylaxis. It is notably difficult to determine the origin and cause of bacteremia. Antibiotics reduce the severity and/or incidence of bacteremia. The European Society of Cardiology and American Heart Association recommend antibiotics prophylaxis for patients at the highest risk undergoing invasive dental procedures [24]. Patients considered at the highest risk of IE are "patients with previous IE, congenital heart disease and rheumatic heart disease and selected heart transplant recipients" [13,24,32]. Several studies have concluded that there is no evidence to suggest that antibiotics prophylaxis is effective or ineffective against IE for patients at the highest risk of IE undergoing invasive dental procedures [33–37]. Furthermore, in 2008 the National Institute for Health and Care Excellence guidelines stated that "antibiotic prophylaxis against IE is not recommended for people undergoing dental procedures" [38]. There is no consensus on the consequences of this guideline issued by the National Institute for Health and Care Excellence [38,39]. Our results indicated that patients diagnosed with IE did not have a higher prevalence of dental treatments. Furthermore, no difference in oral health was observed between the groups in our study. No correlation was found between dental status at the time of [^{18}F]FDG PET/CT and the occurrence of endocarditis, nor between the antecedent of dental care procedures and the occurrence of endocarditis. This may suggest an indication for reducing the prescription of antibiotics prophylaxis.

Some limitations of our study should be addressed. The retrospective design increases the risk of bias. A total of 48 dentists, using their treatment strategy and documentation, supplied dental information (oral hygiene, regularity of dental visits, number of dental treatments, DMFT, and status praesens), which could have resulted in differences in the registration of the severity of dental problems. This is probably most significant for the screening of oral hygiene (plaque index, gingivitis) and periodontal disease, as different screening methods are applied, subject to wide inter-operator variability. Oral hygiene and periodontal disease are the important contributors to the inflammatory oral load.

Furthermore, [^{18}F]FDG PET/CT scans can be influenced by scattering. For example, dental implants or amalgam dental restorations may cause beam hardening and scatter on low-dose CT, which may influence [^{18}F]FDG PET images; therefore, both attenuated and non-attenuated PET scans were visually evaluated.

For future studies, a prospective design that includes the assessment of the severity and extension of periodontal health and acute dental inflammation just before the [^{18}F]FDG PET/CT scan is warranted. Furthermore, a prospective multicenter study with patients receiving a dental check-up just before the [^{18}F]FDG PET/CT scan is warranted if the modification of the antibiotic policy to prevent IE is considered. Another option could be the use of more specific tracers, since [^{18}F]FDG is an aspecific tracer with a high physiological uptake in the oral cavity.

5. Conclusions

The results of this retrospective study suggest that there is no correlation between the [^{18}F]FDG PET/CT uptake in the oral cavity and dental treatments or inflammation/infection reported by the patient's dentist. Furthermore, no correlation between IE and actual oral health status was demonstrated. Based on this study, there is no causal relationship between oral pathogens and the risk of IE. Further studies with proper dental check-up just before the [^{18}F]FDG PET/CT scan are warranted to investigate the relationship between oral inflammations/infections and IE.

Author Contributions: Conceptualization: G.W.D., R.H.J.A.S., L.W.M.v.d.S.; Methodology; G.W.D., R.H.J.A.S., L.W.M.v.d.S.; Validation; G.W.D., R.H.J.A.S., L.W.M.v.d.S.; Formal analysis; G.W.D., R.H.J.A.S., L.W.M.v.d.S., D.V.G.; Investigation; G.W.D., R.H.J.A.S., L.W.M.v.d.S.; Resources; R.H.J.A.S.; Data curation, G.W.D., R.H.J.A.S., L.W.M.v.d.S., D.V.G. Writing—original draft preparation; G.W.D., R.H.J.A.S., L.W.M.v.d.S., A.W.J.M.G., P.A.E., M.W.-B. Writing—review and editing: G.W.D., R.H.J.A.S., L.W.M.v.d.S., A.W.J.M.G., P.A.E., M.W.-B., B.S. Project administration: G.W.D. Supervision: R.H.J.A.S., L.W.M.v.d.S. All authors have read and agreed to the published version of the manuscript.

Ethics Approval: All the procedures performed in this study were in accordance with the ethical standards of the institutional and/or national research committee. Written informed consent was obtained from all the individual participants included in the study.

References

1. Li, X.; Kolltveit, K.M.; Tronstad, L.; Olsen, I. Systemic diseases caused by oral infection. *Clin. Microbiol. Rev.* **2000**, *13*, 547–558. [CrossRef]
2. Loesche, W.J. Association of the oral flora with important medical diseases. *Curr. Opin. Periodontol.* **1997**, *4*, 21–28. [PubMed]
3. Cahill, T.J.; Baddour, L.M.; Habib, G.; Hoen, B.; Salaün, E.; Pettersson, G.B.; Schäfers, H.J.; Prendergast, B.D. Challenges in Infective Endocarditis. *J. Am. Coll. Cardiol.* **2017**, *69*, 325–344. [CrossRef] [PubMed]
4. Lockhart, P.B.; Brennan, M.T.; Thornhill, M.; Michalowicz, B.S.; Noll, J.; Bahrani-Mougeot, F.K.; Sasser, H.C. Poor oral hygiene as a risk factor for infective endocarditis–related bacteremia. *J. Am. Dent. Assoc.* **2009**, *140*, 1238–1244. [CrossRef] [PubMed]

5. Lockhart, P.B.; Brennan, M.T.; Sasser, H.C.; Fox, P.C.; Paster, B.J.; Bahrani-Mougeot, F.K. Bacteremia Associated With Toothbrushing and Dental Extraction. *Circulation* **2008**, *117*, 3118–3125. [CrossRef]
6. Veinot, J.P. Pathologic Findings: Valvular Destruction, Perivalvular Abnormalities, and Extracardiac Findings. In *Endocarditis. Diagnosis and Management*, 2nd ed.; Chan, K.L., Embil, J.M., Eds.; Springer International Publishing: Heidelberg, Germany, 2016; pp. 9–26.
7. Parahitiyawa, N.B.; Jin, L.J.; Leung, W.K.; Yam, W.C.; Samaranayake, L.P. Microbiology of odontogenic bacteremia± beyond endocarditis. *Clin. Microbiol. Rev.* **2009**, *22*. [CrossRef]
8. Glenny, A.-M.; Oliver, R.; Roberts, G.J.; Hooper, L.; Worthington, H. Antibiotics for the prophylaxis of bacterial endocarditis in dentistry. *Cochrane Database Syst. Rev.* **2013**, *10*, CD003813. [CrossRef]
9. Habib, G.; Erba, P.A.; Iung, B.; Donal, E.; Cosyns, B.; Laroche, C.; Popescu, B.A.; Prendergast, B.; Tornos, P.; Sadeghpour, A.; et al. Clinical presentation, aetiology and outcome of infective endocarditis. Results of the ESC-EORP EURO-ENDO (European infective endocarditis) registry: A prospective cohort study. *Eur. Hear. J.* **2019**, *40*, 3222–3232. [CrossRef]
10. Navarro, B.G.; Jané-Salas, E.; Estrugo-Devesa, A.; López, J.L.; Viñas, M. Bacteremia Associated With Oral Surgery: A Review. *J. Évid. Based Dent. Pract.* **2017**, *17*, 190–204. [CrossRef]
11. Cahill, T.J.; Prendergast, B.D. Infective endocarditis. *Lancet* **2016**, *387*, 882–893. [CrossRef]
12. Vogkou, C.T.; Vlachogiannis, N.I.; Palaiodimos, L.; Kousoulis, A.A. The causative agents in infective endocarditis: A systematic review comprising 33,214 cases. *Eur. J. Clin. Microbiol. Infect. Dis.* **2016**, *35*, 1227–1245. [CrossRef] [PubMed]
13. Delahaye, F.; M'Hammedi, A.; Guerpillon, B.; De Gevigney, G.; Boibieux, A.; Dauwalder, O.; Bouchiat, C.; Vandenesch, F. Systematic Search for Present and Potential Portals of Entry for Infective Endocarditis. *J. Am. Coll. Cardiol.* **2016**, *67*, 151–158. [CrossRef] [PubMed]
14. Forner, L.; Larsen, T.; Kilian, M.; Holmstrup, P. Incidence of bacteremia after chewing, tooth brushing and scaling in individuals with periodontal inflammation. *J. Clin. Periodontol.* **2006**, *33*, 401–407. [CrossRef] [PubMed]
15. Almuhaideb, A.; Papathanasiou, N.; Bomanji, J. ^{18}F-FDG PET/CT imaging in oncology. *Ann. Saudi Med.* **2011**, *31*, 3–13. [CrossRef]
16. Mahmood, M.; Kendi, A.T.; Ajmal, S.; Farid, S.; O'Horo, J.C.; Chareonthaitawee, P.; Baddour, L.M.; Sohail, M.R. Meta-analysis of 18F-FDG PET/CT in the diagnosis of infective endocarditis. *J. Nucl. Cardiol.* **2017**, *26*, 922–935. [CrossRef]
17. Heuker, M.; Sijbesma, J.W.A.; Suárez, R.A.; De Jong, J.R.; Boersma, H.H.; Luurtsema, G.; Elsinga, P.H.; Glaudemans, A.W.J.M.; Van Dam, G.M.; Van Dijl, J.M.; et al. In vitro imaging of bacteria using 18F-fluorodeoxyglucose micro positron emission tomography. *Sci. Rep.* **2017**, *7*, 4973. [CrossRef]
18. Carvalho-Sousa, B.; Gomes, F.D.A.; Ferreira, C.M.; Rocha, M.M.D.N.P.; Barros, E.B.; De Albuquerque, D.S. Persistent extra-radicular bacterial biofilm in endodontically treated human teeth: Scanning electron microscopy analysis after apical surgery. *Microsc. Res. Tech.* **2017**, *80*, 662–667. [CrossRef]
19. Irani, S. Orofacial Bacterial Infectious Diseases: An Update. *J. Int. Soc. Prev. Community Dent.* **2017**, *7*, S61–S67. [CrossRef]
20. Yamashiro, K.; Nakano, M.; Sawaki, K.; Okazaki, F.; Hirata, Y.; Takashiba, S. The potential of positron emission tomography/computerized tomography (PET/CT) scanning as a detector of high-risk patients with oral infection during preoperative staging. *Oral Surg. Oral Med. Oral Pathol. Oral Radiol.* **2016**, *122*, 242–249. [CrossRef]
21. Benouaich, V.; Hitzel, A.; Armand, S. Relevance of functional imaging in dental implantology. *J. Clin. Exp. Dent.* **2018**, *10*, e1011–e1016. [CrossRef]
22. Gomes, A.; Glaudemans, A.W.J.M.; Touw, D.J.; Van Melle, J.P.; Willems, T.P.; Maass, A.H.; Natour, E.; Prakken, N.H.J.; Borra, R.J.H.; Van Geel, P.P.; et al. Diagnostic value of imaging in infective endocarditis: A systematic review. *Lancet Infect. Dis.* **2017**, *17*, e1–e14. [CrossRef]
23. Gomes, A.; van Geel, P.P.; Santing, M.; Prakken, N.H.J.; Ruis, M.L.; van Assen, S.; Slart, R.H.J.A.; Sinha, B.; Glaudemans, A.W.J.M. Imaging infective endocarditis: Adherence to a diagnostic flowchart and direct comparison of imaging techniques. *J. Nucl. Cardiol.* **2020**, *27*, 592–608. [CrossRef] [PubMed]

24. Habib, G.; Lancellotti, P.; Antunes, M.J.; Bongiorni, M.G.; Casalta, J.P.; Del Zotti, F.; Dulgheru, R.; El Khoury, G.; Erba, P.A.; Iung, B.; et al. 2015 ESC Guidelines for the management of infective endocarditis: The task force for the management of infective endocarditis of the european society of cardiology (ESC). Endorsed by: European association for cardio-thoracic surgery (EACTS), the European Association of Nuclear Medicine (EANM). *Eur. Heart J.* **2015**, *36*, 3075–3128. [PubMed]
25. Jamar, F.; Buscombe, J.; Chiti, A.; Christian, P.E.; Delbeke, D.; Donohoe, K.J.; Israel, O.; Martin-Comin, J.; Signore, A. EANM/SNMMI Guideline for 18F-FDG Use in Inflammation and Infection. *J. Nucl. Med.* **2013**, *54*, 647–658. [CrossRef] [PubMed]
26. Erba, P.A.; Lancellotti, P.; Vilacosta, I.; Gaemperli, O.; Rouzet, F.; Hacker, M.; Signore, A.; Slart, R.H.J.A.; Habib, G. Recommendations on nuclear and multimodality imaging in IE and CIED infections. *Eur. J. Nucl. Med. Mol. Imaging* **2018**, *45*, 1795–1815. [CrossRef] [PubMed]
27. Shimamoto, H.; Tatsumi, M.; Kakimoto, N.; Hamada, S.; Shimosegawa, E.; Murakami, S.; Furukawa, S.; Hatazawa, J. 18F-FDG accumulation in the oral cavity is associated with periodontal disease and apical periodontitis: An initial demonstration on PET/CT. *Ann. Nucl. Med.* **2008**, *22*, 587–593. [CrossRef]
28. Kito, S.; Koga, H.; Kodama, M.; Yamamoto, N.; Kokuryo, S.; Habu, M.; Matsuo, K.; Nishino, T.; Kubota, K.; Muraoka, K.; et al. Reflection of 18F-FDG accumulation in the evaluation of the extent of periapical or periodontal inflammation. *Oral Surg. Oral Med. Oral Pathol. Oral Radiol.* **2012**, *114*, e62–e69. [CrossRef]
29. Kao, C.-H. Incidental Findings of FDG Uptake in Dental Caries. *Clin. Nucl. Med.* **2003**, *28*, 610. [CrossRef]
30. Pasha, M.A.; Marcus, C.; Fakhry, C.; Kang, H.; Kiess, A.P.; Subramaniam, R.M. FDG PET/CT for Management and Assessing Outcomes of Squamous Cell Cancer of the Oral Cavity. *Am. J. Roentgenol.* **2015**, *205*, W150–W161. [CrossRef]
31. Tubiana, S.; Blotière, P.-O.; Hoen, B.; Lesclous, P.; Millot, S.; Rudant, J.; Weill, A.; Coste, J.; Alla, F.; Duval, X. Dental procedures, antibiotic prophylaxis, and endocarditis among people with prosthetic heart valves: Nationwide population based cohort and a case crossover study. *BMJ* **2017**, *358*, j3776. [CrossRef]
32. Cahill, T.J.; Harrison, J.L.; Jewell, P.; Onakpoya, I.; Chambers, J.B.; Dayer, M.; Lockhart, P.; Roberts, N.; Shanson, D.; Thornhill, M.; et al. Antibiotic prophylaxis for infective endocarditis: A systematic review and meta-analysis. *Heart* **2017**, *103*, 937–944. [CrossRef] [PubMed]
33. Wilson, W.; Taubert, K.A.; Gewitz, M.; Lockhart, P.B.; Baddour, L.M.; Levison, M.; Bolger, A.; Cabell, C.H.; Takahashi, M.; Baltimore, R.S.; et al. Prevention of infective endocarditis: Guidelines from the American heart sssociation. A guideline from the American heart association rheumatic fever, endocarditis and kawasaki disease committee, council on cardiovascular disease in the young, and the council on clinical cardiology, council on cardiovascular surgery and anesthesia, and the quality of care and outcomes research interdisciplinary working group. *J. Am. Dent. Assoc.* **2008**, *139*, 3–24.
34. Rochlen, G.K.; Keenan, A.V. Value of prophylactic antibiotics for invasive dental procedures unclear. *Evid. Based Dent.* **2014**, *15*, 12–13. [CrossRef] [PubMed]
35. Dayer, M.; Thornhill, M. Is antibiotic prophylaxis to prevent infective endocarditis worthwhile? *J. Infect. Chemother.* **2017**, *13*, 1–7. [CrossRef] [PubMed]
36. Thornhill, M.H.; Dayer, M.; Lockhart, P.B.; Prendergast, B. Antibiotic Prophylaxis of Infective Endocarditis. *Curr. Infect. Dis. Rep.* **2017**, *19*, 9. [CrossRef]
37. Scottish Dental Clinical Effectiveness Programme. Drug Prescribing for Dentistry. Dental Clinical Guidance. Bacterial Infections. In *Infective Endocarditis*, 3rd ed.; Dundee Dental Education Centre: Dundee, UK, 2016; p. 29.
38. Thornhill, M.; Dayer, M.J.; Forde, J.M.; Corey, G.R.; Chu, V.H.; Couper, D.; Lockhart, P.B. Impact of the NICE guideline recommending cessation of antibiotic prophylaxis for prevention of infective endocarditis: Before and after study. *BMJ* **2011**, *342*, d2392. [CrossRef]
39. Dayer, M.J.; Jones, S.; Prendergast, B.; Baddour, L.M.; Lockhart, P.B.; Thornhill, M.H. Incidence of infective endocarditis in England, 2000–2013: A secular trend, interrupted time-series analysis. *Lancet* **2015**, *385*, 882–893. [CrossRef]

5

Impact of MRI, CT and Clinical Characteristics on Microbial Pathogen Detection Using CT-Guided Biopsy for Suspected Spondylodiscitis

Alexander Braun [1,*], Thomas Germann [1], Felix Wünnemann [1], Marc-André Weber [2], Marcus Schiltenwolf [3], Michael Akbar [3], Iris Burkholder [4], Hans-Ulrich Kauczor [1] and Christoph Rehnitz [1]

1 Department of Diagnostic and Interventional Radiology, University Hospital Heidelberg, 69120 Heidelberg, Germany; thomas.germann@med.uni-heidelberg.de (T.G.); felix.wuennemann@med.uni-heidelberg.de (F.W.); hans-ulrich.kauczor@med.uni-heidelberg.de (H.-U.K.); christoph.rehnitz@med.uni-heidelberg.de (C.R.)

2 Institute of Diagnostic and Interventional Radiology, Pediatric Radiology and Neuroradiology, University Medicine Rostock, 18057 Rostock, Germany; marc-andre.weber@med.uni-rostock.de

3 Department of Orthopedics and Trauma Surgery, University Hospital Heidelberg, 69118 Heidelberg, Germany; marcus.schiltenwolf@med.uni-heidelberg.de (M.S.); michael.akbar@med.uni-heidelberg.de (M.A.)

4 Department of Nursing and Health, University of Applied Sciences of the Saarland, 66117 Saarbruecken, Germany; iris.burkholder@htwsaar.de

* Correspondence: alexander.braun@med.uni-heidelberg.de

Abstract: Spondylodiscitis accounts for 2–7% of osteomyelitis cases and is characterized by pain, systemic inflammation, and permanent neurological deficits. We aimed to identify imaging characteristics and clinical parameters to successfully predict microbiological pathogens by computed tomography (CT)-guided biopsy in suspected spondylodiscitis cases. Forty consecutive patients (mean age 65.1 years) with suspected spondylodiscitis underwent CT-guided biopsy. CT features (non-sclerotic endplate erosions (NSEs)), magnetic resonance criteria (paravertebral/epidural abscess (PA/EA) formation), and clinical data (C-reactive protein (CRP) > 50 mg/L) were assessed for their predictive potential. NSEs were detected in 6/11 (54.5%) and 1/29(3.4%) patients with positive and negative microbiology, respectively. PA and EA, respectively, were present in 7/11(63.6%) and 3/11 patients with positive microbiology and 7/29 (24.1%) and 2/29 patients with negative microbiology. CRP > 50 was observed in 7/11 (63.6%) and in 7/29 (24.1%) patients with positive and negative microbiology, respectively. Three double combinations possessed near-perfect specificity (PA + NSE, 100%; PA + CRP > 50, 96.6%; NSE + CRP > 50, 96.6%). The top three Youden indices included combinations with NSE. Since CT/magnetic resonance (MR) imaging and CRP are routinely used to evaluate spondylodiscitis, the presented diagnostic criteria and combinations can aid decision-making for biopsy.

Keywords: spondylodiscitis; biopsy; CT; MRI; CRP; microbiology

---

1. Introduction

Spondylodiscitis accounts for 2–7% of osteomyelitis cases and has a reported annual incidence of 1/100,000 to 1/250,000 [1]. Besides intervertebral discs and adjacent vertebral bodies, spondylodiscitis often affects the surrounding paravertebral and epidural spaces. Due to the proximity of key neurological structures, such as the spinal cord and neuroforaminal nerve roots, patients not only suffer from pain and systemic inflammation but also are at risk of suffering permanent neurological deficits [2,3] and in some cases, death [4]. Therefore, a fast induction of targeted antibiotic therapy is critical and may help prevent prolonged and complicated courses [5].

Success rates of pathogen detection by blood culture can vary depending on the patient population and can reportedly be as low as 24.4% [6]. CT-guided biopsy has been used to histopathologically prove the diagnosis of spondylodiscitis and exclude malignancy [7]. Moreover, CT-guided biopsy enables the identification of causative microbiological agents, which is important for determining the appropriate antibiotic therapy. This is especially useful in cases of atypical pathogens, such as (multi-)resistant microbes or tuberculous infection [8,9]. However, CT-guided biopsy of the spine involves risks, such as pain, bleeding, and risk of neurological impairment [10–12]. In addition, it often fails to provide sufficient bioptic yields for pathogen detection, with reported rates of successful microbiological cultivation ranging between 28.1% [13] and 57.1% [14]. This varied success rate depends on the study design and/or preselection of the patient collective.

Several imaging characteristics and clinical/laboratory findings have been studied in order to improve their pathogen detection capabilities. However, currently, there are no defined criteria that are clearly associated with positive/negative pathogen detection and reported assessments have a variable diagnostic performance. For example, while Ahuja et al. suggested c-reactive protein (CRP) levels > 50 mg/L as a positive predictive factor for successful pathogen detection [6], Kasalak et al. reported that CRP levels did in fact not correlate with pathogen detection [8]. Using magnetic resonance imaging (MRI), Spira et al. identified a positive correlation between paravertebral infiltration (with high specificity in cases of simultaneously present paravertebral/epidural abscess (PA/EA)) [15]. In contrast, Kasalak et al. found no significant correlation between MRI features and microbiological yield [8]. Foreman et al. investigated multiple MR/CT variables with regard to pathogen detection, such as lytic and mixed density endplate changes. However, in that study, no CT feature was identified in order to improve pathogen detection [16].

We, therefore, conducted this study in order to identify imaging characteristics, clinical parameters, or a combination thereof, to differentiate between successful and futile detection of microbiological pathogens by CT-guided biopsies in patients with suspected spondylodiscitis.

2. Experimental Section

2.1. Population

This retrospective study was approved by the Ethics Committee of the medical faculty at Heidelberg University (vote S-581/2014). A search of the institution's electronic medical record database from June 2015 to March 2018 was performed for all patients who underwent CT-guided biopsy in cases of suspected spondylodiscitis. General indications for CT-guided biopsy were based on clinical orthopedic examination, laboratory tests, and imaging findings. All patients were screened for infection foci other than the spine, and none of the included patients showed a different focus other than the spine. A suggestion for a CT-guided biopsy was made after a discussion in an interdisciplinary team including orthopedic spine surgeons and senior radiologists. Patients with primary immediate indications for open surgery (for instance patients with neurologic symptoms, highly septic patients) did not undergo a CT-guided biopsy. CT-guided biopsy setting did include patients with relative indications for surgery, who had an increased surgical risk and would, therefore, benefit from the minimally invasive procedure. From an original set of 45 patients, we excluded four patients as their biopsy procedure was terminated before acquisition of sufficient bioptic material. Reasons for premature termination included the patient experiencing falling oxygen levels and intolerable pain during procedure despite optimized analgesia. One patient requested termination without any further documented explanation. Finally, a fifth patient who successfully underwent CT-guided biopsy, but could not undergo MRI examination due to an implanted pacemaker, was also excluded. Therefore, 40 consecutive patients who demonstrated clinical and morphologic findings suggestive of spondylodiscitis and who underwent CT-guided biopsy for pathogen detection, were included for analysis. In 30 of the 40 patients, additional material for histological analysis was obtained. Written informed consent was obtained from the patient or a guardian. The mean patient age was 65.1 years (range 10–89 years). As an institutional standard, in cases involving antibiotic pre-treatment ($n = 11$), antibiotic medication was stopped at least 7 days before CT-guided biopsy to increase the probability of pathogen detection.

2.2. Imaging Parameters

MR imaging: All 40 patients received a pre-interventional contrast-enhanced MRI of the spine and an additional CT for biopsy planning. MRI was performed using a 3.0 tesla system (Magnetom Verio, Siemens Healthineers, Erlangen, Germany). T1-weighted turbospin-echo sequences were obtained with a 700–800 ms repetition time (TR), 12 ms echo time (TE), 150–180° flip angle, and an echo train-length of three. T2-weighted turbo spin-echo sequences were obtained by using a 2.2–7.9/113–119 ms TR/TE, a 150–180° flip angle, and an echo train-length of 19. Short tau inversion recovery sequences were obtained with a 5.1–8.9 ms TR, a 44–45 ms TE, a 210 ms inversion time, a 150–180° flip angle, and an echo train-length of 19. Contrast-enhanced T1-weighted turbo spin-echo sequences were obtained by using a 700–1000/11–12 ms TR/TE, a 150–180° flip angle, and an echo train-length of three. Gadoterate meglumine (Dotarem; Guerbet, Roissy, France) at a dose of 0.1 mmol per kg body weight was used as the intravenous contrast agent.

CT imaging and biopsy: The vertebral level and interventional approach were defined according to the pre-interventional MRI. All patients received moderate intravenous (IV) sedation using 15 mg piritramid (Dipidolor, Hameln, Germany) with continuous monitoring of their vital signs. A CT-guided biopsy was performed using a Somatom Emotion 16-slice-scanner (Siemens Healthineers, Forchheim, Germany). A thin-slice planning CT scan (0.75 mm slice thickness) was conducted in the prone position and multiplanar reconstructions were used to nontraumatically position the biopsy needle. After aseptic preparation of the skin overlying the biopsy needle trajectory, local anesthesia was administered (5–10 mL Carbostesin 0.5%, Astra Zeneca, Wedel, Germany). A small skin incision was made, and the biopsy was performed using a 3.0 mm (11 gauge) biopsy system (Bone Marrow Biopsy Needle, Somatex, Germany or Osteo-Site Ratchet, IZI Medical Products, USA). A transpedicular approach was chosen in 20/40 (50%) patients while a posterolateral/paravertebral approach was chosen in the remaining 20/40 (50%) patients. The choice of approach was based on anatomical considerations and the dominant location of the inflammatory changes. For instance, the paravertebral approach was used in cases where paravertebral inflammation was dominant. When abscesses were biopsied, additional liquefied content was aspirated. A biopsy sample was sent for microbiological examination in 40/40 (100%) patients, and an additional sample was formalin-fixed for histological analysis in 30/40 (75%) patients. Although blood cultures were not systematically performed in the patient cohort in our institution, we additionally retrospectively assessed the proportion of patients in which blood cultures were performed and whether these provided additional information on pathogen detection.

2.3. Evaluation of Imaging and Laboratory Findings

Laboratory findings: We assessed CRP levels using readings obtained as close as possible, but prior, to the time of CT-guided biopsy. Based on the observations by Ahuja et al. [6] we defined a group with CRP levels > 50 and a second < 50 and assessed the pathogen detection rate in both groups. Where applicable, we further assessed the patient's antibiotic treatment regimen, and as an in-house standard, antibiotic therapy was paused at least 7 days before CT-guided biopsy.

Imaging in general: Qualitative image analysis was performed on a standard picture archiving and communication system (Centricity PACS, Version 4.0, GE Healthcare IT solutions, Barrington, IL). It was used to select morphological images, allow coregistration and directly compare anatomic and functional data sets. All images were evaluated in consensus by two reading radiologists with 15 and 3 years of experience in the field of musculoskeletal imaging.

MR imaging: We investigated the presence or absence of PA/EA. An abscess was defined as being iso- or hypo-intense compared to muscle tissue on T1-weighted images, having a fluid-equivalent signal intensity on T2-weighted images, and displaying rim enhancement on contrast-enhanced T1-weighted fat-saturated images [17].

CT imaging: We investigated lesions of the adjacent endplates to evaluate the stage of osteitis evaluating whether non-sclerotic endplate lesions are present, as opposed to sclerotic endplate lesions or absence of any erosions. Non-sclerotic lesions may indicate an earlier stage of osteitis while sclerotic margins indicate the presence of longer-term inflammation [16,18,19]. Non-sclerotic endplate lesions were defined as lytic defects of the endplate without sclerosis of the surrounding bone.

2.4. Statistics

Statistical analysis was performed using the statistical package SAS for Windows Version 9.4 (SAS Institute Inc., North Carolina). All study variables were analyzed descriptively. Continuous variables were summarized using the sample size (n), mean, standard deviation, median, minimum, and maximum. The frequencies and percentages for each level were reported for qualitative variables. The performance of PA/EA, CRP > 50, and non-sclerotic endplate erosions (NSE) in predicting microbial pathogen-proof was described using estimates and exact 95% confidence intervals for sensitivity, specificity, and positive and negative predictive values. In addition, the predictive capacity of several combinations of variables was assessed. As a measure for a descriptive comparison between the performance of the different variables and combinations of variables the Youden Index defined as sensitivity + specificity − 1 together with the 95% confidence intervals was used [20]. The Youden Index treats false negative and false positive errors as equally undesirable. The minimal value of the Youden Index is 0 indicating that the diagnostic test reports the same proportion of positive tests for diseased and control group. If the diagnostic test produces no false positives nor false negatives, then the Youden Index reaches the maximal value 1.

3. Results

3.1. Microbiology, Histology, and Follow-Up

Causative pathogens were detected in 11/40 patients (27.5%), including *Escherichia coli* ($n = 3$; 7.5%), *Staphylococcus* ($n = 6$; 15%), and *Streptococcus* species. ($n = 2$; 5.0%). A causative fungal agent was not detected in any of the biopsy samples. Histological analysis was performed for $n = 30$ samples and it revealed signs of acute inflammation in 9/30 patients (30.0%), chronic inflammation in 16/30 patients (53.3%), and nonspecific results in 5/30 samples (16.7%). Malignancy was excluded in all patients by either histological analysis ($n = 30$; 75.0%) or observing the improvement of symptoms and inflammatory changes in follow-up examinations ($n = 10$; 25%). In 12/40 (30%) patients additional blood cultures were performed. In 3/12 (25%) a pathogen was detected. Two detected pathogens correlated with results from CT-guided biopsy while one additional pathogen was detected in a patient with negative microbiologic result following CT-guided biopsy. This patient received targeted antibiotics and responded. Additional 16s RNA polymerase chain reaction (PCR) analyses were not performed. Empiric antibiotics were given in all culture-negative cases, three of which required additional surgical therapy. At the time of discharge from the hospital patient records and available follow-up imaging documented an improvement.

3.2. Laboratory Findings

CRP levels above 50 mg/L were found in 7/11 (63.6%) patients with positive microbiology but only in 7/29 (24.1%) samples with negative microbiology (Table 1). The mean CRP for all patients was 51.2 mg/L (SD 62.9). Mean CRP for patients with positive microbiology ($n = 11$) was 84.6 mg/L (SD 73.3) and for those without was 38.4 mg/L (SD 51.9).

Table 1. The performance of single variables in predicting positive microbiology from a biopsy (TP = true positive, TN = true negative, FP = false positive, FN = false negative).

Biopsy Phenotype	Sensitivity TP/(TP + FN)	Specificity TN/(TN + FP)	PPV TP/(TP + FP)	NPV TN/(TN + FN)
Paravertebral abscess	7/11 = 63.6% (30.8%–89.1%)	22/29 = 75.9% (56.5%–89.7%)	7/14 = 50.0% (23.0%–77.0%)	22/26 = 84.6% (65.1%–95.6%)
Epidural abscess	3/11 = 27.3% (6.0%–61.0%)	27/29 = 93.1% (77.2%–99.2%)	3/5 = 60.0% (14.7%–94.7%)	27/35 = 77.1% (59.9%–89.6%)
Non-sclerotic vertebral endplate erosion	6/11 = 54.6% (23.4%–83.3%)	28/29 = 96.6% (82.2%–99.9%)	6/7 = 85.7% (42.1%–99.6%)	28/33 = 84.9% (68.1%–94.9%)
CRP > 50	7/11 = 63.6% (30.8%–89.1%)	22/29 = 75.9% (56.5%–89.7%)	7/14 = 50.0% (23.0%–77.0%)	22/26 = 84.6% (65.1%–95.6%)

3.3. Imaging Findings

MRI: PA (Figure 1) was observed in 7/11 (63.6%) patients with positive microbiology compared to only 7/29 samples (24.1%) with negative microbiology. EA (Figures 2 and 3) was present in 3/11 (27.3%) patients with positive microbiology but only in 2/29 (6.9%) samples with negative microbiology. EA was also present in all patients featuring PA.

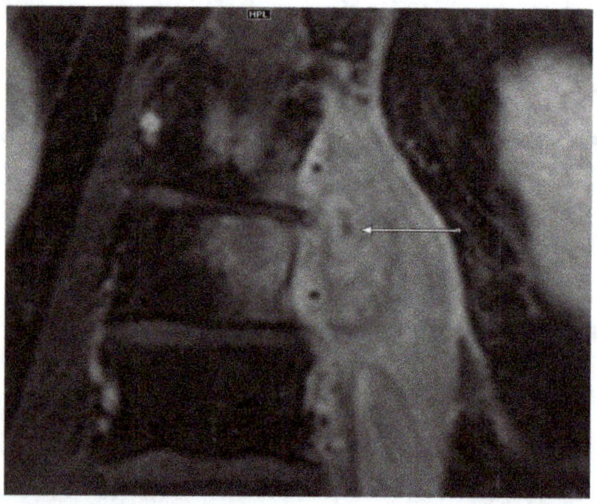

Figure 1. Coronal T1 weighted, fat-saturated, contrast-enhanced magnetic resonance (MR) image of the lumbar spine at the level L1-L3. A paravertebral abscess in the left psoas muscle of a 53-year old patient is present (arrow). The detected pathogen after computed CT-guided biopsy was *Staphylococcus aureus*.

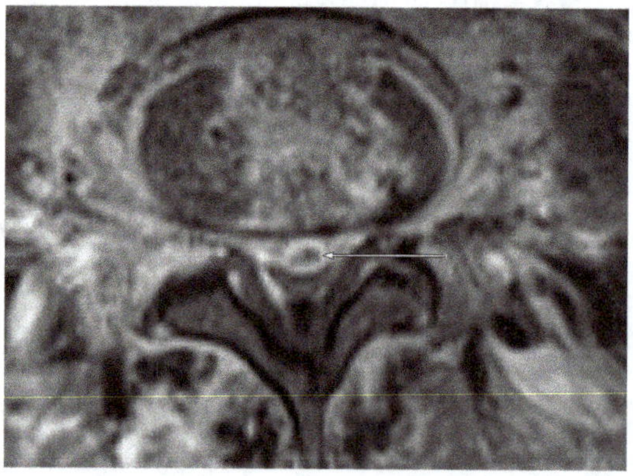

Figure 2. Transversal T1 weighted, fat-saturated, contrast-enhanced image of the lumbar spine level L5/L6 in a 52-year old patient. An epidural abscess is present (arrow). The detected pathogen after CT-guided biopsy was *E. coli*.

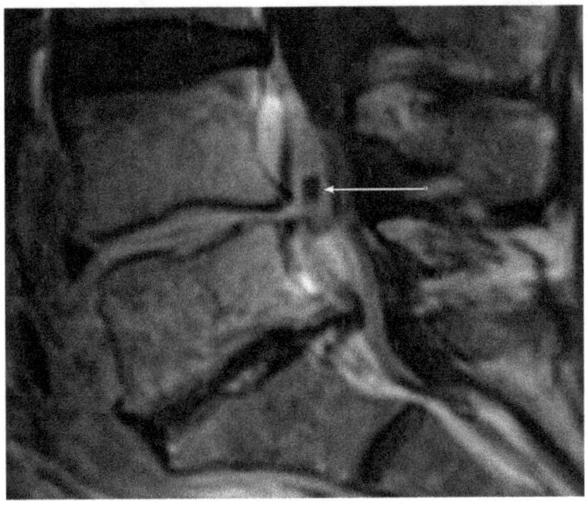

Figure 3. Sagittal T1 weighted, fat-saturated, contrast-enhanced image of the lumbar spine level L5-S1 in the same patient as shown in Figure 2. The epidural abscess in the spinal canal is marked with an arrow.

CT: NSE (Figure 4, sclerotic erosion for better differentiation in Figure 5) was observed in 6/11 (54.5%) patients with positive microbiology but only in 1/29 (3.4%) samples with negative microbiology.

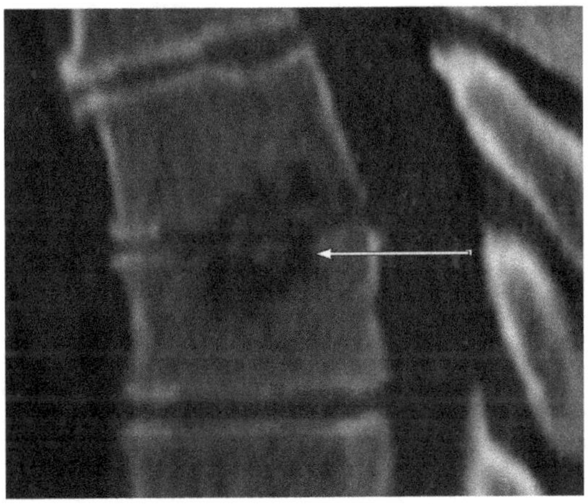

Figure 4. CT scan (sagittal reconstruction) of thoracic spine level Th6-Th7 showing non-sclerotic erosions of adjacent endplates of the thoracic spine in 55-year old patient. The detected pathogen after CT-guided biopsy was *E. coli*.

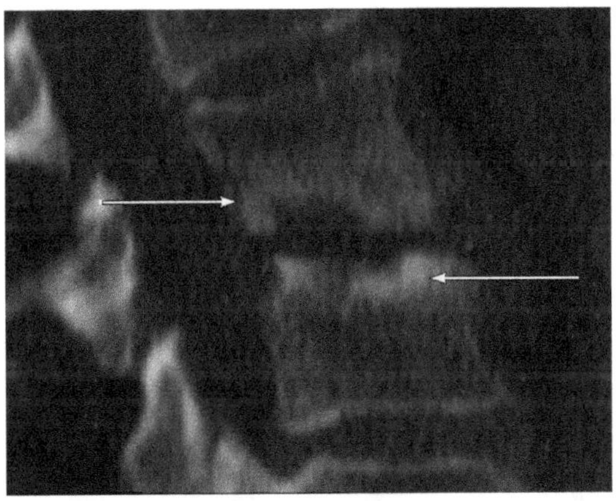

Figure 5. CT scan (sagittal reconstruction) of lumbar spine level L2-L3. As opposed to Figure 4 showing marginally sclerotic erosions of adjacent endplates of the lumbar spine in 77-year old patient. No detected pathogen after CT-guided biopsy.

The investigated variables varied in their respective statistical performance for predicting positive microbiological results. Sensitivity, specificity, positive predictive value (PPV), and negative predictive value (NPV) with accompanying confidence intervals for each variable are listed in Table 1. In particular, EA and NSE displayed high specificity for the prediction of positive microbiological results.

3.4. Combination of Variables

Double and triple combinations of included variables were tested for their sensitivity, specificity, PPV, and NPV as shown in Table 2. EA was not included as all patients with EA also exhibited PA. Performance, with respect to sensitivity, specificity, PPV, NPV, and the Youden Index, varied across the various combination of variables. Perfect specificity and PPV were achieved for the combination of PA and NSE (i.e., (PA and NSE)). Excellent specificity was achieved when using a combination of PA and CRP > 50, or CRP > 50 and NSE (i.e., (PA and CRP > 50), (CRP > 50 and NSE)). The presence of either PA or CRP > 50 resulted in very high NPV and sensitivity (i.e., (PA or CRP > 50)). The top three Youden indices included combinations with NSE. The predictive performance of all assessed variables and their combinations, as determined by calculating the Youden index, is presented in ascending order in Table 3.

Table 2. The performance of variable combinations in predicting positive microbiology from a biopsy. (TP = true positive, TN = true negative, FP = false positive, FN = false negative)

	Sensitivity TP/(TP + FN)	Specificity TN/(TN + FP)	PPV TP/(TP + FP)	NPV TN/(TN + FN)
Paravertebral abscess and non-sclerotic erosion	4/11 = 36.4% (10.9%–69.2%)	29/29 = 100.0% (88.1%–100.0%)	4/4 = 100.0% (39.8%–100.0%)	29/36 = 80.6% (64.0%–91.8%)
Paravertebral abscess or non-sclerotic erosion	9/11 = 81.8% (48.2%–97.7%)	21/29 = 72.4% (52.8%–87.3%)	9/17 = 52.9% (27.8%–77.0%)	21/23 = 91.3% (72.0%–98.9%)
Paravertebral abscess and CRP > 50	6/11 = 54.6% (23.4%–83.3%)	28/29 = 96.6% (82.2%–99.9%)	6/7 = 85.7% (42.1%–99.6%)	28/33 = 84.8% (68.1%–94.9%)
Paravertebral abscess or CRP > 50	8/11 = 72.7% (39.0%–94.0%)	16/29 = 55.2% (35.7%–73.6%)	8/19 = 38.1% (18.1%–61.6%)	16/21 = 84.2% (60.4%–96.6%)
CRP > 50 and non-sclerotic erosion	3/11 = 27.3% (6.0%–61.0%)	28/29 = 96.6% (82.2%–99.9%)	3/4 = 75.0% (19.4%–99.4%)	28/36 = 77.8% (60.9%–89.9%)
CRP > 50 or non-sclerotic erosion	10/11 = 90.9% (58.7%–99.8%)	22/29 = 75.9% (56.5%–89.7%)	10/17 = 58.8% (32.9%–81.6%)	22/23 = 95.7% (78.1%–99.9%)
Paravertebral abscess and non-sclerotic erosion and CRP > 50	3/11 = 27.3% (6.0%–61.0%)	29/29 = 100.0% (88.1%–100.0%)	3/3 = 100.0% (29.2%–100.0%)	29/37 = 78.4% (61.8%–90.2%)
Paravertebral abscess or non-sclerotic erosion or CRP > 50	10/11 = 90.9% (58.7%–99.8%)	16/29 = 55.2% (35.7%–73.6%)	10/23 = 43.5% (23.2%–65.5%)	16/17 = 94.1% (71.3%–99.9%)

Table 3. The Youden Index calculated for combinations of variables in predicting positive microbiology from a biopsy in ascending order.

	Youden Index	95% Confidence Interval
Paravertebral abscess	0.201	(0.0–0.543)
Epidural abscess	0.204	(0.0–0.483)
CRP > 50 and non-sclerotic erosion	0.239	(0.0–0.510)
Paravertebral abscess and non-sclerotic erosion and CRP > 50	0.273	(0.010–0.536)
Paravertebral abscess or CRP > 50	0.279	(0.0–0.598)
Paravertebral abscess and non-sclerotic erosion	0.364	(0.080–0.648)
CRP > 50	0.395	(0.071–0.719)
Paravertebral abscess or non-sclerotic erosion or CRP > 50	0.461	(0.213–0.709)
Non-sclerotic vertebral endplate erosion	0.512	(0.210–0.814)
Paravertebral abscess and CRP > 50	0.512	(0.210–0.814)
Paravertebral abscess or non-sclerotic erosion	0.542	(0.262–0.822)
CRP > 50 or non-sclerotic erosion	0.668	(0.437–0.899)

4. Discussion

Endeavors to identify both clinical variables and imaging features predictive of microbiological pathogen detection in spondylodiscitis patients have been undertaken by several studies [6,8,15,16,21]. However, results were, in part conflicting and there still exists no consensus in the issue. Concrete diagnostic criteria and clear clinical decision-making pathways for performing CT-guided biopsies are not yet defined. In our study, we investigated the efficacy of individual CT and MRI features as well as laboratory findings (i.e., CRP > 50) and a combination of features to predict positive pathogen detection following CT-guided biopsy. As diagnostic work-up in spondylodiscitis patients in most institutions routinely include CT and MR imaging and CRP tests, the combination of these tests alongside the presented criteria, may ease and aid in further therapeutic decision-making processes.

Since in a clinical setting not every proposed feature may be present simultaneously, we investigated a variety of combinations. Thus, for a given patient, depending on the clinical features present, physicians can tailor their decision-making based on the individual patient's circumstances and the probability of successful pathogen detection via CT-guided biopsy. NSE and EA exhibited very high specificities as individual variables. Both features, if present, will produce very few futile CT-guided biopsies. Thus, from a clinical perspective, if either or both features are present, a biopsy can be considered under the knowledge of a potentially higher probability of pathogen detection. This holds true even more so for the combinations of PA and CRP > 50 and CRP > 50 and NSE, both of which demonstrate excellent specificity. On the other hand, the CRP > 50 or NSE combination demonstrates a high NPV and consecutively, successful pathogen detection is very unlikely in the absence of both. The combination of PA and NSE led to perfect specificity and PPV, and therefore, any patient displaying these features simultaneously might benefit from a CT-guided biopsy. The top three Youden indices included NSE as a variable. Thus, NSE can be regarded as an important feature both as a single variable and in a combination. In contrast, if NSE is not present, i.e., if the erosions were sclerosed or absent, the probability of successful pathogen detection is low. This is in line with the pathophysiologic consideration of NSE representing a more acute, active stage of osteitis while surrounding sclerosis is associated with more chronic and less active stages [18]. Foreman et al. investigated multiple MR/CT variables with regard to pathogen detection, including lytic and mixed density endplate changes [16]. Although these patterns were more frequent in the group with positive microbiology, no CT imaging parameter was identified in order to improve the prediction of microbiologic or histologic outcomes using a multivariable regression model. The authors, therefore, stated that a dedicated CT scan does not provide any additional predictive information for the biopsy result if an MRI scan is already available. Differences in our study may be explained, in part, by differences in the study population, the assessment methods, and technical differences. However, based on our results, we regard NSE as a decisive pattern, suggestive of a positive pathogen outcome. Thus, we recommend performing a CT and thoroughly evaluating the presence of NSE or on the other hand sclerotic margins/absence or erosions.

In line with our results, Spira et al. observed that epidural infiltration and paravertebral abscesses also had high specificities of 83.3% and 90.9%, respectively [15]. In our study, only a small percentage of patients featured EA and thus, EA may not represent a robust predictor for positive microbiology despite its high specificity.

Previously published studies on the predictive value of CRP levels are controversial with Kasalak et al. dismissing CRP as a reliable predictor and Ahuja et al. suggesting CRP > 50 mg/L to be linked with positive microbiological yields. Our findings support the observation from Ahuja et al. as positive pathogen detection was significantly higher in patients with CRP levels > 50 mg/L. With our own results showing solid specificity and good NPV for CRP as a single variable, such contradictory results may be attributed to divergence in the investigated patient populations or the inclusion of cases with other causes of altered CRP levels, including previous antibiotics or the time between the last antibiotic dose and the CT-guided biopsy. In our setting and as a clinical standard in our institution, we used an interval of at least 7 days between the last antibiotic dose and CT biopsy, which may also have contributed to such differences.

None of the investigated features or combinations therein had perfect diagnostic performance values and could, therefore, be used to completely rule out the possibility for positive microbiological results. The decision to perform a biopsy should always be made in the clinical context of each individual patient. Moreover, Figure 6 presents a simplified decision-support pathway regarding CT-guided biopsy in suspected spondylodiscitis based on our results. This figure provides different probabilities of pathogen detection depending on the investigated laboratory and imaging findings in a simplified manner highlighting our main results. However, it should not be used as a final therapy-decision tool in an individual patient.

Our study had several limitations. It has to be clearly stated that this is a retrospective study based on a relatively small patient group from a single center. This study does not intend to inform clinical decision making on an individual basis. Therefore, the presented results should not be used to finally judge about performing or not performing CT-biopsies in spondylodiscitis cases without further confirmatory validation studies. Prospective studies with larger patient cohorts performed in different centers with cross-validation of the findings are needed to confirm our findings. These prospective studies might also include a multivariate analysis to investigate the weighting and interaction of each factor and predict the likelihood of having positive microbiology. We did not calculate every possible variable combination that might be associated with positive or negative biopsy yields; thus, other combinations might also be helpful in decision making. Additionally, our patient preselection, which was performed within the university-clinical setting, may vary from other possible settings (e.g., a community setting with lower frequencies of spondylodiscitis and a possibly differing spectrum of pathogens). False-positive microbiological results due to contamination with non-pathogen germ contamination cannot be ruled out with absolute certainty; however, they seem very unlikely in a scenario where clinical presentation, laboratory findings, and imaging features are all concordant with spondylodiscitis. It must also be stated that a negative pathogen detection using CT-guided biopsy does not exclude infection and should not be used as an argument to refuse antibiotic treatment. To validate our findings, further prospective studies with a larger patient cohort are needed, especially those including rare disease subgroups, such as specific spondylodiscitis. However, our study is strengthened by the fact that all data pertaining to variables used in this study are acquired prior to, or during treatment, in almost every case. Thus, the implementation of our findings into the clinical routine could prove beneficial.

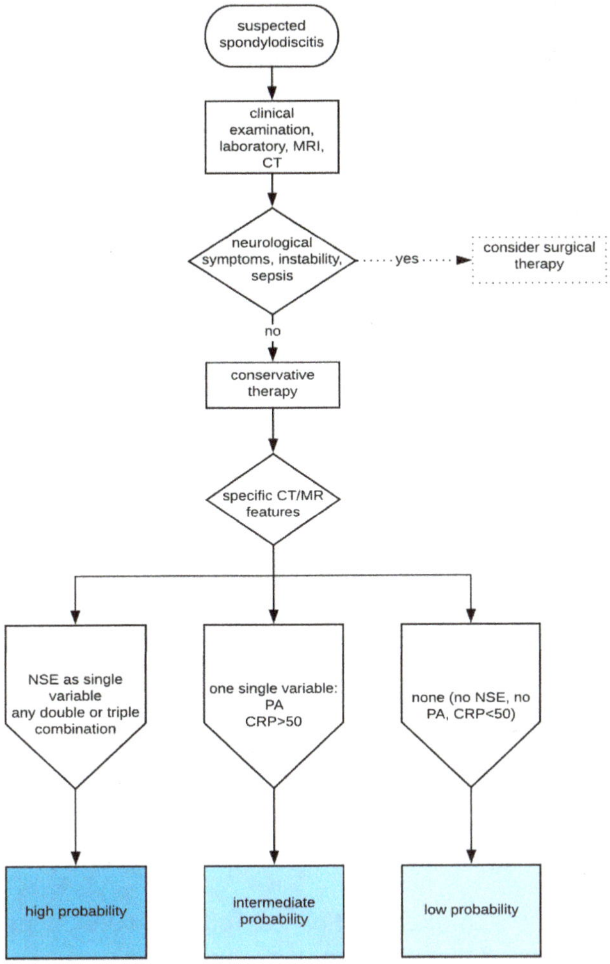

Figure 6. Simplified decision-support pathway regarding probability of pathogen detection following CT-guided biopsy based on imaging and laboratory findings in suspected spondylodiscitis.

5. Conclusions

NSE, CRP > 50, and PA/EA were associated with positive pathogen detection. A double combination of any three had near perfect specificities. If NSE, CRP > 50, and PA/EA were absent the probability of pathogen detection was low. The highest diagnostic performances were exhibited by combinations with NSE. CT evaluation for presence of NSE and sclerosed margins of erosions or absence of erosions as counterparts is therefore very informative. If these features are confirmed in future prospective studies these might support clinicians in the decision to perform or avoid a CT-guided biopsy in specific settings based on CRP, MRI, and CT. However, we would like to stress that, at the present stage, individual therapy decisions should not be based on the presented results as they have to be confirmed in future validation studies.

Author Contributions: Conceptualization: C.R. and A.B.; methodology: A.B., C.R., I.B., M.A.; validation: C.R. and M.-A.W.; formal analysis: I.B., A.B. and C.R.; data interpretation: A.B., C.R., I.B., H.-U.K., M.S., M.A., T.G., F.W. and M.-A.W.; writing—original draft preparation, A.B. and C.R.; writing—review and editing, A.B., C.R., I.B., H.-U.K., M.S., M.A, T.G., F.W. and M.-A.W. All authors have read and agreed to the published version of the manuscript.

Acknowledgments: We would like to thank Oyunbileg von Stackelberg for her organizational support.

References

1. Petkova, A.S.; Zhelyazkov, C.B.; Kitov, B.D. Spontaneous Spondylodiscitis—Epidemiology, Clinical Features, Diagnosis and Treatment. *Folia Med.* **2017**, *59*, 254–260. [CrossRef]
2. Akalan, N.; Ozgen, T. Infection as a cause of spinal cord compression: A review of 36 spinal epidural abscess cases. *Acta Neurochir.* **2000**, *142*, 17–23. [CrossRef]
3. Eismont, F.J.; Bohlman, H.H.; Soni, P.L.; Goldberg, V.M.; Freehafer, A.A. Pyogenic and fungal vertebral osteomyelitis with paralysis. *J. Bone Jt. Surg.* **1983**, *65*, 19–29. [CrossRef]
4. Dragsted, C.; Aagaard, T.; Ohrt-Nissen, S.; Gehrchen, M.; Dahl, B. Mortality and health-related quality of life in patients surgically treated for spondylodiscitis. *J. Orthop. Surg.* **2017**, *25*. [CrossRef]
5. Lestin-Bernstein, F.; Tietke, M.; Briedigkeit, L.; Heese, O. Diagnostics and antibiotic therapy for spondylodiscitis. *J. Med. Microbiol.* **2018**, *67*, 757–768. [CrossRef]
6. Ahuja, N.; Sharma, H. The effectiveness of computed tomography-guided biopsy for the diagnosis of spondylodiscitis: An analysis of variables affecting the outcome. *Eur. Rev. Med. Pharmacol. Sci.* **2017**, *21*, 2021–2026. [PubMed]
7. Iwata, E.; Scarborough, M.; Bowden, G.; McNally, M.; Tanaka, Y.; Athanasou, N.A. The role of histology in the diagnosis of spondylodiscitis: Correlation with clinical and microbiological findings. *Bone Jt. J.* **2019**, *101*, 246–252. [CrossRef] [PubMed]
8. Kasalak, Ö.; Wouthuyzen-Bakker, M.; Adams, H.J.A.; Overbosch, J.; Dierckx, R.A.J.O.; Jutte, P.C.; Kwee, T.C. CT-guided biopsy in suspected spondylodiscitis: Microbiological yield, impact on antimicrobial treatment, and relationship with outcome. *Skelet. Radiol.* **2018**, *47*, 1383–1391. [CrossRef] [PubMed]
9. Enoch, D.A.; Cargill, J.S.; Laing, R.; Herbert, S.; Corrah, T.W.; Brown, N.M. Value of CT-guided biopsy in the diagnosis of septic discitis. *J. Clin. Pathol.* **2008**, *61*, 750–753. [CrossRef]
10. Metzger, C.S.; Johnson, D.W.; Donaldson, W.F. Percutaneous biopsy in the anterior thoracic spine. *Spine* **1993**, *18*, 374–378. [CrossRef]
11. Olscamp, A.; Rollins, J.; Tao, S.S.; Ebraheim, N.A. Complications of CT-guided biopsy of the spine and sacrum. *Orthopedics* **1997**, *20*, 1149–1152. [CrossRef] [PubMed]
12. Sucu, H.K.; Bezircioglu, H.; Ciçek, C.; Erşahin, Y. Computerized tomography-guided percutaneous transforaminodiscal biopsy sampling of vertebral body lesions. *J. Neurosurg.* **2003**, *99*, 51–55. [CrossRef] [PubMed]
13. Michel, S.C.; Pfirrmann, C.W.; Boos, N.; Hodler, J. CT-guided core biopsy of subchondral bone and intervertebral space in suspected spondylodiskitis. *AJR Am. J. Roentgenol.* **2006**, *186*, 977–980. [CrossRef] [PubMed]
14. Rieneck, K.; Hansen, S.E.; Karle, A.; Gutschik, E. Microbiologically verified diagnosis of infectious spondylitis using CT-guided fine needle biopsy. *APMIS* **1996**, *104*, 755–762. [CrossRef] [PubMed]
15. Spira, D.; Germann, T.; Lehner, B.; Hemmer, S.; Akbar, M.; Jesser, J.; Weber, M.A.; Rehnitz, C. CT-Guided Biopsy in Suspected Spondylodiscitis—The Association of Paravertebral Inflammation with Microbial Pathogen Detection. *PLoS ONE* **2016**, *11*, e0146399. [CrossRef] [PubMed]
16. Foreman, S.C.; Schwaiger, B.J.; Gempt, J.; Jungmann, P.M.; Kehl, V.; Delbridge, C.; Wantia, N.; Zimmer, C.; Kirschke, J.S. MR and CT Imaging to Optimize CT-Guided Biopsies in Suspected Spondylodiscitis. *World Neurosurg.* **2017**, *99*, 726–734. [CrossRef] [PubMed]
17. Chandnani, V.P.; Beltran, J.; Morris, C.S.; Khalil, S.N.; Mueller, C.F.; Burk, J.M.; Bennett, W.F.; Shaffer, P.B.; Vasila, M.S.; Reese, J.; et al. Acute experimental osteomyelitis and abscesses: Detection with MR imaging versus CT. *Radiology* **1990**, *174*, 233–236. [CrossRef] [PubMed]
18. Vorbeck, F.; Morscher, M.; Ba-Ssalamah, A.; Imhof, H. Infectious spondylitis in adults. *Radiologe* **1996**, *36*, 795–804. [CrossRef]
19. Ahlhelm, F.; Kelm, J.; Naumann, N.; Shariat, K.; Grunwald, I.; Reith, W.; Nabhan, A. Spondylitis/spondylodiscitis. *Radiologe* **2006**, *46*, 480–485. [CrossRef]
20. Youden, W.J. Index for rating diagnostic tests. *Cancer* **1950**, *3*, 32–35. [CrossRef]
21. Heyer, C.M.; Brus, L.J.; Peters, S.A.; Lemburg, S.P. Efficacy of CT-guided biopsies of the spine in patients with spondylitis—An analysis of 164 procedures. *Eur. J. Radiol.* **2012**, *81*, e244–e249. [CrossRef] [PubMed]

6

Diagnostic Value of ^{18}F-FDG-PET/CT in Patients with FUO

Stamata Georga [1,*], Paraskevi Exadaktylou [1], Ioannis Petrou [1], Dimitrios Katsampoukas [1], Vasilios Mpalaris [1], Efstratios-Iordanis Moralidis [1], Kostoula Arvaniti [2], Christos Papastergiou [3] and Georgios Arsos [1]

1 3rd Department of Nuclear Medicine, Aristotle University of Thessaloniki Medical School, Papageorgiou General Hospital, 56403 Thessaloniki, Greece; voulaexadaktylou@hotmail.com (P.E.); giannispetrou@hotmail.com (I.P.); katsampoukas@hotmail.com (D.K.); vmpalaris@yahoo.gr (V.M.); emoral@auth.gr (E.-I.M.); garsos@auth.gr (G.A.)

2 ICU and Antimicrobial Stewardship Unit, Papageorgiou General Hospital, 56403 Thessaloniki, Greece; arvanitik@hotmail.com

3 Department of Radiology, Papageorgiou General Hospital, 56403 Thessaloniki, Greece; christospapastergiou65@gmail.com

* Correspondence: matageorga@gmail.com

Abstract: Conventional diagnostic imaging is often ineffective in revealing the underlying cause in a considerable proportion of patients with fever of unknown origin (FUO). The aim of this study was to assess the diagnostic value of fluorine-18 fluorodeoxyglucose positron emission tomography/computed tomography (^{18}F-FDG-PET/CT) in patients with FUO. We retrospectively reviewed ^{18}F-FDG-PET/CT scans performed on 50 consecutive adult patients referred to our department for further investigation of classic FUO. Final diagnosis was based on histopathological and microbiological findings, clinical criteria, or clinical follow-up. Final diagnosis was established in 39/50 (78%) of the patients. The cause of FUO was infection in 20/50 (40%), noninfectious inflammatory diseases in 11/50 (22%), and malignancy in 8/50 (16%) patients. Fever remained unexplained in 11/50 (22%) patients. ^{18}F-FDG-PET/CT scan substantially contributed to the diagnosis in 70% of the patients, either by identifying the underlying cause of FUO or by directing to the most appropriate site for biopsy. Sensitivity, specificity, accuracy, positive predictive value (PPV) and negative predictive value (NPV) of ^{18}F-FDG-PET/CT for active disease detection in patients with FUO were 94.7%, 50.0%, 84.0%, 85.7%, and 75.0%, respectively. In conclusion, whole-body ^{18}F-FDG-PET/CT is a highly sensitive method for detection of the underlining cause of FUO or for correctly targeting suspicious lesions for further evaluation.

Keywords: fever of unknown origin; FUO; PET/CT; ^{18}F-FDG-PET/CT

---

1. Introduction

Despite the immense progress of laboratory and imaging modalities, fever of unknown origin (FUO) remains a diagnostic challenge. FUO was originally defined by Petersdorf and Beeson in 1961 as body temperature higher than 38.3 °C, on at least three occasions over a period of at least three weeks, with no diagnosis made despite one week of inpatient investigation [1]. The initial definition of FUO was subsequently modified by Durack and Street in 1991 by removing the requirement of inpatient investigation and also by excluding immunocompromised patients as they may require an entirely different diagnostic approach [2]. Later, the quantitative criterion of uncertain diagnosis after a period of time was proposed to be replaced by a qualitative criterion of a number of obligatory investigations that should be performed to qualify the condition as FUO [3–5].

The differential diagnosis of FUO includes a wide spectrum of highly heterogeneous diseases, which is traditionally subdivided into four categories: infections, malignancies, non-infectious inflammatory diseases (NIID), and miscellaneous causes, with their incidence strongly affected by the local epidemiology [6,7]. Expectedly, the proportion of undiagnosed cases of FUO ranged from 7% to 53% in various studies, thus indicating that the diagnostic investigation of FUO still remains a challenge [7,8].

Structural cross-sectional imaging modalities such as computed tomography (CT) and magnetic resonance imaging (MRI) can be used to detect focal pathologies, but they may be less accurate in the early stages of infectious and inflammatory diseases. Furthermore, distinction of active inflammation from healing or treated infection or postoperative changes and maturing scar tissue is often hardly achievable by radiological modalities [9].

Conversely, nuclear medicine modalities are capable of early detection of disease activity at a cellular or even molecular level, preceding morphological alterations, and also to distinguish between active and inactive disease and between infection and aseptic inflammation or malignancy [10]. In the few past decades, a variety of specific and non-specific radiopharmaceuticals have been proposed for imaging infection and inflammation [11]. ^{67}Ga (gallium) citrate scintigraphy has been widely used in the past to investigate FUO [12–14] due to its accumulation in both infections and acute or chronic inflammations and neoplasms. However, its low specificity and suboptimal imaging characteristics, along with the introduction of newer radiopharmaceuticals for imaging of infection and inflammation like labeled leucocytes and ^{18}F-fluorodeoxyglucose (^{18}F-FDG) have dramatically reduced its use in most clinical indications, including FUO.

Labeled leucocyte scintigraphy is a highly specific method for imaging infection because labeled leucocytes migrate actively into infectious foci [15]. However, it is not a very helpful modality in patients with FUO, because infections account for only a portion of FUO cases, ranging from 11% to 57% in various studies [6–8].

^{18}F-FDG, the most commonly used radiotracer for positron emission tomography/computed tomography (PET/CT), accumulates avidly in most viable neoplasms and has been extensively studied in patients with malignancies for diagnosis, staging, and treatment response assessment [16]. Since Tahara et al. first showed high ^{18}F-FDG uptake in abdominal abscesses in 1989 [17], evidence is growing on the usefulness of ^{18}F-FDG-PET/CT in the diagnosis and management of several inflammatory and infectious diseases [18] based on the high glucose uptake by activated inflammatory cells, related to their increased glycolytic activity and overexpression of glucose transporters (GLUT), especially GLUT 1 and GLUT 3. Shorter procedure duration and higher resolution and sensitivity are the comparative advantages of ^{18}F-FDG-PET over conventional scintigraphy, making ^{18}F-FDG-PET an appealing modality for imaging infection and inflammation especially since the emergence of PET/CT [19].

Several studies indicate the potential contributory role of both ^{18}F-FDG-PET alone [12,13,20–23] and ^{18}F-FDG-PET/CT [24–28] in the management of patients of FUO. However, the representativeness of the populations studied may be questionable as in the majority of the Northwestern European studies NIID is the leading causes of FUO, whereas in those coming from Asia, infections are more common, with tuberculosis predominating. As far as we know, only limited data are available regarding Southern Europe and Mediterranean countries. For example, to the best of our knowledge, there are only two previous studies on FUO in Greece [29,30], none of them dealing with the role of ^{18}F-FDG-PET/CT imaging in the diagnosis of FUO.

We performed a retrospective study at a tertiary academic general hospital in Northern Greece in order to assess the diagnostic value of ^{18}F-FDG-PET/CT in patients presenting with FUO.

2. Experimental Section

2.1. Patient Population

Fifty consecutive immunocompetent adult patients of Caucasian origin were studied retrospectively. Patients were admitted to the PET/CT department of Papageorgiou General Hospital in Northern Greece, between November 2016 and July 2019, for further classic FUO investigation.

All patients enrolled in the study fulfilled the revised Petersdorf's criteria of FUO [3]. Patients with nosocomial infections or known immunodeficiency (e.g., neutropenia, HIV-associated infection, hypogammaglobulinemia or on systemic corticosteroids) were excluded from the study.

The initial diagnostic work-up of all patients included a comprehensive medical history, physical examination, routine hematological, biochemical, and serological tests, blood and urine cultures and plain chest radiographies. Concerning the inflammatory blood markers, values higher than 20 mm/h, 0.8 mg/dL, and 0.5 ng/mL were considered as indicative of abnormally elevated erythrocyte sedimentation rate (ESR), C-reactive protein (CRP) level, and procalcitonin (PCT), respectively. Computed tomography (CT), MRI and echocardiography had been performed in the vast majority of the patients prior to ^{18}F-FDG-PET/CT imaging, while invasive investigations such as endoscopies and parenchymal organs, bone marrow, or temporal artery biopsies had been occasionally conducted.

Underlying pathologies that could be related to the cause of the fever or might affect the interpretation of the ^{18}F-FDG-PET/CT scan were recorded for all patients. The presence of diabetes mellitus along with relevant blood glucose lowering drugs was recorded. Antibiotic or corticosteroid treatment prior to ^{18}F-FDG-PET/CT imaging or chemotherapy in the last 6 months was also recorded.

2.2. ^{18}F-FDG-PET/CT Imaging

All ^{18}F-FDG-PET/CT scans were performed using a 16-slice integrated PET/CT scanner (Discovery 710; GE Healthcare).

Patients fasted for at least 12 h before intravenous injection of ^{18}F-FDG at a dose of 4 MBq/kg of body weight. In patients carrying cardiovascular implantable electronic devices (CIED) or prosthetic cardiac valves, suspected of cardiac infection as the cause of FUO, a preparation protocol for suppression of myocardial glucose metabolism was applied, consisting of a high fat–low carbohydrate diet started three days before imaging followed by a prolonged ($\approx$18 h) fasting. The target serum glucose levels at the time of ^{18}F-FDG administration was less than 150 mg/dL.

Skull base to mid-thigh PET/CT imaging started 60 min after intravenous injection of ^{18}F-FDG, at a 3 min per bed position rate in a three-dimensional mode. On clinical suspicion of the involvement of lower extremities, a whole-body scan including the legs was performed. Delayed regional images were additionally obtained in cases of ambiguous findings. Low-dose helical CT without contrast enhancement (30–300 mA automatically adjusted to tissue depth, 120 kV, slice thickness of 3.75 mm) was performed for attenuation correction of PET emission data and anatomic mapping.

PET sections were obtained by an iterative reconstruction algorithm (ordered subset expectation maximization (OSEM)) and corrected for attenuation by the corresponding CT attenuation maps. Maximum intensity projection (MIP) images and reconstructed sections (low-dose CT, attenuation corrected PET, and fused PET/CT) were then displayed for analysis in the standard axial, coronal, and sagittal planes.

2.3. Image Analysis

All ^{18}F-FDG-PET/CT images were reviewed by two experienced nuclear medicine physicians and a radiologist aware of the clinical data. Disagreement between the readers were resolved by consensus. Image interpretation was based on visual inspection of the body for areas of abnormally high ^{18}F-FDG uptake. In addition, in cases of hypermetabolic PET foci adjacent to hyperdense CT findings (e.g., prosthetic cardiac valves or heavy coronary vessel calcification), the non-attenuation corrected (NAC) sections were thoroughly inspected, to exclude PET false positivity resulting from attenuation overcorrection.

Studies were considered as positive for active disease if increased ^{18}F-FDG uptake, focal or diffuse, other than normal or otherwise explainable was observed. The pattern (focal, linear, or diffuse) and the intensity of ^{18}F-FDG uptake were visually assessed. Conversely, studies with a normal or otherwise explainable ^{18}F-FDG pattern of distribution throughout the body were classified as negative for active disease processes.

A positive study was classified as "true positive" (TP) when abnormal ^{18}F-FDG uptake in an organ or tissue corresponded to the cause of fever, as confirmed by additional investigations, and as "false positive" (FP) when it was proven unrelated to the cause of fever or when the fever remained undiagnosed during the follow-up period.

A negative study was classified as "true negative" (TN) when no cause of fever was identified during the clinical follow-up for at least 6 months or the fever resolved spontaneously without specific treatment, and as "false negative" (FN) when a focal infection, inflammation, or malignancy was eventually identified as the cause of fever within 6 months or fever persisted throughout the follow-up period or the patient died febrile without a definite diagnosis.

Follow-up was accomplished by reviewing the patients' medical records or by contacting the referring physician or the patients themselves.

Final diagnosis was based on histopathological and microbiological findings, on fulfillment of widely acceptable diagnostic criteria or clinical follow-up. The duration of follow-up exceeded 6 months in all patients without a definite diagnosis.

An ^{18}F-FDG-PET/CT scan was considered as contributory to the diagnosis if it directly identified the underlying cause of FUO or correctly suggested the site for a diagnostic biopsy. In all other situations, it was considered as non-contributory to the diagnosis.

^{18}F-FDG uptake by suspect lesions was also semi-quantitatively evaluated by means of the maximum standardized uptake value (SUVmax). SUVmax was derived using properly sized spherical volumes of interest (VOIs) according to current EANM (European Association of Nuclear Medicine) guidelines [31]. In case of multiple hypermetabolic foci, the highest relevant SUVmax value was recorded.

2.4. Statistical Analysis

Sensitivity, specificity, accuracy, positive predictive value (PPV), and negative predictive value (NPV) of ^{18}F-FDG-PET/CT scan for the detection of active disease were calculated as per standard definitions. Continuous variables were expressed either as means ± standard deviation (SD), or as medians and interquartile range, as appropriate. Categorical variables were expressed as number and proportions and the between-groups differences were tested by means of Pearson's X^2 test (or Fisher's exact test where applicable). Differences of the continuous variables between patient groups were tested for significance using either *t*-test for normally distributed variables or the nonparametric Mann–Whitney U tests as appropriate. Statistical significance was accepted for $p < 0.05$. Statistical analysis was accomplished using the IBM SPSS 23.0 statistic software package (IBM Corp., Armonk, NY, USA).

3. Results

From November 2016 to July 2019, fifty-four patients were referred to our PET/CT facility installed in a 700-bed academic general hospital, for classic FUO investigation. The majority of the patients were mainly coming from the Internal Medicine or Infectious Diseases departments of other hospitals in the area. Four patients were excluded from the study; one was 16 years old, two were lost to follow-up, and one with an ^{18}F-FDG-PET/CT scan highly suspicious for lymphoma who died shortly after without a definite diagnosis. Thus, 50 adult patients all having ^{18}F-FDG-PET/CT scan for classic FUO investigation were eventually included in the study.

3.1. Patients Characteristics and Final Diagnoses

The main demographic and clinical characteristics of the patients enrolled in the study are summarized in Table 1.

Table 1. Demographic and clinical characteristics of the study group.

Characteristic	*n* (%)	Median (IQR, Min–Max)
Number of patients	50	
Gender (male/female)	28/22 (56%/44%)	
Age (years)		59 (25, 17–85)
Concomitant Diseases/Conditions	50 (100%)	
Malignancies	8 (16%)	
Breast/ AML/H&N/URO/CR/WM	2/2/1/1/1/1	
Diabetes Mellitus	7 (14%)	
Chronic kidney desease	7 (14%)	
Cardiovascular devices	6 (12%)	
Vascular grafts/Prosthetic valves/CIED	4/1/1	
Bowel diversions	4 (8%)	
Thyroid diseases	3 (6%)	
Multinodular goiter, Hashimoto thyroiditis	2/1	
Prosthetic joints	3 (6%)	
Spinal surgery	2 (4%)	
Miscellaneous	3 (6%)	
SLE/AS/Meningioma	1/1/1	
Duration of fever (days)		40 (60, 21–365)
Common clinical/radiological findings		
Lymphadenopathy	16 (32%)	
Splenomegaly	10 (20%)	
Elevated blood inflammatory markers (ESR, CRP, PCT)	31 (62%)	
Medications	17 (34%)	
Antibiotics	13 (26%)	
Corticosteroids	1 (2%)	
Chemotherapy (last dose 4 months ago)	3 (6%)	

n, number of patients; IQR, interquartile range; AML, acute myeloid leukemia; H&N, head and neck cancer; URO, urothelial cancer; CR, colorectal cancer; WM, Waldenstrom macroglobulinemia; CIED, cardiac implantable electronic device; SLE, systemic lupus erythematosus; AS, ankylosing spondylitis; ESR, erythrocyte sedimentation rate; CRP, C-reactive protein; PCT, procalcitonin.

Because of the varying origin of the patients and the retrospective nature of the study, a uniform diagnostic work-up before ^{18}F-FDG-PET/CT imaging was missing. However, after the initial diagnostic work-up and before ^{18}F-FDG-PET/CT scan, almost all of them (49/50) had been submitted to several advanced investigations (median 3, min–max 0–8). The advanced investigations performed prior to the ^{18}F-FDG-PET/CT scan on our patients are listed in Table 2.

A final diagnosis was established in 39/50 (78%) patients and was classified into 4 categories: infection, malignancy, non-infectious inflammatory diseases (NIID), and undiagnosed fever. The cause of FUO was infection in 20 patients (40%), malignancy in 8 patients (16%), NIID in 11 patients (22%), while the fever remained unexplained in 11 patients (22%). The final diagnoses for the 50 patients studied are listed in Table 3.

Table 2. Advanced investigations performed prior to PET/CT scan.

Investigation	*n* (%)
Echocardiography	20 (40%)
Computed tomography (CT)	
Thoracic CT	39 (78%)
Abdominal CT	36 (72%)
Cervical CT	8 (16%)
Cerebral CT	7 (14%)
Magnetic Resonance Imaging (MRI)	
Abdominal MRI	7 (14%)
Lumbar spine MRI	4 (8%)
Cerebral MRI	3 (6%)
Cervical spine MRI	1 (2%)
Endoscopy	
Gastroscopy	4 (8%)
Colonoscopy	4 (8%)
Bronchoscopy	3 (6%)
Nuclear medicine procedures	
^{99m}Tc-MDP bone scan	2 (4%)
^{99m}Tc-HMPAO-labeled leucocyte scan	1 (2%)
^{99m}Tc-pertechnetate thyroid scan	1 (2%)
^{99m}Tc-MAG-3 Renogram	1 (2%)
Biopsies	
Lymph node or parenchymal organ biopsy	7 (14%)
Bone marrow biopsy	9 (18%)
Temporal artery biopsy	3 (6%)

n, number of patients; MDP, methylene diphosphonate; HMPAO, hexamethylpropylene-amine oxime; MAG-3, mercapto-acetyl-triglycine. PET/CT, fluorodeoxyglucose positron emission tomography/computed tomography.

Table 3. Final diagnoses of 50 patients with fever of unknown origin (FUO).

Diagnostic Categories	*n* (%)
Infections	20 (40%)
Abdominal abscesses	4
Infectious cyst in polycystic renal disease	3
Pneumonia/inflammation of bronchiectasis cysts	3
Vascular graft infection	3
Tuberculous spondylitis	1
Bacterial spondylodiscitis	1
Pulmonary tuberculosis	1
CIED-associated infection	1
Infectious lymphadenopathy	1
Cryptococcosis	1
Leishmaniasis	1
Malignancy	8 (16%)
Non-Hodgkin's lymphoma	5
Hodgkin's disease	1
Lung cancer	1
Relapse of urinary tract carcinoma	1

Table 3. *Cont.*

Diagnostic Categories	*n* (%)
Non-infectious Inflammatory diseases (NIID)	11 (22%)
Large vessel vasculitis/Takayasu's arteritis	3
Adult-onset Still's disease	2
Sarcoidosis	1
Polymyalgia rheumatica	1
Inflammatory bowel disease	1
Familial Mediterranean fever	1
Neo-esophagus inflammation from gastroesophageal reflux	1
Subacute thyroiditis	1
Undiagnosed fever	11 (22%)
Spontaneous recovery of fever	7
Recovery of fever with corticosteroids or NSAIDs	3
Recurrent fever until death	1

n, number of patients; CIED, cardiac implantable electronic device; NSAIDs, non-steroidal anti-inflammatory drugs.

3.2. ^{18}F-FDG-PET/CT Results

The standard preparation protocol for ^{18}F-FDG-PET/CT imaging was applied to 45 of the 50 patients studied, whereas five patients successfully followed the preparation protocol for cardiac imaging. Among them, in 4 patients, the fever was found unrelated to cardiac infection, while in one patient the cause of fever was CIED associated infection; however, in this patient, the ^{18}F-FDG-PET/CT scan was false negative.

Mean serum glucose levels of the patients at the time of ^{18}F-FDG administration was 96.7 ± 20.2 mg/dL (min–max 63–155 mg/dL) and did not differ between patients with contributory and non-contributory scans (94.8 ± 17.8 mg/dL vs. 101.3 ± 25.1 mg/dL), respectively ($p = 0.077$).

^{18}F-FDG-PET/CT scan was abnormal in 42/50 (84%) patients studied, showing single or multiple hypermetabolic foci compatible with active disease, while the scan was negative for active disease in 8 patients (16%).

Of the 42 positive ^{18}F-FDG-PET/CT scans, 36 were considered as true positive (TP) scans and 6 as false positive (FP) scans. Thus, a definite diagnosis was established in 85.7% of patients with positive scans. The TP scans included 19 cases of infections, 8 cases of malignancy, and 9 cases of non-infectious inflammatory diseases. The TP scans in the group of infections included all the cases of infectious diseases listed in Table 3, except of one case of CIED-associated infection, in which the ^{18}F-FDG-PET/CT scan was false negative.

All the 8 patients with a final diagnosis of malignancy (5 newly diagnosed non-Hodgkin's lymphomas, 1 Hodgkin's disease, 1 lung cancer, and 1 urinary tract carcinoma relapse) had a true positive ^{18}F-FDG-PET/CT scan. Among them, there was only one with recurrence of a previous malignancy (recurrence of urinary tract carcinoma initially diagnosed 1 years ago) and another with aggressive transformation of a previous hematological malignancy (Waldenstrom macroglobulinemia diagnosed 5 years ago, now diagnosed with non-Hodgkin's lymphomas). Of the 6 other patients, 5 had no history of malignancy, and 1 had a history of a different malignant disease (breast cancer diagnosed 6 years ago).

The 9 TP scans in the group with NIID included three patients with large vessel vasculitis and one of each of the following: sarcoidosis, polymyalgia rheumatica, familial Mediterranean fever, adult-onset Still's disease, subacute thyroiditis, and exacerbation of inflammatory bowel disease.

There were 6 FP scans; they included 4 cases of undiagnosed fever with spontaneous resolution during the follow-up period, one case of adult-onset Still's disease, and a case of neo-esophagus inflammation from gastroesophageal reflux.

Eight out of fifty patients studied had a negative ^{18}F-FDG-PET/CT scan. Six of them were considered true negative (TN); in five of these cases the fever resolved spontaneously with no evidence of disease during the at least 6-month follow-up period, while in one case the fever resolved after corticosteroid administration. Finally, there were two false negative (FN) scans; the first case was an elderly patient with recurrent febrile episodes until death a year later with a possible diagnosis of viral encephalitis and the second one was a febrile patient who was eventually diagnosed, according to clinical criteria and echocardiography, with CIED-associated infection, whose fever resolved after the CIED removal. The last patient was on antibiotic treatment for prostatitis for two weeks before the ^{18}F-FDG-PET/CT scan without remission of the fever. Thus, among the patients with negative scans, a definite diagnosis was established in only one (12%).

^{18}F-FDG-PET/CT results according to the category of final diagnosis are depicted in Table 4. Nineteen of twenty patients in the group of infections had a true positive scan. The final diagnoses in patients with false (positive or negative) ^{18}F-FDG-PET/CT scans are presented in Table 5.

Table 4. ^{18}F-FDG-PET/CT scan results according to the category of final diagnosis.

Categories	TP	FP	TN	FN	*N*
Infections	19	0	0	1	20
Malignancies	8	0	0	0	8
Non-infectious inflammatory diseases	9	2	0	0	11
Undiagnosed fever	0	4	6	1	11
Total (%)	36 (72%)	6 (12%)	6 (12%)	2 (4%)	50

The median SUVmax [IQR] was higher in malignant diseases (16.9 [18.7]) followed by that in infections (9.1 [6.1]), NIID (6.2 [6.6]) and in undiagnosed fever (5.9 [6.3]). The median SUVmax [IQR] was significantly higher in malignant diseases than in all the other diagnoses together (16.9 [18.7] vs. 7.1 [6.2], $p = 0.01$). Similarly, the median SUVmax [IQR] was significantly higher in contributory than in non-contributory ^{18}F-FDG-PET/CT scans (9.2 [7.1] vs. 4.9 [5.7], $p = 0.01$). ^{18}F-FDG uptake quantified by SUVmax in different groups of final diagnosis is graphically presented in Figure 1.

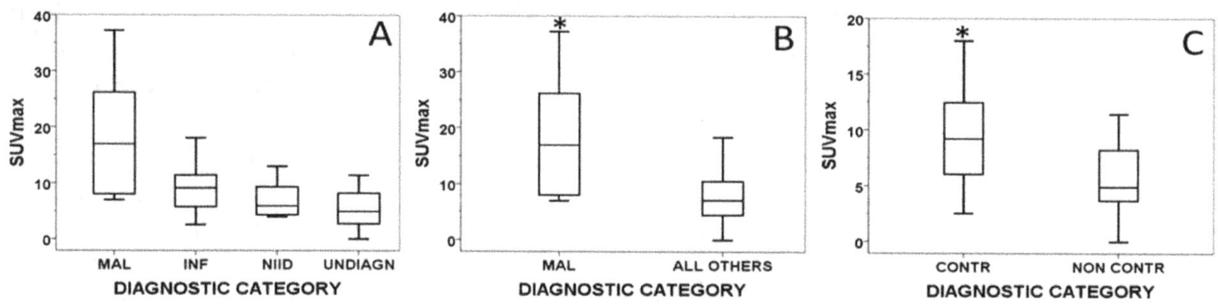

Figure 1. Box plot graphs showing SUVmax distribution in various diagnostic categories. Across the four groups of final diagnosis (**A**); between malignancy and non-malignancy (**B**) and between contributory and non-contributory scans (**C**). SUVmax, maximum-standardized uptake value; NIID, non-infectious inflammatory disease; MAL, malignant; INF, infectious; NIID, non-infectious inflammatory disease; UNDIAGN, undiagnosed; CONTR, contributory; NONCONTR, non-contributory; * $p < 0.05$.

Table 5. Final diagnosis in patients with false positive or false negative ^{18}F-FDG-PET/CT scans.

Gender, Age	Underlying Conditions	^{18}F-FDG-PET/CT Result	Final Diagnosis	Outcome
M, 81 years	COPD, recurrent respiratory infections, prosthetic AoV	FN	No diagnosis; possible viral encephalitis	Death
M, 78 years	CIED	FN	CIED-associated infection	Fever remission after CIED removal
M, 70 years	Recurrent episodes of aspiration pneumonia; neo-esophagus due to gastrointestinal bleeding	FP: possible pulmonary aspergillosis; diffuse hypermetabolic activity along neo-esophagus	Inflammation of the neo-esophagus from gastroesophageal reflux	Spontaneous recovery
F, 57 years	THA, SLE	FP: active axillary and subclavicular lymphadenopathy (d.d. lymphoma, sarcoidosis, non-specific inflammation)	No diagnosis	Lymph node biopsy without pathological findings; spontaneous recovery
M, 49 years	Lymphadenopathy	FP: extensive (intrapelvic, inguinal, axillary), moderately active lymphadenopathy and splenic involvement; overall impression in favor of lymphoproliferative disease, (d.d. inflammatory/granulomatous etiology)	No diagnosis	Lymph node biopsy without pathological findings; recovery after antibiotics
M, 54 years	AML	FP: multiple, diffuse hypermetabolic liver lesions (d.d. infectious lesions/infiltration from hematological disease)	No diagnosis	Spontaneous recovery
M, 56 years	L3–L4 spondylodiscitis	FP: increased prostate uptake, possible prostate abscess	Adult-onset Still's disease	Recovery with steroids
F, 63 years	Multinodular goiter, TB	FP: finding compatible with moderately active pericarditis, inactive granulomatous lung disease	No diagnosis	Recovery with steroids

M, male; F, female; FP, false positive; FN, false negative; d.d., differential diagnosis; COPD, chronic obstructive pulmonary disease; CIED, cardiac implantable electronic device; THA, total hip arthroplasty; SLE, systemic lupus erythematosus; AML, acute myeloid leukemia; TB, tuberculosis.

The overall sensitivity, specificity, accuracy, positive predictive value (PPV), and negative predictive value (NPV) of ^{18}F-FDG-PET/CT for active disease detection in our patients were 94.7%, 50.0%, 84.0%, 85.7%, and 75.0%, respectively. The sensitivity of ^{18}F-FDG-PET/CT for diagnosing active disease processes was higher in the group of malignancies where all of the scans were true positive (sensitivity of 100%) followed by the group of infections where the ^{18}F-FDG-PET/CT scans were true positive in 19/20 patients and false negative in 1/20, giving a sensitivity of 95%. However, due to the relatively small number of patients in the different groups of diagnoses, no further analysis of the diagnostic performance of ^{18}F-FDG-PET/CT in each group of patients was undertaken.

The ^{18}F-FDG-PET/CT scan was considered contributory to the diagnosis in 35/50 (70%) of the patients, either by identifying the underlying cause of FUO (causal diagnosis in 25 patients) or by correctly directing to the most appropriate site for successful biopsy leading to an accurate diagnosis (biopsy site selection in 10 patients). All the TP ^{18}F-FDG-PET/CT scans, but one, were considered as contributory to the diagnosis, and this was the case of a patient with a true positive scan but diagnosis of adult-onset Still's disease based on exclusion criteria of other diseases, thus allocating the PET/CT scan to the not contributory to the diagnosis category. The true negative ^{18}F-FDG-PET/CT scans as well as the false positive and false negative scans were considered as non-contributory to the diagnosis.

Some representative cases of the diagnostic contribution of ^{18}F-FDG-PET/CT scan in patients with FUO are shown in Figures 2–6.

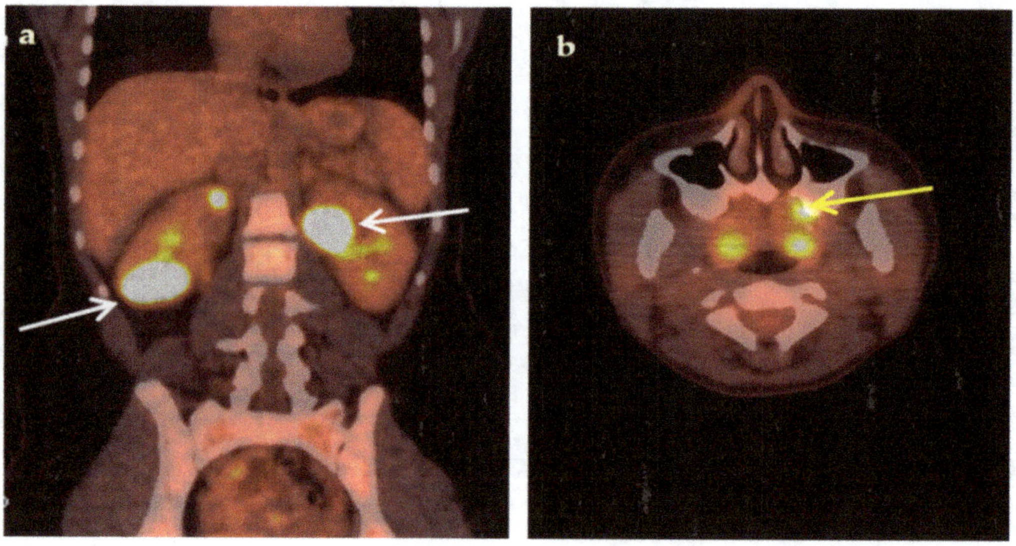

Figure 2. An 18-year-old woman presented with a 3-week fever, elevated inflammatory blood markers (ESR 77 mm/h, CRP 9.3 mg/dL) and an abdominal CT scan suggestive of possible renal abscesses. Coronal fused ^{18}F-FDG-PET/CT image (**a**), demonstrated multiple hypodense, highly hypermetabolic lesions in both kidneys, the largest (white arrows) in the lower pole of the right kidney (SUVmax 35.3) and in the upper pole of the left kidney (SUVmax 34.4), compatible with renal abscesses, confirmed by biopsy. Transaxial fused ^{18}F-FDG-PET/CT image (**b**) demonstrated high ^{18}F-FDG paradental uptake in the left maxilla (yellow arrow) raising concern for hematogenous spread of dental infection. Complementary focused interrogation revealed a history of a painful, undertreated dental condition of the left maxilla preceding fever.

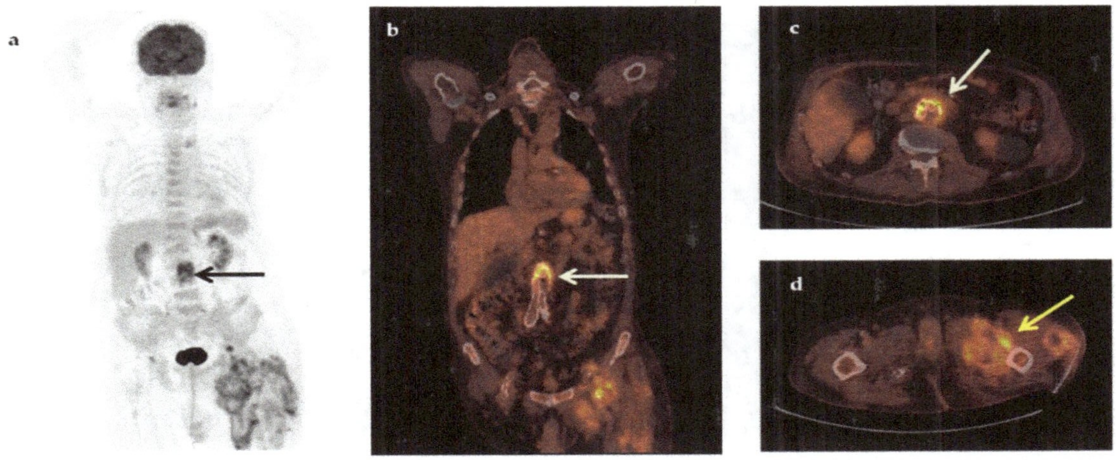

Figure 3. A 74-year-old man with a medical history of aortobiiliac vascular prosthesis because of an asymptomatic aneurysm 5 months ago, presented with a 2-month fever, increased inflammatory blood markers (ESR 83 mm/h, CRP 19.2 mg/dL) and intramuscular fluid collections in the left thigh, (revealed in a CT for localized pain). Maximum intensity projection ^{18}F-FDG-PET (**a**), coronal fused (**b**) and transaxial fused ^{18}F-FDG-PET/CT images at the level of the L3 vertebra (**c**), demonstrated increased metabolic activity in the wall of the abdominal aneurysm (arrows) at that level (SUVmax 7.0), suspicious of infection. In addition, transaxial fused FDG-PET/CT image at the level of thighs (**d**) revealed intramuscular hypermetabolic collections with air bubbles in the left thigh, suspicious of abscesses (yellow arrow). Vascular graft infection was confirmed by histopathology after removal of the aortic graft (*Klebsiella pneumoniae*, *Pseudomonas aeruginosa*).

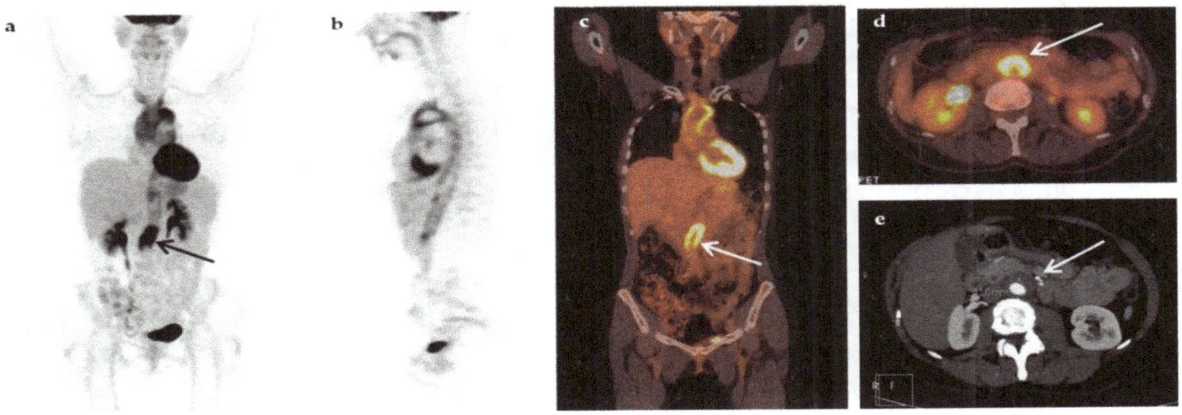

Figure 4. A 52-year-old woman presented with prolonged fever (over 6 months) and increased inflammatory blood markers (ESR 76 mm/h, CRP 9.3 mg/dL). The patient had a medical history of breast cancer seven years ago. Maximum-intensity projection ^{18}F-FDG-PET (**a**), sagittal ^{18}F-FDG-PET (**b**), coronal fused ^{18}F-FDG-PET/CT (**c**), and transaxial fused FDG-PET/CT images at the level of the renal vessels (**d**) demonstrated increased metabolic activity within the wall of the thoracic and abdominal aorta, extending to the subclavian arteries, more intense at the root of the aorta and above the aortic bifurcation (arrows). The findings were compatible with vasculitis of large- and medium-sized arteries, mainly affecting the aorta (panaortitis). Transverse section of the CT angiography at the level of renal vessels (**e**) showed thickening of the aorta wall, more pronounced at the level below the renal vessels (arrow), but with no evidence of narrowing of the aortic lumen. A diagnosis of large vessel vasculitis/Takayasu's arteritis was made, and fever resolved after treatment with corticosteroids.

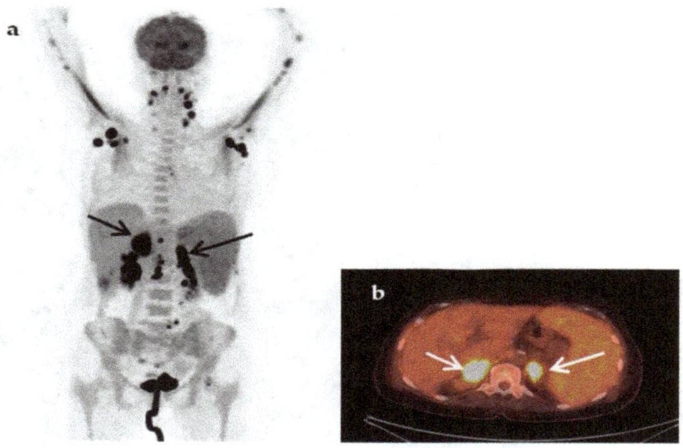

Figure 5. A 75-year-old woman presented with a 4-week fever associated with malaise and weight loss. The abdominal CT revealed splenomegaly and adrenal masses. Maximum-intensity projection (MIP) ^{18}F-FDG-PET (**a**) showed extensive highly hypermetabolic lymphadenopathy, cervical, axillary (SUVmax 22.7) and abdominal and hypermetabolic (SUVmax 16.8) adrenal masses (fused transaxial ^{18}F-FDG-PET/CT image (**b**), arrows), hypermetabolic hepatic lesions (at least two) and multiple hypermetabolic bone metastases and splenomegaly with diffuse homogeneously increased metabolic activity. The findings were suspicious of lymphoma. A diagnosis of non-Hodgkin's lymphoma was confirmed by histopathology after biopsy of an axillary lymph node.

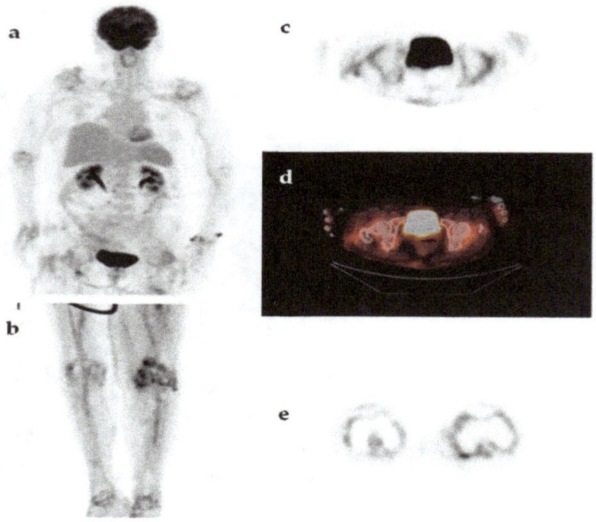

Figure 6. An 85-year-old woman presented with a 2-month fever. The patient had a history of total left knee arthroplasty with no signs of loosening or infection. MIP ^{18}F-FDG-PET image (**a**,**b**), transaxial ^{18}F-FDG-PET and ^{18}F-FDG-PET/CT images at the level of hips (**c**,**d**) and transaxial ^{18}F-FDG-PET image at the level of knees (**e**) demonstrated diffuse, symmetric, moderately increased ^{18}F-FDG uptake, in the large peripheral joints (shoulders, hips, knees) accompanied by increased ^{18}F-FDG uptake along the medium-sized arteries (axillary, humeral, femoral, and tibial arteries). The findings were compatible with polymyalgia rheumatica and the fever resolved upon treatment with corticosteroids.

3.3. Baseline Patient Characteristics in Contributory and Non-Contributory Scans

A detailed comparison of many clinical (age, gender, fever duration, prior antibiotic administration, lymphadenopathy, splenomegaly, presence of diabetes mellitus) and laboratory (number of prior advanced investigations and levels of elevated inflammatory blood markers) characteristics showed no

The overall sensitivity and specificity of ^{18}F-FDG-PET/CT for active disease detection calculated in our study were 94.7% and 50.0%, respectively, in accordance with two recent meta-analyses supporting the diagnostic role of ^{18}F-FDG-PET/CT in patients with FUO. The first of them published in 2016, including 42 studies with 2058 patients with FUO reported a pooled sensitivity and specificity of ^{18}F-FDG-PET/CT of 86% and 52%, respectively [45]. The second one, published in 2018, including 23 studies with 1927 patients concluded that ^{18}F-FDG-PET/CT was very helpful for recognizing and for excluding, as well, diseases as causes of FUO with a pooled sensitivity and specificity of 84% and 63%, respectively [39]. The sensitivity of ^{18}F-FDG-PET/CT in our study was higher in the group of malignancies where all of the scans were true positive reaching a sensitivity of 100%, followed by the group of infections with true positive scans in 95% of patients, missing only one case of infectious disease. This was in agreement with previous studies highlighting the superior clinical efficacy of ^{18}F-FDG-PET/CT in populations with higher proportions of patients with infections and malignancies [27,28,37,45].

However, in the setting of FUO, comparison of different studies in terms of sensitivity and specificity may be misleading for a number of reasons, including variation in FUO definition, patient characteristics, diagnostic work-up sequence, and diagnostic gold standard multiplicity. In an attempt to overcome these problems, the estimation of the clinical helpfulness of PET scan in the diagnosis of FUO has been suggested instead of the formal sensitivity and specificity [10]. During the last two decades, several studies have explored the diagnostic contribution of stand-alone ^{18}F-FDG-PET [12,13,20–23] and more recently of the ^{18}F-FDG-PET/CT scans [24–28,33–36] in patients of FUO, concluding clinical helpfulness varying widely between 16% and 69% for the stand-alone ^{18}F-FDG-PET studies and between 38% and 75% for the ^{18}F-FDG-PET/CT studies.

In the present study, ^{18}F-FDG-PET/CT was helpful and substantially contributed to the diagnosis in 70% of patients, either by identifying the underlying cause of FUO or by correctly targeting suspicious lesions for diagnostic biopsy. Only the true positive scans were considered as contributory to the diagnosis in our study. All the other scans, including the true negative ones were considered as non-contributory to the diagnosis. Similarly, the majority (12/14) of studies included in a recent meta-analysis [40] considered only the positive ^{18}F-FDG-PET and ^{18}F-FDG-PET/CT scans as helpful to the diagnosis. However, this approach has been questioned, as in a recent meta-analysis of 13 studies [43] it was concluded that the diagnostic yield of ^{18}F-FDG-PET/CT in patients with FUO should take into account not only the positive cases but also the true negative ones claiming that patients with a negative ^{18}F-FDG-PET/CT scans are more likely to have a favorable course. Although it may be true for a considerable fraction of patients with undiagnosed fever, we have not allocated the true negative scans to the contributory to the diagnosis ones in our study, because a negative ^{18}F-FDG-PET/CT scan did not actually explain the cause of the fever, which may remain virtually undiagnosed until its, often spontaneous, remission.

In our study, a definite diagnosis was established in a high percentage of patients with positive scans (PPV of 85.7%), in accordance with previous studies [12,20,23,24,35]. A meta-analysis of 14 studies showed that an abnormal ^{18}F-FDG-PET scan is associated with increased likelihood of definite diagnosis, thus, favoring the adoption of ^{18}F-FDG-PET as a first-line investigation in FUO [40]. On the other hand, in our study, a definite diagnosis was established in a very low percentage of patients with negative scans, in particular in only one out of the 8 patients with negative scans (12%). A presumptive diagnosis could explain the fever in another case while the remaining 6 cases with negative scans were considered as true negatives given a high enough NPV of 75%. High NPV of ^{18}F-FDG-PET or ^{18}F-FDG-PET/CT in the context of FUO had also been steadily reported in previous studies [12,20,23,24].

Regarding patient characteristics tested for a possible correlation with contributory PET/CT scans, in contrast to previous studies [4,27,32,33,36], we did not find any significant differences in any of the variables tested (age, gender, prior antibiotic administration, presence of lymphadenopathy or splenomegaly, presence of diabetes mellitus, number of advanced diagnostic tests performed before

PET/CT scan, serum glucose level at the time of ^{18}F-FDG administration, or inflammatory blood markers) between patients with contributory and not contributory scans.

In particular, the duration of the fever before the ^{18}F-FDG-PET/CT scan, did not differ significantly in our study between patients with contributory and non-contributory ^{18}F-FDG-PET/CT CT scans, although the duration of the fever was shorter in patients with contributory scans. This finding might be in contrast with those of previous studies [4,27,32,36] reporting a positive correlation between short fever duration and a positive scan.

Many studies investigating the clinical value of ^{18}F-FDG-PET/CT scan in patients with FUO have already reported an elevated CRP as a significant predictor for a positive scan [21,25,32,33,36,46]. In accordance with these studies, an increased CRP level was observed in 22 patients; all of them had a positive ^{18}F-FDG-PET/CT scan, which was true positive in 90.9% of them. In fact, most of these patients (65%) were eventually diagnosed with infection.

In contrast to its established use in oncology, the standardized uptake value (SUV) has not been adequately assessed as a semi-quantitative measure of the severity of inflammation and infection and there is no cutoff value suggested to avoid false positive results [16]. Therefore, its calculation in infection and inflammation is not a standard practice, although it may be helpful in repeated studies for response to treatment. In our study, the SUVmax value was significantly higher in malignancies than in all the other diagnoses. This was not a surprise as SUV values are generally higher in malignant lesions compared to benign lesions. In a large Chinese multi-center retrospective study including 376 patients with FUO and inflammation of unknown origin (IUO) [47], ^{18}F-FDG uptake, estimated by either SUVmax or by visual inspection scoring was significantly higher in malignant compared to non-malignant diseases. Moreover, a significantly higher SUVmax in the contributory scans compared to the non-contributory ones was observed in our study. Our findings on SUVmax, taken together, suggest that a high SUVmax found in the context of FUO investigation may be indicative of underlying malignancy as a cause of FUO and may be also associated with a better diagnostic performance of the ^{18}F-FDG-PET/CT scan.

The main limitation of the present study is its retrospective nature, closely associated with the lack of a uniform diagnostic work-up before ^{18}F-FDG-PET/CT imaging. Both the diagnostic tests performed prior to ^{18}F-FDG-PET/CT scan, and the timing of the scan itself, were conducted at the discretion of the referring physicians, widely varying among the patients. Nevertheless, they all had sufficient basic diagnostic work up, met the criteria to qualify as FUO, and most of them (49/50) had also submitted to multiple (median 3) advanced investigations. Another limitation has been the absence of an indisputable diagnostic gold standard, an obstacle common to most studies involving patients with heterogeneous nosologic background. Finally, the small sample sizes of the particular diagnostic subgroups of the present study represent an additional limitation. In order to minimize selection bias, we included consecutive adult patients with a stereotypic referral indication of FUO. Therefore, the present study aims to be representative of the cases investigated as FUO in a PET/CT academic facility of a general tertiary hospital in Greece in recent years.

Nevertheless, larger, prospective studies with more stringent referral criteria are warranted in order to further elucidate the role and timing of ^{18}F-FDG-PET/CT scan in the investigation of FUO.

5. Conclusions

Our findings show that ^{18}F-FDG-PET/CT scan is highly sensitive in either detecting causes of FUO, undetected by conventional imaging or in correctly targeting suspected lesions for successful diagnostic biopsy. The ^{18}F-FDG-PET/CT contributed substantially to the diagnosis of FUO in a high percentage (70%) of our patients. Our results further support the use of ^{18}F-FDG-PET/CT in the assessment of FUO.

Author Contributions: Conceptualization, S.G.; formal analysis, S.G. and G.A.; investigation, S.G., P.E., I.P., and D.K.; methodology, S.G. and G.A.; resources, V.M., K.A., and C.P.; supervision, G.A.; visualization, S.G.; writing—original draft, S.G. and P.E.; writing—review and editing, S.G., E.-I.M., and G.A. All authors have read and agreed to the published version of the manuscript.

References

1. Petersdorf, R.G.; Beeson, P.B. Fever of unexplained origin: Report on 100 cases. *Medicine* **1961**, *40*, 1–30. [CrossRef] [PubMed]
2. Durack, D.T.; Street, A.C. Fever of unknown origin—Reexamined and redefined. *Curr. Clin. Top. Infect. Dis.* **1991**, *11*, 35–51. [PubMed]
3. Petersdorf, R.G. Fever of unknown origin. An old friend revisited. *Arch. Intern. Med.* **1992**, *152*, 21–22. [CrossRef]
4. de Kleijn, E.M.; Vandenbroucke, J.P.; van der Meer, J.W. Fever of unknown origin (FUO). I. A prospective multicenter study of 167 patients with FUO, using fixed epidemiologic entry criteria. The Netherlands FUO Study Group. *Medicine* **1997**, *76*, 392–400. [CrossRef] [PubMed]
5. Knockaert, D.C.; Vanderschueren, S.; Blockmans, D. Fever of unknown origin in adults: 40 years on. *J. Intern. Med.* **2003**, *253*, 263–275. [CrossRef] [PubMed]
6. Horowitz, H.W. Fever of unknown origin or fever of too many origins? *N. Eng. J. Med.* **2013**, *368*, 197–199. [CrossRef] [PubMed]
7. Mourad, O.; Palda, V.; Detsky, A.S. A comprehensive evidence-based approach to fever of unknown origin. *Arch. Intern. Med.* **2003**, *163*, 545–551. [CrossRef]
8. Mulders-Manders, C.; Simon, A.; Bleeker-Rovers, C. Fever of unknown origin. *Clin. Med.* **2015**, *15*, 280–284. [CrossRef]
9. Kouijzer, I.J.E.; Bleeker-Rovers, C.P.; de Geus-Oei, L.-F. Nuclear medicine imaging of fever of unknown origin. In *Nuclear Medicine in Infectious Diseases*; Signore, A., Glaudemans, A.W.J.M., Eds.; Springer Nature Switzerland AG: Cham, Switzerland, 2020; pp. 199–214. [CrossRef]
10. Meller, J.; Sahlmann, C.O.; Scheel, A.K. 18F-FDG PET and PET/CT in fever of unknown origin. *J. Nucl. Med.* **2007**, *48*, 35–45.
11. Goldsmith, S.J.; Vallabhajosula, S. Clinically proven radiopharmaceuticals for infection imaging: Mechanisms and applications. *Semin. Nucl. Med.* **2009**, *39*, 2–10. [CrossRef]
12. Meller, J.; Altenvoerde, G.; Munzel, U.; Jauho, A.; Behe, M.; Gratz, S.; Luig, H.; Becker, W. Fever of unknown origin: Prospective comparison of [18F]FDG imaging with a double-head coincidence camera and gallium-67 citrate SPET. *Eur. J. Nucl. Med.* **2000**, *27*, 1617–1625. [CrossRef] [PubMed]
13. Blockmans, D.; Knockaert, D.; Maes, A.; De Caestecker, J.; Stroobants, S.; Bobbaers, H.; Mortelmans, L. Clinical value of [(18)F]fluoro-deoxyglucose positron emission tomography for patients with fever of unknown origin. *Clin. Infect. Dis.* **2001**, *32*, 191–196. [CrossRef] [PubMed]
14. Knockaert, D.C.; Mortelmans, L.A.; De Roo, M.C.; Bobbaers, H.J. Clinical value of gallium-67 scintigraphy in evaluation of fever of unknown origin. *Clin. Infect. Dis.* **1994**, *18*, 601–605. [CrossRef] [PubMed]
15. Signore, A.; Jamar, F.; Israel, O.; Buscombe, J.; Martin Comin, J.; Lazzeri, E. Clinical indications, image acquisition and data interpretation for white blood cells and anti-granulocyte monoclonal antibody scintigraphy: An EANM procedural guideline. *Eur. J. Nucl. Med. Mol. Imaging* **2018**, *45*, 1816–1831. [CrossRef]
16. Jamar, F.; Buscombe, J.; Chiti, A.; Christian, P.E.; Delbeke, D.; Donohoe, K.J.; Israel, O.; Martin-Comin, J.; Signore, A. EANM/SNMMI Guideline for 18F-FDG Use in Inflammation and Infection. *J. Nucl. Med.* **2013**, *54*, 647–658. [CrossRef]
17. Tahara, T.; Ichiya, Y.; Kuwabara, Y.; Otsuka, M.; Miyake, Y.; Gunasekera, R.; Masuda, K. High [18F]-fluorodeoxyglucose uptake in abdominal abscesses: A PET study. *J. Comput. Assist. Tomogr.* **1989**, *13*, 829–831. [CrossRef]
18. Glaudemans, A.W.J.M.; de Vries, E.F.J.; Galli, F.; Dierckx, R.A.J.O.; Slart, R.H.J.A.; Signore, A. The use of 18F-FDG-PET/CT for diagnosis and treatment monitoring of inflammatory and infectious diseases. *Clin. Dev. Immunol.* **2013**, *2013*, 623036. [CrossRef]

19. Al-Zaghal, A.; Raynor, W.Y.; Seraj, S.M.; Werner, T.J.; Alavi, A. FDG-PET imaging to detect and characterize underlying causes of fever of unknown origin: An unavoidable path for the foreseeable future. *Eur. J. Nucl. Med. Mol. Imaging* **2019**, *46*, 2–7. [CrossRef]
20. Bleeker-Rovers, C.P.; de Kleijn, E.M.H.A.; Corstens, F.H.M.; van der Meer, J.W.M.; Oyen, W.J.G. Clinical value of FDG PET in patients with fever of unknown origin and patients suspected of focal infection or inflammation. *Eur. J. Nucl. Med. Mol. Imaging* **2004**, *31*, 29–37. [CrossRef]
21. Bleeker-Rovers, C.P.; Vos, F.J.; Mudde, A.H.; Dofferhoff, A.S.M.; de Geus-Oei, L.F.; Rijnders, A.J.; Krabbe, P.F.M.; Corstens, F.H.M.; van der Meer, J.W.M.; Oyen, W.J.G. A prospective multi-centre study of the value of FDG-PET as part of a structured diagnostic protocol in patients with fever of unknown origin. *Eur. J. Nucl. Med. Mol. Imaging* **2007**, *34*, 694–703. [CrossRef]
22. Kjaer, A.; Lebech, A.-M.; Eigtved, A.; Hojgaard, L. Fever of unknown origin: Prospective comparison of diagnostic value of 18F-FDG PET and 111In-granulocyte scintigraphy. *Eur. J. Nucl. Med. Mol. Imaging* **2004**, *31*, 622–626. [CrossRef] [PubMed]
23. Lorenzen, J.; Buchert, R.; Bohuslavizki, K.H. Value of FDG PET in patients with fever of unknown origin. *Nucl. Med. Commun.* **2001**, *22*, 779–783. [CrossRef] [PubMed]
24. Keidar, Z.; Gurman-Balbir, A.; Gaitini, D.; Israel, O. Fever of unknown origin: The role of 18F-FDG PET/CT. *J. Nucl. Med.* **2008**, *49*, 1980–1985. [CrossRef] [PubMed]
25. Balink, H.; Collins, J.; Bruyn, G.A.; Gemmel, F. F-18 FDG PET/CT in the diagnosis of fever of unknown origin. *Clin. Nucl. Med.* **2009**, *34*, 862–868. [CrossRef]
26. Buch-Olsen, K.M.; Andersen, R.V.; Hess, S.; Braad, P.E.; Schifter, S. 18F-FDG-PET/CT in of unknown origin: Clinical value. *Nucl. Med. Commun.* **2014**, *35*, 955–960. [CrossRef]
27. Gafter-Gvili, A.; Raibman, S.; Grossman, A.; Anvi, T.; Paul, M.; Leibovici, L.; Tadmor, B.; Groshar, D.; Bernstine, H. [18F]FDG-PET/CT for the diagnosis of patients with fever of unknown origin. *Q J. Med* **2015**, *108*, 289–298. [CrossRef]
28. Singh, N.; Kumar, R.; Malhotra, A.; Bhalla, A.S.; Kumar, U.; Sood, R. Diagnostic utility of fluorodeoxyglucose positron emission tomography/computed tomography in pyrexia of unknown origin. *Indian J. Nucl. Med.* **2015**, *30*, 204–212. [CrossRef]
29. Efstathiou, S.P.; Pefanis, A.V.; Tsiakou, A.G.; Skeva, I.I.; Tsioulos, D.I.; Achimastos, A.D.; Mountokalakis, T.D. Fever of unknown origin: Discrimination between infectious and non-infectious causes. *Eur. J. Intern. Med.* **2010**, *21*, 137–143. [CrossRef]
30. Spernovasilis, N.; Tsioutis, C.; Markaki, L.; Zafeiri, M.; Soundoulounaki, S.; Gikas, A. Fever of unknown origin caused by infectious diseases in the era of migrant and refugee crisis. *Travel Med. Infect. Dis.* **2020**, *33*, 101425. [CrossRef]
31. Boellaard, R.; Delgado-Bolton, R.; Oyen, W.J.G.; Giammarile, F.; Tatsch, K.; Eschner, W.; Verzijlbergen, F.J.; Barrington, S.F.; Pike, L.C.; Weber, W.A.; et al. FDG PET/CT: EANM procedure guidelines for tumour imaging: Version 2.0. *Eur. J. Nucl. Med. Mol. Imaging* **2015**, *42*, 328–354. [CrossRef]
32. Bleeker-Rovers, C.P.; Vos, F.J.; de Kleijn, E.M.H.A.; Mudde, A.H.; Dofferhoff, T.S.M.; Richter, C.; Smilde, T.J.; Krabbe, P.F.M.; Oyen, W.J.G.; van der Meer, J.W.M. A prospective multicenter study on fever of unknown origin: The yield of a structured diagnostic protocol. *Medicine* **2007**, *86*, 26–38. [CrossRef] [PubMed]
33. Crouzet, J.; Boudousq, V.; Lechiche, C.; Pouget, J.P.; Kotzki, P.O.; Collombier, L.; Lavigne, J.P.; Sotto, A. Place of (18)F-FDG-PET with computed tomography in the diagnostic algorithm of patients with fever of unknown origin. *Eur. J. Clin. Microbiol. Infect. Dis.* **2012**, *31*, 1727–1733. [CrossRef]
34. Kouijzer, I.J.E.; Mulders-Manders, C.M.; Bleeker-Rovers, C.P.; Oyen, W.J.G. Fever of Unknown Origin: The Valueof FDG-PET/CT. *Semin. Nucl. Med.* **2018**, *48*, 100–107. [CrossRef]
35. Jaruskova, M.; Belohlavek, O. Role of FDG-PET and PET/CT in the diagnosis of prolonged febrile states. *Eur. J. Nucl. Med. Mol. Imaging* **2006**, *33*, 913–918. [CrossRef] [PubMed]
36. Wang, W.-X.; Cheng, Z.-T.; Zhu, J.-L.; Xing, M.-Y.; Zheng, C.-F.; Wang, S.-J.; Xie, N.-N.; XianYu, Z.-Q.; Song, J.-X. Combined clinical parameters improve the diagnostic efficacy of 18F-FDG PET/CT in patients with fever of unknown origin (FUO) and inflammation of unknown origin (IUO): A prospective study in China. *Int. J. Infect. Dis.* **2020**, *93*, 77–83. [CrossRef] [PubMed]
37. Kubota, K.; Nakamoto, Y.; Tamaki, N.; Kanegae, K.; Fukuda, H.; Kaneda, T.; Kitajima, K.; Tateishi, U.; Morooka, M.; Ito, K.; et al. FDG-PET for the diagnosis of fever of unknown origin: A Japanese multi-center study. *Ann. Nucl. Med.* **2011**, *25*, 355–364. [CrossRef] [PubMed]

38. Lee, S.-W.; Kim, S.-J.; Seo, Y.; Jeong, S.Y.; Ahn, B.-C.; Lee, J. F-18 FDG PET for assessment of disease activity of large vessel vasculitis: A systematic review and meta-analysis. *J. Nucl. Cardiol.* **2019**, *26*, 59–67. [CrossRef]
39. Kan, Y.; Wang, W.; Liu, J.; Yang, J.; Wang, Z. Contribution of 18F-FDG PET/CT in a case-mix of fever of unknown origin and inflammation of unknown origin: A meta-analysis. *Acta Radiol.* **2018**, *60*, 716–725. [CrossRef]
40. Besson, F.L.; Chaumet-Riffaud, P.; Playe, M.; Noel, N.; Lambotte, O.; Goujard, C.; Prigent, A.; Durand, E. Contribution of 18F-FDG PET in the diagnostic assessment of fever of unknown origin (FUO): A stratification-based meta-analysis. *Eur. J. Nucl. Med. Mol. Imaging* **2016**, *43*, 1887–1895. [CrossRef]
41. Balink, H.; Tan, S.S.; Veeger, N.J.G.M.; Holleman, F.; van Eck-Smit, B.L.F.; Bennink, R.J.; Verberne, H.J. 18F-FDG PET/CT in inflammation of unknown origin: A cost-effectiveness pilot-study. *Eur. J. Nucl. Med. Mol. Imaging* **2015**, *42*, 1408–1413. [CrossRef]
42. Knockaert, D.C.; Dujardin, K.S.; Bobbaers, H.J. Long-term follow-up of patients with undiagnosed fever of unknown origin. *Arch. Intern. Med.* **1996**, *156*, 618–620. [CrossRef] [PubMed]
43. Takeuchi, M.; Nihashi, T.; Gafter-Gvili, A.; García-Gómez, J.M.; Andres, E.; Blockmans, D.; Iwata, M.; Terasawa, T. Association of 18F-FDG PET or PET/CT results with spontaneous remission in classic fever of unknown origin: A systematic review and meta-analysis. *Medicine* **2018**, *97*, e12909. [CrossRef] [PubMed]
44. Suhrcke, M.; Stuckler, D.; Suk, J.E.; Desai, M.; Senek, M.; McKee, M.; Tsolova, S.; Basu, S.; Abubakar, I.; Hunter, P.; et al. Impact of Economic Crises on Communicable Disease Transmission and Control: A Systematic Review of the Evidence. *PLoS ONE* **2011**, *6*, e20724. [CrossRef]
45. Takeuchi, M.; Dahabreh, I.J.; Nihashi, T.; Iwata, M.; Varghese, G.M.; Terasawa, T. Nuclear Imaging for Classic Fever of Unknown Origin: Meta-Analysis. *J. Nucl. Med.* **2016**, *57*, 1913–1919. [CrossRef] [PubMed]
46. Balink, H.; Veeger, N.J.G.M.; Bennink, R.J.; Slart, R.H.J.A.; Holleman, F.; van Eck-Smit, B.L.F.; Verberne, H.J. The predictive value of C-reactive protein and erythrocyte sedimentation rate for 18F-FDG PET/CT outcome in patients with fever and inflammation of unknown origin. *Nucl. Med. Commun.* **2015**, *36*, 604–609. [CrossRef]
47. Wang, Q.; Li, Y.-M.; Li, Y.; Hua, F.-C.; Wang, Q.-S.; Zhang, X.-L.; Cheng, C.; Wu, H.; Yao, Z.-M.; Zhang, W.-F.; et al. 18F-FDGPET/CT in fever of unknown origin and inflammation of unknown origin: A Chinese multi-center study. *Eur. J. Nucl. Med. Mol. Imaging* **2019**, *46*, 159–165. [CrossRef]

7

Imaging Modalities for the Diagnosis of Vascular Graft Infections: A Consensus Paper amongst Different Specialists

Chiara Lauri [1,2,*], Roberto Iezzi [3], Michele Rossi [4], Giovanni Tinelli [5], Simona Sica [5], Alberto Signore [1,2], Alessandro Posa [3], Alessandro Tanzilli [3], Chiara Panzera [6], Maurizio Taurino [6], Paola Anna Erba [2,7] and Yamume Tshomba [5]

1. Nuclear Medicine Unit, Department of Medical-Surgical Sciences and of Translational Medicine, "Sapienza" University of Rome, 00161 Rome, Italy; alberto.signore@uniroma1.it
2. Department of Nuclear Medicine and Molecular Imaging, University of Groningen, University Medical Center Groningen, 9700 Groningen, The Netherlands; paola.erba@unipi.it
3. Radiology Unit, Fondazione Policlinico Universitario A. Gemelli IRCCS, Roma-Università Cattolica del Sacro Cuore, 00168 Rome, Italy; roberto.iezzi@unicatt.it (R.I.); alessandro.posa@gmail.com (A.P.); alessandrotanzilli93@gmail.com (A.T.)
4. Radiology Unit, Department of Medical-Surgical Sciences and Translational Medicine, Faculty of Medicine and Psychology, Sant'Andrea Hospital, "Sapienza" University of Rome, 00161 Rome, Italy; michele.rossi@uniroma1.it
5. Unit of Vascular Surgery, Fondazione Policlinico Universitario Gemelli IRCCS, Roma-Università Cattolica del Sacro Cuore, 00168 Rome, Italy; giovanni.tinelli@policlinicogemelli.it (G.T.); simonasica1@gmail.com (S.S.); yamume.tshomba@policlinicogemelli.it (Y.T.)
6. Vascular Surgery Unit, Department of Clinical and Molecular Medicine, Faculty of Medicine and Psychology, Sant'Andrea Hospital, "Sapienza" University of Rome, 00161 Rome, Italy; chiara.panzera1@gmail.com (C.P.); maurizio.taurino@uniroma1.it (M.T.)
7. Nuclear Medicine, Department of Translational Research and New Technology in Medicine, University of Pisa, 56123 Pisa, Italy

* Correspondence: chialau84@hotmail.it

Abstract: Vascular graft infection (VGI) is a rare but severe complication of vascular surgery that is associated with a bad prognosis and high mortality rate. An accurate and prompt identification of the infection and its extent is crucial for the correct management of the patient. However, standardized diagnostic algorithms and a univocal consensus on the best strategy to reach a diagnosis still do not exist. This review aims to summarize different radiological and Nuclear Medicine (NM) modalities commonly adopted for the imaging of VGI. Moreover, we attempt to provide evidence-based answers to several practical questions raised by clinicians and surgeons when they approach imaging in order to plan the most appropriate radiological or NM examination for their patients.

Keywords: infection; vascular graft; multimodality imaging; WBC scintigraphy; FDG-PET/CT; angio-CT; personalized medicine

---

1. Introduction

Vascular graft infection (VGI) is a rare condition, representing one of the most life-threatening complications in vascular surgery. The incidence ranges from 1.5% to 6%, mainly depending on the anatomic location of the graft, and clinical characteristics are highly variable and are related to the site of the implant, causative pathogen, and time after surgery [1].

Location categories for VGI include extracavitary (primarily in the groin—80%, or lower extremities—20%) and intracavitary (primarily in the abdomen—70%, or less commonly within the thorax—30%) sites. Extracavitary infections usually occur when there is a wound infection in the groin or intraoperative contamination, while intracavitary infections are due to intraoperative contamination, mechanical erosion in the bowel, genitourinary system or skin seeding by bacteremia, or involvement in contiguous infectious processes such as spondylodiscitis.

According to the time of onset after surgery, VGIs may be classified in "early" infections if they occur within 4 months after implantation and they usually show systemic signs and symptoms of infection (as fever); or "late" infections when they occur after 4 months from surgery and, in this case, signs and symptoms could be absent [2,3].

Patient related risk factors are diabetes, malnutrition, chronic renal impairment/failure, liver disease/failure or cirrhosis, previous radiotherapy or chemotherapy, malignancy, autoimmune disorders, long term corticosteroid use [4].

Diagnosis of VGI is complex, being related to clinical presentation, laboratory studies and imaging, so quick and correct diagnosis of VGIs can be challenging.

Standard laboratory tests are usually non-specific: typical findings include leukocytosis (left shift) and a high erythrocyte sedimentation rate. Cultures from wounds or perigraft fluid can be collected in VGI-suspected patients in order to diagnose and guide antibiotic therapy [5].

The Management of Aortic Graft Infection Collaboration (MAGIC) depicted major and minor criteria for VGI diagnosis, based on clinical/surgical, laboratory and radiological data: aortic graft infection (AGI) can be suspected when there is one major criterion, or two minor criteria from two different categories, whereas diagnosis is certain if there is one major criterion plus any other criterion (both minor or major) from another category [6].

A prompt identification of the infection and its extent is crucial for prognostication of the patient and for planning the correct treatment. Although there is general agreement that the diagnosis of VGI derives from a combination of clinical, radiological, nuclear medicine (NM) and laboratory findings, an univocal consensus on the diagnostic criteria for imaging modalities still does not exist.

This review aims to provide an updated overview of radiologic and NM strategies for the diagnosis of VGI.

2. Surgical Management of VGI: How Can Imaging Be Helpful?

The management of VGI is extremely complex, and the centralization of the patient is crucial. The treatment needs to be evaluated on a case-by-case basis. Antimicrobial therapy is an integral part of VGI treatment. In the acute phase, intensive antimicrobial therapy with (broad range) antibiotics, directed against the most likely infecting organisms, is indicated to control infection and sepsis [7]. However, when possible, surgical therapy must be attempted. Recently, the European Society for Vascular Surgery (ESVS) 2020 Clinical Practice Guidelines on the Management of Vascular Graft and Endograft Infections recommended the complete excision of all graft material and infected tissue for fit patients (Class I, Level B) [7]. Historically, the gold standard surgical approach was the total removal of the infected graft, extensive debridement of the infected area, and extra-anatomic reconstruction (EAR) outside the infected field. However, this approach has higher 30-day mortality (26.7%) and lowest one-year survival (54.3%) rates compared to in situ repair (ISR) [8]. Indeed, nowadays, most surgeons prefer the second approach. Like the original gold standard, ISR includes complete removal of the graft, aggressive debridement of the infected tissues, but, unlike EAR, ISR also provides arterial reconstruction with suturing in the healthy, non-infected aorta (Figure 1). A video about graft removal is available in supplementay materials (Video S1).

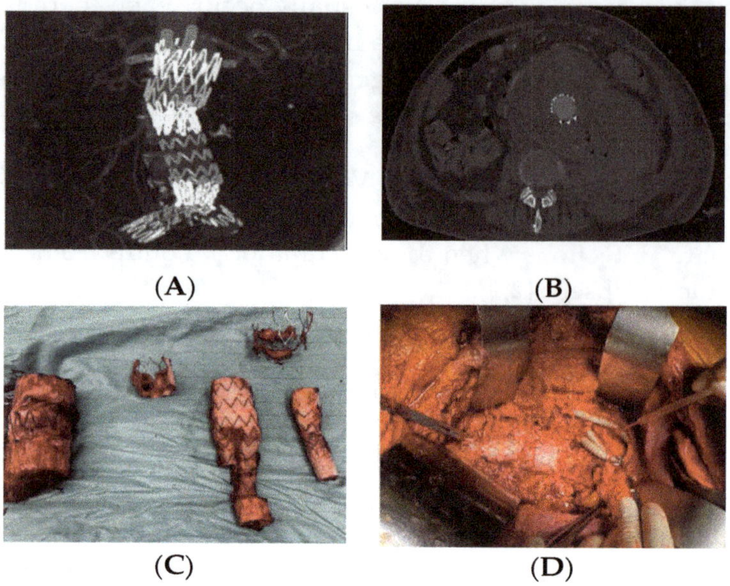

Figure 1. (**A**,**B**) Pre-operative computed tomography (CT) scan showing graft disruption, perigraft fluid and air in a 72-year-old man with an infected abdominal endograft; (**C**) explanted graft after in situ repair (ISR) with visceral debranching: aorto-mesenteric bypass, right renal artery Y graft, aorto-left renal artery bypass. The reconstruction has been completed with lower extremity revascularization with extra-anatomic reconstruction (EAR) axillo-bifemoral; (**D**) final result after EAR.

Different graft materials may be used for reconstruction, including autologous veins, cryopreserved allografts, rifampicin-bonded or silver-coated synthetic grafts, and xenogenous grafts, and they seem to show similar rates of infection (veins 2%, cryopreserved allografts 9%, rifampicin bonded or silver coated prosthesis 11%) [9].

Imaging plays a key role in confirming the diagnosis of VGI and guiding the treatment. In particular, it is useful in investigating the position and the structural integrity of the graft or endograft (Figure 1), it may confirm or exclude peri-graft inflammation, and delineate its extent; it may reveal the presence or absence of perigraft fluid or gas, anastomotic leakage or pseudoaneurysms, the grade of graft involvement and the presence of graft-enteric erosion/a fistula. Moreover, imaging is fundamental to plan a strategy for revascularization, and for imaging-guided perigraft fluid aspiration.

3. Radiological Modalities for Imaging VGI

3.1. *Ultrasonography (US)*

Ultrasonography (US) is the first-choice imaging modality for assessing vascular diseases due to its well-known advantages, represented by repeatability, availability, cost-effectiveness, safety profile; moreover, it is non-invasive and easy to perform. However, it is operator dependent, and is hampered by patient habitus (obesity, intestinal gas or ascites) and the patient's level of collaboration. In addition, it doesn't offer a detailed anatomic roadmap like other imaging modalities. US can be useful in the evaluation of perigraft fluid collections or abscesses, and can distinguish a fluid collection from a hematoma or a pseudoaneurysm. It can also be used for US-guided aspiration [10]. Contrast-Enhanced Ultrasonography (CEUS) is not routinely used for the diagnosis of VGI, due to its unproven ability to improve diagnostic performance [11].

3.2. *Computed Tomography (CT)—CT–Angiography (CTA)*

Computed tomography (CT) is the first-choice and gold-standard imaging modality, particularly in intracavitary VGI. A recent meta-analysis showed that CT–angiography (CTA) has an overall pooled sensitivity of 67% and an overall pooled specificity of 63% [12]. In particular, previous studies depicted a difference in the diagnostic performance of CTA between low- and high-grade VGI.

CT in low-grade infections has high false negative rates, resulting in a sensitivity of only 55.5% [6], since it can be very difficult to differentiate early/low-grade VGI findings from para-physiological ones (e.g., the postoperative local residues as small fluid collection or gas). It is not clearly defined at what time after surgery the presence of gas or fluid can be considered to represent suspected/positive VGI (Figure 2). On the other hand, CT has better accuracy in advanced or complex VGI (e.g., aorto-enteric erosion/fistula), with a sensitivity and specificity of about 85–94% [6,12].

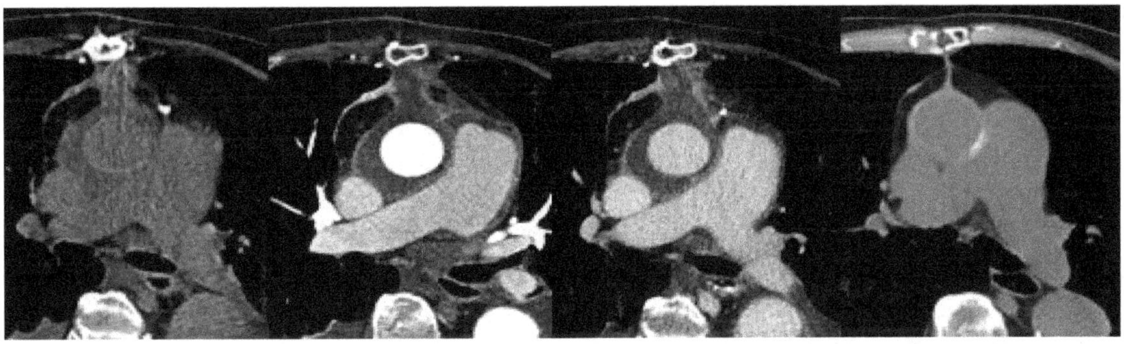

Figure 2. Post-surgical ascending aortic repair (Bentall procedure) 1-month CT scan. From left panel to right: unenhanced CT, arterial phase and late phase CT images show aortic graft patency with perigraft fluid and stranding. These findings can be considered a typical post-operative appearance as confirmed by their disappearance in the 3-month unenhanced CT image (right image).

However, radiological follow-up could be mandatory for increasing diagnostic accuracy in VGI. In detail, on serial CTA follow-up, a suspect can be posed if there are new findings, or the perigraft fluid/gas collection increases over time or persists beyond three months from the surgery, or there is a rapid dimensional increase in the aneurysm sac [13–15].

MAGIC minor criteria alone are not sufficient for the diagnosis of VGI, due to their subjective nature; these minor criteria include perigraft soft tissue alterations, like fat stranding (pathological increase in fat tissue attenuation) and phlegmon (diffuse inflammation of the soft or connective tissue) [16,17]. Infection spreading to adjacent structures can cause hydronephrosis, psoas abscess, focal bowel thickening, and discitis/osteomyelitis, but the presence of a major criterion is required to confirm the VGI [18,19] (Figure 3).

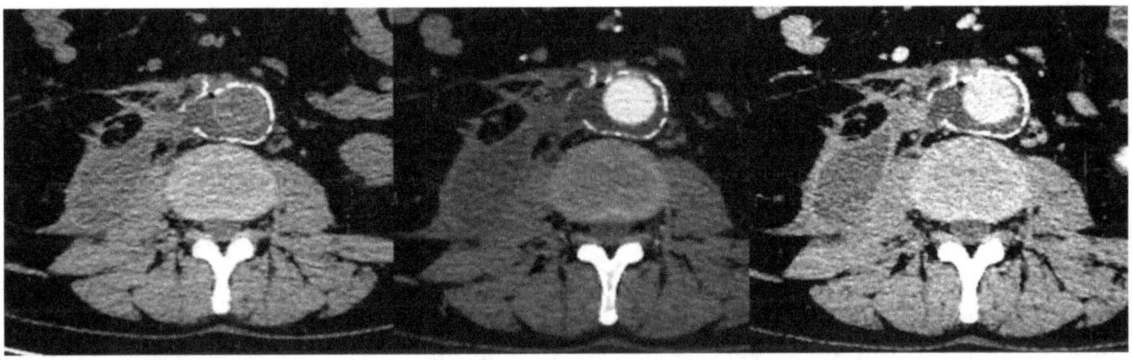

Figure 3. Open surgical repair of abdominal aortic aneurysm (65-year-old male). From left panel to right: unenhanced and enhanced (arterial phase and late phase) CT scans 4 months after treatment show aortic graft patency with perigraft fluid and air, enhancing the soft tissue around the graft and abscess near the right psoas muscle. These findings are consistent with perigraft infection, as also confirmed by fluid aspiration.

Pseudoaneurysm formation is a recognized finding in VGI, but it may also be present in a non-infective setting, particularly following the focal dehiscence of a vascular suture. Septic emboli from the infected graft can be a threatening occurrence, leading to vascular occlusions and the distal spread of the infection [20].

VGI must not be confused with the primary vasculitis of large vessels, even though these two entities are unlikely to be similar, the latter not usually being localized around the graft and being associated with wall-thickening [21]. Chapman et al. reported the case of a VGI mimicking hypertrophic osteoarthropathy [22]. Imaging alone, however, can be deceitful, due to the presence of some diagnostic pitfall conditions (mostly iatrogenic) that can mimic VGI. In more detail, in patients who underwent periaortic fluid aspiration or in patients with an aortic endograft and a recent type-II endoleak embolization with the direct puncture of the aneurysmatic sac, gas-like images could represent diagnostic pitfalls, mimicking graft infections. For these reasons, an adequate clinical history knowledge, including all procedures performed, is mandatory to avoid false-positive diagnosis. Performing nonenhanced imaging is particularly important in this postoperative setting, as surgical or embolic devices (glue, coils, or other high-attenuation materials) may be most conspicuous at this phase. Furthermore, some bioabsorbable hemostatic agents such as gelatin or cellulose may also appear as an ill-defined, gas-filled heterogeneous mass, sometimes with rim enhancement, potentially mimicking abscesses, hematomas, or retained foreign bodies (Figure 4). In selected cases, CT can be also used to guide the percutaneous aspiration of perigraft fluid collections.

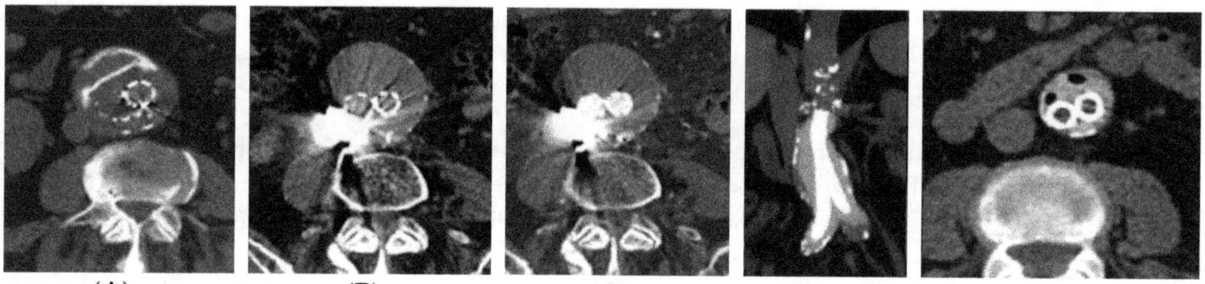

(A) (B) (C) (D) (E)

Figure 4. In patients with aortic stent grafts who underwent embolization for type II endoleak, diagnostic pitfalls need to be considered and known. They could be represented by hyperdense structures/materials, represented by glue/liquid embolics or coils (**A–C**), or also by intra-sac gas, in the case of percutaneous puncture/embolization, or new endografts with polymer-filled endobags (**D–E**).

3.3. Magnetic Resonance Imaging (MRI)

Magnetic resonance imaging (MRI) has not been evaluated as extensively as CT for the diagnosis of VGI, but has demonstrated good positive and negative predictive values (95% and 80% respectively) [11]. MRI has some advantages compared to CT examination, due to the absence of radiation exposure, the use of noniodinated contrast media, and the possible application of advanced imaging techniques (e.g., functional and dynamic imaging). However, it has some disadvantages like a longer examination time, less availability, and higher costs. Moreover, a high magnetic field strength is required with an increase in ferromagnetic artifacts due to metallic stents. When considering safety issues, it is well known that risk of incompatibility is quite low, as MR-compatible materials have been increasingly used since the mid-1990s. Most vascular grafts are mainly made of stainless steel or nitinol, are non-ferromagnetic, or contain variable amounts of platinum, cobalt alloy, gold, tantalum, making them weakly ferromagnetic. Furthermore, implantation against the vessel wall provides sufficient stability, reducing the risk of dislodgement. Data from the literature allow us to conclude that MRI can be performed in patients after vascular graft implantation without significant risk at any time, but the risk of incompatibility must be well known and properly checked. Claustrophobia, pacemakers or patients not compliant with sedation (<5%) are contraindications to MRI. MRI, with its high contrast resolution, can easily demonstrate small perigraft fluid collections but, like CT, it is not able to distinguish the para-physiological perigraft fluid in the early postoperative period from an infected perigraft fluid collection. MRI imaging does not allow for the differentiation of the signal void produced by calcifications of the aortic wall from that of air bubbles in the perigraft infection [23]. In the case of graft infection, MRI can show eccentric fluid collection with low to medium signal intensity on T1-weighted images and high signal intensity on T2-weighted ones.

MRI is able to better distinguish perigraft fluid from inflammation and fibrosis than CT [18]. The use of contrast-enhanced T1-weighted fat acquisitions may also help in detecting the surroundings of tissue edema and inflammatory alteration that are indicative but non specific findings of infection.

3.4. Digital Subtraction Angiography (DSA)

DSA has a role for revascularization in selected patients (e.g., in case of distal limb or splanchnic ischemia, occlusive disease or graft thrombosis), and to better define inflow and outflow targets for the surgical bypass. It is mandatory for interventional procedures, whereas it has almost no use in VGI diagnosis.

4. Nuclear Medicine Imaging of VGI

Functional hybrid imaging offers the possibility to study a process from a molecular point of view and it is able to identify pathophysiological signs that can occur before morphological changes become detectable.

Different radiopharmaceuticals and modalities are available for imaging infection and inflammation. In particular, in suspected VGI, two procedures are currently applied, radiolabeled white blood cells (WBC) scintigraphy and ^{18}F-fluorodeoxyglucose positron emission tomography/computed tomography ([^{18}F]FDG PET/CT).

4.1. Gamma-Camera Imaging for VGI

The role of radiolabeled WBC scintigraphy in the field of infection is nowadays well consolidated. The possibility to specifically investigate granulocyte migration in tissues represents a surrogate marker of infections [24]. It provides an accurate differentiation between infection and sterile inflammation. This imaging modality is, therefore, considered the gold standard for the diagnosis of several infective diseases [25].

Granulocytes can be easily radiolabeled with both ^{111}In and ^{99m}Tc, with the latter being the preferred isotope for both physical characteristics and dosimetric issues.

The European Society of Nuclear Medicine (EANM) provided several guidelines to address the standardization of WBC labeling, acquisition protocols and interpretation criteria [25–27]. In particular, for the assessment of VGI, a dynamic scan within the first 5 min is suggested in order to visualize the vascular tree and aneurisms. Static images acquired, with times corrected for the isotope decay, at 30 min–1 h (early images) post injection (p.i.) and delayed images (2–4 h p.i.), might be sufficient to provide the diagnosis. However, late images (20–24 h p.i.) are strongly recommended in equivocal cases, low grade/chronic infection and follow-up studies [25,28] when positive single-photon emission computed tomography (SPECT)/CT images are mandatory for the exact localization of the infection (soft tissue only, graft, or both) and for the evaluation of its extent (7) (Figure 5), since their use has been demonstrated as increasing the diagnostic accuracy [25,28].

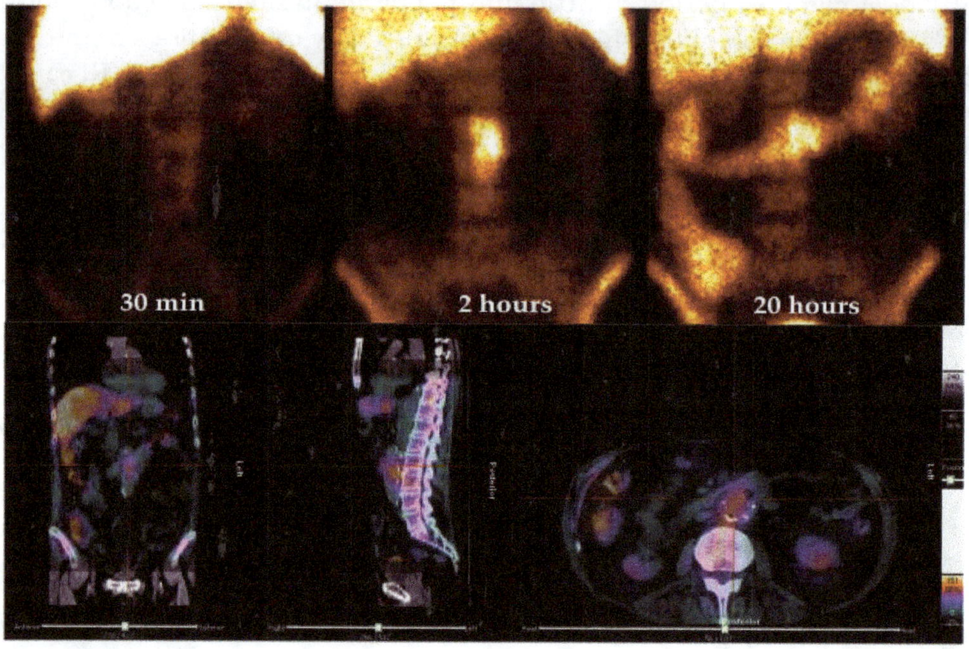

Figure 5. An example of ^{99m}Tc-labeled white blood cell (WBC) scintigraphy acquired with times corrected for isotope decay at 30 min, 2 and 20 h p.i. in a patient with suspected abdominal vascular graft infection (VGI). Planar anterior images show an increased uptake in abdominal region that was consistent for an infection (upper panel). Dingle-photon emission computed tomography (SPECT)/CT images (bottom) acquired 2 h p.i. allowed the correct localization of the uptake in the inner of abdominal aortic graft.

A whole-body scan at 2–4 h p.i. is strongly suggested in order to detect any additional sites of infection or septic embolism.

Once correctly acquired and displayed, the correct interpretation is derived from the comparison of uptake extent and intensity between late and delayed images. By following these recommendations, we can easily differentiate between an infection from sterile inflammation, which is an infection characterized by an increased uptake over time in terms of extent and/or intensity, and sterile inflammation characterized by a decreased or stable uptake over time [25,29,30].

Data from the literature are inconsistent, with different accuracies being reported, depending on the population sample and the different method and gold standard used. However, if we take into account the few existing meta-analyses and systematic reviews on this imaging modality, the authors all conclude that radiolabeled WBC is a powerful tool in diagnosing a VGI [12,31] (Table 1).

In particular, comparing ^{99m}Tc-WBC scintigraphy with ^{111}In-WBC scintigraphy and CT, Annovazzi et al. [31] reported higher sensitivity (97.7% vs. 84.1% vs. 75%), specificity (88.6% vs. 79.4% vs. 56.6%), diagnostic accuracy (94.6% vs. 81.5% vs. 78.6), positive predictive value (PPV) (90% vs. 85% vs. 100%) and negative predictive value (NPV) (100% vs. 93.8% vs. 82%) for the ^{99m}Tc-WBC scan. More recently, in another meta-analysis, WBC SPECT/CT demonstrated the highest diagnostic performance in VGI diagnosis [12] (Table 1). Indeed, the added value of SPECT/CT over planar images has been clearly shown by several authors. In the study performed by Bar-Shalom and co-workers, ^{111}In-WBC SPECT/CT was able to improve diagnosis, better localize and evaluate the extent of the disease in 67% of patients with suspected VGI [32]. These results were further confirmed in the retrospective study performed by Khaja and colleagues on 20 patients with suspected VGI where the use of SPECT/CT resulted in improved sensitivity, diagnostic accuracy and NPV compared to the planar images and standalone CT [33].

Similarly, in 55 patients with suspected late and low-grade VGI, ^{99m}Tc-WBC SPECT/CT showed a specificity and sensitivity of 100%, far superior to planar images, SPECT stand alone and ultrasounds

(US), reducing false positive results in 37% of patients [28]. The estimated sensitivity of WBCS (without SPECT/CT) in diagnosing VGEI in the most recent meta-analysis was 0.90 (95% CI 0.85 to 0.94) with a specificity of 0.88 (95% CI 0.81 to 0.94) [12]. When WBCS was combined with SPECT/CT, the sensitivity increased to 0.99 (95% CI 0.92 to 1.00), with a specificity of 0.82 (95% CI 0.57 to 0.96) (Table 1).

Several factors, unfortunately, limit the routine use of radiolabeled WBC in clinical practice—the labeling procedure is time consuming and it requires the manipulation of potentially infected blood. For these reasons, the labeling procedure must be performed by trained personnel in dedicated environments (with isolators, laboratories equipped with hoods and centrifuges). Moreover, multiple timepoints are necessary for the acquisitions, thus requiring the patient to come back to the NM Department the day after in order to conclude the exam. Because of the aforementioned limitations and limited availability, the recent European Society for Vascular Surgery 2020 Clinical Practice Guidelines on the Management of Vascular Graft and Endograft Infections does not recommended WBCs as the first imaging modality in diagnosing VGI [7].

Scintigraphy with radiolabeled anti-granulocyte antibodies (AGA) has been investigated in alternative WBC scintigraphy.

In VGI, some series reported a sensitivity of 92–100% and a specificity ranging from 62.5% to 100% [34–37]. The in vivo labeling procedure of a murine AGA is easier and quicker compared to the in vitro labeling of WBC. However, the main drawback of this approach is related to the possibility to induce human anti-murine antibodies (HAMA) after the administration of these molecules, thus limiting their use in follow-up. Moreover, the data available in the literature on the use of radiolabeled AGA in the assessment of VGI are based only on small series without standardized protocols of acquisition and interpretation. Therefore, there is no convincing evidence supporting their superiority over autologous leucocytes.

Table 1. Summary of the most relevant reviews and meta-analysis on Nuclear Medicine (NM) modalities for imaging.

Paper	Imaging Modality	Sensitivity	Specificity
Annovazzi 2005 [31]	^{99m}Tc-WBC ^{111}In-WBC CT	97.7% 84.1% 75%	88.6% 79.4% 56.6%
Reinders Folmer 2018 [12]	[^{18}F]FDG PET [^{18}F]FDG PET/CT WBC (planar) WBC SPECT/CT CTA	94% 95% 90% 99% 67%	70% 80% 88% 82% 63%
Khaja 2013 [33]	^{99m}Tc-WBC ^{111}In-WBC [^{18}F]FDG PET/CT	83.7% 83% 93.7%	97.5% 87% 75%
Kim 2019 [38]	[^{18}F]FDG PET/CT	96%	74%
Rojoa 2019 [39]	[^{18}F]FDG PET/CT: 1. graded uptake 2. focal uptake 3. SUVmax 4. T/B ratio 5. DTPI	 89% 93% 98% 57% 100%	 61% 78% 80% 76% 88%

White blood cell (WBC); computed tomography (CT); ^{18}F-fluorodeoxyglucose positron emission tomography/computed tomography ([^{18}F]FDG PET/CT); single-photon emission computed tomography (SPECT); computed tomography–angiography (CTA).

4.2. [^{18}F]FDG PET/CT Imaging of VGI

In the last decades, [^{18}F]FDG PET/CT has gained an important role in the field of infection and inflammation, as summarized in the guidelines published in 2013 by EANM and the Society of Nuclear Medicine and Molecular Imaging (SNMMI) [40].

[^{18}F]FDG PET/CT offers several advantages over labeled WBC: the presence of a CT co-registration that does not require any change in the patient's position and which allows a more precise localization of the uptake and higher quality images than gamma camera isotopes. Moreover, the length of scan is shorter (2–3 h vs. 20 h) and it provides a whole-body study without the need for blood manipulation.

Despite a high sensitivity, a major drawback of [^{18}F]FDG is its relatively low specificity. False positive results may be observed in post-surgical flogosis, especially within the first 6–8 weeks, and in foreign-body reaction induced by the synthetic materials of the graft, characterized by a low-grade inflammation [41,42]. Therefore, to limit the rate of false positive results, specific interpretation criteria need to be applied.

Table 1 summarizes the results of the most recent meta-analyses evaluating [^{18}F]FDG PET/CT in the work-up of VGI [12,38,39]. The most recent one [38] reports a pooled sensitivity of 96%, ranging between 81% [43] and 100% [42,44–46], and a pooled specificity of 74%, ranging between 29% [47] and 92% [48].

Several interpretation criteria for [^{18}F]FDG PET/CT have been proposed and they mainly consider the pattern of uptake, the tissue to background (T/B) ratio, the visual grading scale and the calculated maximum standardized uptake value (SUVmax). The [^{18}F]FDG pattern can be classified as "focal" or "diffuse", "homogeneous" or "inhomogeneous", "mild" or "intense".

Spacek et al., studying 96 low-grade prostheses, defined focal uptake as the most valid diagnostic parameter, leading to a very high specificity (92.7%) and PPV (93.5%). Conversely, mild inhomogeneous uptake must be interpreted with caution, being consistent with both low-grade infection and sterile inflammation around the foreign body. The co-registered CT assessment for the definition of graft borders (irregular vs. smooth) is also of paramount importance in this manuscript: the presence of irregular borders associated to focal [^{18}F] FDG uptake is highly predictive of VGI [41].

Focal uptake as major sign of VGI, compared to the diffuse homogeneous uptake found in up to 92% of non-infected grafts and most frequently observed in Dacron prostheses (Figure 6), has also been reported by Keidar et al. [49].

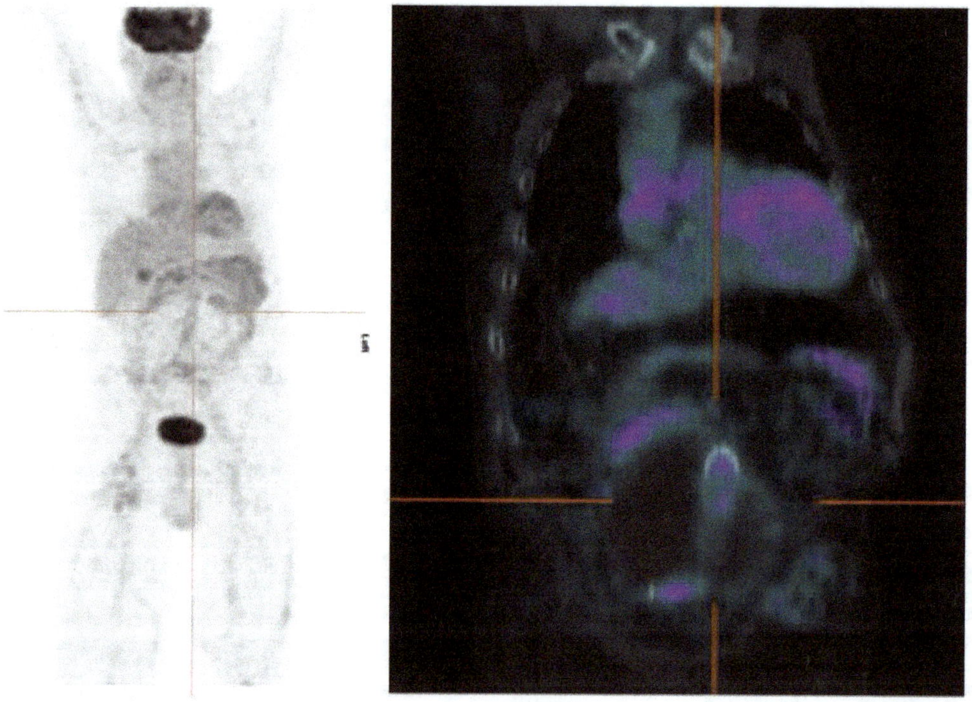

Figure 6. An example of negative [^{18}F]FDG PET/CT scan in a patient with suspected infection of abdominal graft implanted 2 years before for the exclusion of a large aneurysm. The images show mild (SUVmax 2.4), homogeneous uptake along the whole tract of the prosthesis without any focal uptake.

A four- or five-point visual scale was also proposed to diagnose VGI, with the presence of grades 3 or 4 being indicative of infection [50,51]. In grade 0, [^{18}F]FDG uptake is similar to background uptake; in grade 1, [^{18}F]FDG uptake is similar to that which occurs in the inactive muscles and fat (low [^{18}F]FDG uptake); in grade 2, [^{18}F]FDG uptake is higher than in inactive muscles (moderate [^{18}F]FDG uptake); in grade 3, [^{18}F]FDG uptake is less than the physiologic uptake shown by the bladder (strong [^{18}F]FDG uptake) and in grade 4, [^{18}F]FDG uptake is comparable to physiologic urinary uptake (very strong [^{18}F]FDG uptake).

The contributions of SUVmax and T/B ratio in the qualitative evaluation have also been examined.

Several thresholds of SUVmax have been proposed, but they are not universally recognized. Some authors suggested a SUVmax > 8 in the perigraft area as cut-off value for distinguishing infected graft from non-infected graft [42,50]. The use of this cut-off was associated with 100% of specificity and 80% of sensitivity. However, since it is well known that SUVmax evaluation is affected by several technical factors that may differ among the centers, T/B ratio is maybe a more reproducible parameter. Saleem et al. proposed a cut-off of 5.9 ± 2.7 for infections (vs. 4.1 ± 2.1 in non-infected grafts) [50], but, of course, these findings need to be further confirmed by larger studies and they need to be validated and standardized. At the moment, SUV and TBR analyses seem to have limited value in the assessment of VGI.

In a recently published meta-analysis exploring the accuracy and the efficacy of [^{18}F]FDG PET/CT, the authors analyzed five different methods of interpretation of a PET/CT scan [39]. The sensitivity and specificity of qualitative assessment, using a five-point visual scale, were 89% and 61%, respectively; for focal uptake, they were 93% and 78%, respectively; for SUVmax, they were 98% and 80%; 57% and 76% for T/B ratio, respectively, and 100% and 88% for dual timepoint imaging (DTPI). However, only one paper investigated the added value of DTPI with additional delayed acquisitions and calculation of percentages of SUVmax change between initial and delayed images [44]. Despite the limitations of SUVmax, from this meta-analysis, it emerges that focal uptake and SUVmax are the most reliable tools for the interpretation of a PET/CT scan. Nevertheless, larger prospective and retrospective studies are needed to support these findings.

5. Consensus Statements from Round Table of 3rd European Congress of Infection and Inflammation

During the 3rd European Congress of Infection and Inflammation organized in Rome in December 2019, several specialists evaluating patients with VGI gave lectures on this topic from different points of view. Final discussions and a round table were carried out by the representatives of each specialty (C.L., R.I., M.R., G.T., A.S., M.T., P.A.E., Y.T), who also contributed to the present review. Although not officially endorsed by the respective European Societies of NM (EANM), Radiology (ESR) and Vascular Surgery (ESVS), here we summarize several statements that emerged from the round table of the Congress and that reached an oral consensus among these different specialists, aiming to provide evidence-based answers to the most frequent clinical questions.

5.1. In Case of a Partial Resection Graft for a Fragile Patient Unfit for a Total VGI Explantation, the Exact Infection Graft Location Could Be Useful for the Surgical Strategy. Which Radiological Integration Is More Precise in This Diagnosis?

Once a WBC scintigraphy or a [^{18}F]FDG PET/CT scan clearly demonstrates that infection is not extended to the entire graft and perigraft tissues, a partial explanation is taken into consideration by surgeons if invasiveness limitation is advisable. What the surgeons need to know is the graft patency, the exact location of perigraft tissue alterations, the extent of fluid collection, and whether it would be possible to perform ligations or surgical bypass. All of this information is easily and can currently be obtained with CTA. There is almost no role for MRI. Only in selected cases could it be necessary to resort to DSA and endovascular interventions like embolization or stent grafting before surgery.

5.2. Does CTA Still Play a Role in Diagnosing Vascular Graft Infections or Should It Be Considered Obsolete, Replaced by NM Imaging?

CTA is requested by clinicians as the first-choice imaging modality in cases of suspected VGI. The main role is still to be considered for excluding this eventuality. A lack of significant peri-prosthetic fluid collections or bubbles (and also other information) could be collected, such as structural graft alterations, angulations or thrombosis. In these cases, a "wait and see" strategy can be adopted. In the case of persistent symptoms and more founded suspicions, a second CTA is still indicated to ascertain the evolution of the previous findings. In the case of endografts, CTA is the best imaging modality for demonstrating ruptures, disconnections, displacements and endoleaks, which are conditions often associated with infections. Last but not least, fluid collection aspiration for biological tests and cultures is almost exclusively performed by interventional radiologists under CT guidance. Therefore, CTA still plays a critical role in the diagnosis of VGI as the first diagnostic imaging modality [7]. NM modalities are complementary and may be useful to map the extent of the infection. Therefore, for patients with a clinical suspicion of vascular graft/endograft infection and with non-convincing findings on CTA, the use of WBC scintigraphy or [^{18}F]FDG PET/CT is recommended as an additional imaging modality to improve diagnostic accuracy.

5.3. Does Antibiotic Therapy Affect NM Exams Accuracy? Should Antibiotic Therapy Be Stopped before NM Exams? If Yes, How Long before?

The influence of ongoing antimicrobial treatment on the different NM modalities and, in particular, on radiolabeled WBC scintigraphy, is still a matter of debate. Although the use of antibiotics is frequently reported in several papers, the duration of treatment is not always mentioned and it is not linked to the outcome of WBC scintigraphy or [^{18}F]FDG PET/CT. Moreover, data regarding VGI do not exist, therefore a definitive conclusion on this topic cannot be provided.

From other clinical contexts mainly focused on musculoskeletal infections, some authors suggested that antibiotic treatment does not affect the accuracy of radiolabeled WBC; however, it is well known that antimicrobial treatment may reduce the chemiotaxis of leukocytes, thus resulting in lower migration into infected sites. Therefore, when antimicrobial therapy is ongoing, it should be considered during the scan interpretation, whereas, if the patient is at the end of antibiotic treatment, it is a common practice in the NM department to delay the execution of WBC scintigraphy after 2 weeks of therapy withdrawal.

Although antimicrobial treatment is known to decrease the intensity of [^{18}F]FDG uptake, in a recently published retrospective study aiming to assess whether [^{18}F]FDG PET/CT performance for the diagnosis of infective processes could be affected by ongoing antibiotic therapy, no false negative cases were detected in the group of patients receiving the treatment, thus demonstrating that the accuracy of this modality is not influenced by antibiotic administration [52].

5.4. Is It Reasonable to Perform an [^{18}F]FDG-PET/CT after a Positive WBC Scintigraphy?

The answer to this question may be extracted in the meta-analysis of Reinders Folmer, where pre and post-test probabilities of having VGI have been calculated for CTA, [^{18}F]FDG PET, [^{18}F]FDG PET/CT, WBC scintigraphy with only planar images and WBC scintigraphy with planar images + SPECT/CT [12]. Of these modalities, WBC scintigraphy combined with SPECT/CT acquisitions scored best in terms of positive post-test probability (96%), followed by WBC scintigraphy with only planar images (94%), [^{18}F]FDG PET/CT (83%), CTA (80%) and standalone [^{18}F]FDG PET (78%). It means that, after positive WBC scintigraphy + SPECT/CT, a patient suspected of having a VGI has a 96% probability of being infected. This is not surprising considering the high number of true positives detected by this modality, which is, of course, superior to the number of true positives identified by [^{18}F]FDG PET/CT.

Therefore, we can assume that a positive WBC scintigraphy, especially if correctly acquired with SPECT/CT and interpreted by following EANM recommendations, is sufficient for the diagnosis and does not require an additional study with [^{18}F]FDG PET/CT.

5.5. Which Imaging Modality Is Recommended Within the First 3 Months after Surgery in the Suspicion of Early Infection?

It is well known that inflammatory changes, such as non-infected hematoma or lymphocele, may occur and persist for months after surgery, especially in more invasive approaches, and may result in false positive cases at both [^{18}F]FDG PET/CT scans and, more rarely, at WBC scintigraphy, thus impacting on their accuracy. Moreover, synthetic graft material (Dacron or Gore-Tex) induces a foreign-body reaction which may present [^{18}F]FDG uptake, thus representing a frequent pitfall in the interpretation of a PET scan. Indeed, after surgery, some inflammatory cells, mainly macrophages and fibroblasts, may use glucose as a source of energy for completing the healing process; for this reason, [^{18}F]FDG is taken up by the healing tissue.

In a large retrospective study performed by Keidar, as previously mentioned, the authors explored the [^{18}F]FDG uptake in 107 non-infected grafts in relation to graft material and time elapsed from surgery for a follow-up of up to 16 years. In this wide interval of time, they found no substantial reduction in the metabolic activity shown by synthetic grafts, thus meaning that post-surgical flogosis could be detectable after many years following surgery [49]. However, the pattern could be helpful in differentiating a sterile inflammation from an infection, since diffuse homogeneous uptake is usually observed in the first condition, reflecting a low-grade inflammation. On the contrary, infections usually show focal uptake. These findings were also confirmed by Wassèlius and colleagues in 10 out of 12 grafts implanted in open surgery and one out of four patients who underwent an endovascular procedure (mean time interval from surgery: 5.8 years). Notably, only one of the 16 patients had an infection based on biochemical and clinical data [46].

In terms of the usefulness of radiolabeled WBC in the post-surgical period, it is well known that this modality has higher specificity and accuracy in differentiating a sterile flogosis from an infection, compared with [^{18}F]FDG PET/CT. In 2006, Liberatore et al. found no false positive results in patients studied within 1 month after surgery, concluding that this modality is reliable to assess an infection in the earlier stages after endovascular surgery [53]. Of course, this conclusion could be affected by the type of population studied and, in particular, by the probability of having an infection or not, and larger studies are needed to confirm this finding.

In conclusion, we can state that the perfect timing to perform an NM examination mainly depends on the type of surgery (open vs. endovascular approach), clinical indication and pre-test probability of infection. After surgery, the presence of aseptic flogosis must always be taken into consideration, especially in the interpretation of an [^{18}F]FDG PET/CT scan and, therefore, the evaluation of the pattern of uptake and CT abnormalities must be accurate in order to correctly interpret the exam.

Larger multicenter studies are needed in order to provide an evidence-based answer to this question.

6. Conclusions

Accurate diagnosis of VGI is challenging and requires a multimodality and multidisciplinary approach in order to ensure the best management of these patients. Several radiological and NM modalities are available, each one with its pros and cons. US is usually used for extracavitary graft infection, while CT/CTA is the first-choice imaging modality for intracavitary graft infection. However, CTA may present some limitations, particularly in low-grade infections. In cases of equivocal CTA, WBC scintigraphy or [^{18}F]FDG PET/CT are recommended in order to improve diagnostic accuracy, but the use of appropriate interpretation criteria is mandatory.

The best diagnostic option would be to combine anatomical/radiological and functional imaging in order to obtain an earlier and more effective diagnosis, which should be mandatory for decision making and for defining the best treatment options.

Many efforts still need to be directed towards the definition of accurate algorithms that aim to make diagnostic approaches more uniform among different centers.

Author Contributions: Conceptualization, C.L.; methodology, C.L. and A.S.; resources, C.L., R.I., G.T., S.S., A.S., A.P., A.T., C.P., M.T., P.A.E. and Y.T.; writing—original draft preparation, C.L., R.I., G.T., S.S., A.S., A.P., A.T., C.P., M.T., P.A.E. and Y.T.; writing—review and editing, C.L.; supervision, R.I., G.T., M.R., S.S., A.S., A.P., A.T., C.P., M.T., P.A.E. and Y.T. All authors have read and agreed to the published version of the manuscript.

References

1. Wilson, W.R.; Bower, T.C.; Creager, M.A.; Amin-Hanjani, S.; O'Gara, P.T.; Lockhart, P.B.; Darouiche, R.O.; Ramlawi, B.; Derdeyn, C.P.; Bolger, A.F.; et al. Vascular Graft Infections, Mycotic Aneurysms, and Endovascular Infections: A Scientific Statement from the American Heart Association. *Circulation* **2016**, *134*, e412–e460. [CrossRef]
2. Gharamti, A.; Kanafani, Z.A. Vascular Graft Infections An update. *Infect. Dis. Clin. N. Am.* **2018**, *32*, 789–809. [CrossRef]
3. Kilic, A.; Arnaoutakis, D.J.; Reifsnyder, T.; Black, J.H., 3rd; Abularrage, C.J.; Perler, B.A.; Lum, Y.W. Management of infected vascular grafts. *Vasc. Med.* **2016**, *21*, 53–60. [CrossRef] [PubMed]
4. Fitzgerald, S.F.; Kelly, C.; Humphreys, H. Diagnosis and treatment of prosthetic aortic graft infections: Confusion and inconsistency in the absence of evidence or consensus. *J. Antimicrob. Chemother.* **2005**, *56*, 996–999. [CrossRef] [PubMed]
5. Andercou, O.; Marian, D.; Olteanu, G.; Stancu, B.; Cucuruz, B.; Noppeney, T. Complex treatment of vascular prostheses infections. *Medicine* **2018**, *97*, e11350. [CrossRef] [PubMed]
6. Lyons, O.T.; Baguneid, M.; Barwick, T.D.; Bell, R.E.; Foster, N.; Homer-Vanniasinkam, S.; Hopkins, S.; Hussain, A.; Katsanos, K.; Modarai, B.; et al. Diagnosis of Aortic Graft Infection: A Case Definition by the Management of Aortic Graft Infection Collaboration (MAGIC). *Eur. J. Vasc. Endovasc. Surg.* **2016**, *52*, 758–763. [CrossRef]
7. Chakfé, N.; Diener, H.; Lejay, A.; Assadian, O.; Berard, X.; Caillon, J.; Fourneau, I.; Glaudemans, A.W.J.M.; Koncar, I.; Lindholt, J.; et al. Editor's Choice—European Society for Vascular Surgery (ESVS) 2020 Clinical Practice Guidelines on the Management of Vascular Graft and Endograft Infections. *Eur. J. Vasc. Endovasc. Surg.* **2020**, *59*, 339–384. [CrossRef]
8. Post, I.C.J.H.; Vos, C.G. Systematic Review and Meta-Analysis on the Management of Open Abdominal Aortic Graft Infections. *Eur. J. Vasc. Endovasc. Surg.* **2019**, *58*, 258–281. [CrossRef]
9. Batt, M.; Feugier, P.; Camou, F.; Coffy, A.; Senneville, E.; Caillon, J.; Calvet, B.; Chidiac, C.; Laurent, F.; Revest, M.; et al. A meta-analysis of outcomes after in situ reconstructions for aortic graft infection. *Angiology* **2018**, *69*, 370–379. [CrossRef]
10. Antonello, R.M.; D'Oria, M.; Cavallaro, M.; Dore, F.; Cova, M.A.; Ricciardi, M.C.; Comar, M.; Campisciano, G.; Lepidi, S.; De Martino, R.R.; et al. Management of abdominal aortic prosthetic graft and endograft infections. A multidisciplinary update. *J. Infect. Chemother.* **2019**, *25*, 669–680. [CrossRef]
11. Rafailidis, V.; Partovi, S.; Dikkes, A.; Nakamoto, D.A.; Azar, N.; Staub, D. Evolving clinical applications of contrast-enhanced ultrasound (CEUS) in the abdominal aorta. *Cardiovasc. Diagn. Ther.* **2018**, *8*, S118–S130. [CrossRef] [PubMed]
12. Reinders Folmer, E.I.; Von Meijenfeldt, G.C.I.; Van der Laan, M.J.; Glaudemans, A.W.J.M.; Slart, R.H.J.A.; Saleem, B.R.; Zeebregts, C.J. Diagnostic Imaging in Vascular Graft Infection: A Systematic Review and Meta-Analysis. *Eur. J. Vasc. Endovasc. Surg.* **2018**, *56*, 719–729. [CrossRef] [PubMed]
13. Bruggink, J.L.M.; Slart, R.H.J.A.; Pol, J.A.; Reijnen, M.M.P.J.; Zeebregts, C.J. Current role of imaging in diagnosing aortic graft infections. *Semin. Vasc. Surg.* **2011**, *24*, 182–190. [CrossRef] [PubMed]
14. Heikkinen, L.; Valtonen, M.; Lepäntalo, M.; Saimanen, E.; Järvinen, A. Infrarenal endoluminal bifurcated stent graft infected with Listeria monocytogenes. *J. Vasc. Surg.* **1999**, *29*, 554–556. [CrossRef]
15. Mantoni, M.; Neergaard, K.; Christoffersen, J.K.; Lambine, T.L.; Baekgaard, N. Longterm computed tomography follow-up after open surgical open surgical repair of abdominal aortic aneurysms. *Acta Radiol.* **2006**, *47*, 549–553. [CrossRef]

16. Thornton, E.; Mendiratta-Lala, M.; Siewert, B.; Eisenberg, R.L. Patterns of fat stranding. *Am. J. Roentgenol.* **2011**, *197*, W1–W14. [CrossRef]
17. Adam, A.D.A.; Dixon, A.K.; Gillard, J.; Schaefer-Prokop, C.; Grainger, R.; Allison, D. *Grainger & Allison's Diagnostic Radiology*; Churchill Livingstone: Edinburgh, Scotland, 2014; ISBN 978-0702042959.
18. Orton, D.F.; LeVeen, R.F.; Saigh, J.A.; Culp, W.C.; Fidler, J.L.; Lynch, T.J.; Goertzen, T.C.; McCowan, T.C. Aortic prosthetic graft infections: Radiologic manifestations and implications for management. *Radiographics* **2000**, *20*, 977–993. [CrossRef]
19. Macedo, T.A.; Stanson, A.W.; Oderich, G.S.; Johnson, C.M.; Panneton, J.M.; Tie, M.L. Infected aortic aneurysms: Imaging findings. *Radiology* **2004**, *231*, 250–257. [CrossRef]
20. Gazzani, S.E.; Bianchini Massoni, C.; Marcato, C.; Paladini, I.; Rossi, C. Endovascular treatment of iliac artery rupture after septic embolization. *Acta Biomed.* **2019**, *90*, 339–342. [CrossRef]
21. Kissin, E.Y.; Merkel, P.A. Diagnostic imaging in Takayasu arteritis. *Curr. Opin. Rheumatol.* **2004**, *16*, 31–37. [CrossRef]
22. Chapman, S.A.; Delgadillo, D., 3rd; MacGuidwin, E.; Greenberg, J.I.; Jameson, A.P. Graft Infection Masquerading as Rheumatologic Disease: A Rare Case of Aortobifemoral Graft Infection Presenting as Hypertrophic Osteoarthropathy. *Ann. Vasc. Surg.* **2017**, *41*, 283.e11–283.e18. [CrossRef] [PubMed]
23. Auffermann, W.; Olofsson, P.A.; Rabahie, G.N.; Tavares, N.J.; Stoney, R.J.; Higgins, C.B. Incorporation versus infection of retroperitoneal aortic grafts: MR imaging features. *Radiology* **1989**, *172*, 359–362. [CrossRef] [PubMed]
24. Signore, A.; Lauri, C.; Galli, F. Radiolabelled probes targeting infection and inflammation for personalized medicine. *Curr. Pharm. Des.* **2014**, *20*, 2338–2345. [CrossRef] [PubMed]
25. Signore, A.; Jamar, F.; Israel, O.; Buscombe, J.; Martin-Comin, J.; Lazzeri, E. Clinical indications, image acquisition and data interpretation for white blood cells and anti-granulocyte monoclonal antibody scintigraphy: An EANM procedural guideline. *Eur. J. Nucl. Med. Mol. Imaging* **2018**, *45*, 1816–1831. [CrossRef]
26. de Vries, E.F.; Roca, M.; Jamar, F.; Israel, O.; Signore, A. Guidelines for the labelling of leucocytes with 99mTc-HMPAO. Inflammation/Infection Taskgroup of the European Association of Nuclear Medicine. *Eur. J. Nucl. Med. Mol. Imaging* **2010**, *37*, 842–848. [CrossRef]
27. Roca, M.; de Vries, E.F.; Jamar, F.; Israel, O.; Signore, A. Guidelines for the labelling of leucocytes with 111In-oxine. Inflammation/Infection Taskgroup of the European Association of Nuclear Medicine. *Eur. J. Nucl. Med. Mol. Imaging* **2010**, *37*, 835–841. [CrossRef]
28. Erba, P.A.; Leo, G.; Sollini, M.; Tascini, C.; Boni, R.; Berchiolli, R.N.; Menichetti, F.; Ferrari, M.; Lazzeri, E.; Mariani, G. Radiolabelled leucocyte scintigraphy versus conventional radiological imaging for the management of late, low-grade vascular prosthesis infections. *Eur. J. Nucl. Med. Mol. Imaging* **2014**, *41*, 357–368. [CrossRef]
29. Glaudemans, A.W.; de Vries, E.F.; Vermeulen, L.E.; Slart, R.H.; Dierckx, R.A.; Signore, A. A large retrospective single-centre study to define the best image acquisition protocols and interpretation criteria for white blood cell scintigraphy with 99m Tc-HMPAO-labelled leucocytes in musculoskeletal infections. *Eur. J. Nucl. Med. Mol. Imaging* **2013**, *40*, 1760–1769. [CrossRef]
30. Erba, P.A.; Glaudemans, A.W.; Veltman, N.C.; Sollini, M.; Pacilio, M.; Galli, F.; Dierckx, R.A.; Signore, A. Image acquisition and interpretation criteria for 99mTc-HMPAO-labelled white blood cell scintigraphy: Results of a multicenter study. *Eur. J. Nucl. Med. Mol. Imaging* **2014**, *41*, 615–623. [CrossRef]
31. Annovazzi, A.; Bagni, B.; Burroni, L.; D'Alessandria, C.; Signore, A. Nuclear medicine imaging of inflammatory/infective disorders of the abdomen. *Nucl. Med. Commun.* **2005**, *26*, 657–664. [CrossRef]
32. Bar-Shalom, R.; Yefremov, N.; Guralnik, L.; Keidar, Z.; Engel, A.; Nitecki, S.; Israel, O. SPECT/CT using 67Ga and 111In-labeled leukocyte scintigraphy for diagnosis of infection. *J. Nucl. Med.* **2006**, *47*, 587–594. [PubMed]
33. Khaja, M.S.; Sildiroglu, O.; Hagspiel, K.; Rehm, P.K.; Cherry, K.J.; Turba, U.C. Prosthetic vascular graft infection imaging. *Clin. Imaging* **2013**, *37*, 239–244. [CrossRef] [PubMed]
34. Roll, D.; Hierholzer, M.; Hepp, W.; Langer, M.; Zwicker, C.; Felix, R. Diagnostic evaluation of radioimmunoscintigraphy (RIS) using 123I-labeled monoclonal antibodies against human granulocytes (Mab-47) for the detection of prosthetic vascular graft infection. *Nucl. Med. Biol.* **1991**, *18*, 135–140. [CrossRef]

35. Cordes, M.; Hepp, W.; Langer, R.; Pannhorst, J.; Hierholzer, J.; Felix, R. Vascular graft infection: Detection by 123I-labeled antigranulocyte antibody (anti-NCA95) scintigraphy. *Nucl. Med.* **1991**, *30*, 173–177.
36. Cordes, M.; Hepp, W.; Barzen, G.; Langer, R. Diagnostic evaluation of radioimmunoscintigraphy (RIS) with use of iodine 123-labeled antibodies against human granulocytes (123I-anti-NCA95) for the detection of prosthetic vascular graft infection. *J. Vasc. Surg.* **1991**, *14*, 703–704. [CrossRef]
37. Tronco, G.G.; Love, C.; Rini, J.N.; Yu, A.K.; Bhargava, K.K.; Nichols, K.J.; Pugliese, P.V.; Palestro, C.J. Diagnosing prosthetic vascular graft infection with the antigranulocyte antibody 99mTc-fanolesomab. *Nucl. Med. Commun.* **2007**, *28*, 297–300. [CrossRef]
38. Kim, S.J.; Lee, S.W.; Jeong, S.Y.; Pak, K.; Kim, K. A systematic review and meta-analysis of (18)F-fluorodeoxyglucose positron emission tomography or positron emission tomography/computed tomography for detection of infected prosthetic vascular grafts. *J. Vasc. Surg.* **2019**, *70*, 307–313. [CrossRef]
39. Rojoa, D.; Kontopodis, N.; Antoniou, S.A.; Ioannou, C.V.; Antoniou, G.A. 18F-FDG PET in the Diagnosis of Vascular Prosthetic Graft Infection: A Diagnostic Test Accuracy Meta-Analysis. *Eur. J. Vasc. Endovasc. Surg.* **2019**, *57*, 292–301. [CrossRef]
40. Jamar, F.; Buscombe, J.; Chiti, A.; Christian, P.E.; Delbeke, D.; Donohoe, K.J.; Israel, O.; Martin-Comin, J.; Signore, A. EANM/SNMMI guideline for 18F-FDG use in inflammation and infection. *J. Nucl. Med.* **2013**, *54*, 647–658. [CrossRef]
41. Spacek, M.; Belohlavek, O.; Votrubova, J.; Sebesta, P.; Stadler, P. Diagnostics of "non-acute" vascular prosthesis infection using 18F-FDG PET/CT: Our experience with 96 prostheses. *Eur. J. Nucl. Med. Mol. Imaging* **2009**, *36*, 850–858. [CrossRef]
42. Tokuda, Y.; Oshima, H.; Araki, Y.; Narita, Y.; Mutsuga, M.; Kato, K.; Usui, A. Detection of thoracic aortic prosthetic graft infection with 18F-fluorodeoxyglucose positron emission tomography/computed tomography. *Eur. J. Cardiothorac. Surg.* **2013**, *43*, 1183–1187. [CrossRef] [PubMed]
43. Berger, P.; Vaartjes, I.; Scholtens, A.; Moll, F.L.; De Borst, G.J.; De Keizer, B.; Bots, M.L.; Blankensteijn, J.D. Differential FDG-PET Uptake Patterns in Uninfected and Infected Central Prosthetic Vascular Grafts. *Eur. J. Vasc. Endovasc. Surg.* **2015**, *50*, 376–383. [CrossRef] [PubMed]
44. Chang, C.Y.; Chang, C.P.; Shih, C.C.; Yang, B.H.; Cheng, C.Y.; Chang, C.W.; Chu, L.S.; Wang, S.J.; Liu, R.S. Added Value of Dual-Time-Point 18F-FDG PET/CT with Delayed Imaging for Detecting Aortic Graft Infection: An Observational Study. *Medicine* **2015**, *94*, e1124. [CrossRef] [PubMed]
45. Sah, B.R.; Husmann, L.; Mayer, D.; Scherrer, A.; Rancic, Z.; Puippe, G.; Weber, R.; Hasse, B. VASGRA Cohort. Diagnostic performance of 18F-FDG-PET/CT in vascular graft infections. *Eur. J. Vasc. Endovasc. Surg.* **2015**, *49*, 455–464. [CrossRef] [PubMed]
46. Wassélius, J.; Malmstedt, J.; Kalin, B.; Larsson, S.; Sundin, A.; Hedin, U.; Jacobsson, H. High 18F-FDG Uptake in synthetic aortic vascular grafts on PET/CT in symptomatic and asymptomatic patients. *J. Nucl. Med.* **2008**, *49*, 1601–1605. [CrossRef]
47. Guenther, S.P.; Cyran, C.C.; Rominger, A.; Saam, T.; Kazmierzcak, P.M.; Bagaev, E.; Pichlmaier, M.; Hagl, C.; Khaladj, N. The relevance of 18F-fluorodeoxyglucose positron emission tomography/computed tomography imaging in diagnosing prosthetic graft infections post cardiac and proximal thoracic aortic surgery. *Interact. Cardiovasc. Thorac. Surg.* **2015**, *21*, 450–458. [CrossRef]
48. Keidar, Z.; Engel, A.; Hoffman, A.; Israel, O.; Nitecki, S. Prosthetic vascular graft infection: The role of 18F-FDG PET/CT. *J. Nucl. Med.* **2007**, *48*, 1230–1236. [CrossRef]
49. Keidar, Z.; Pirmisashvili, N.; Leiderman, M.; Nitecki, S.; Israel, O. 18F-FDG uptake in noninfected prosthetic vascular grafts: Incidence, patterns, and changes over time. *J. Nucl. Med.* **2014**, *55*, 392–395. [CrossRef]
50. Saleem, B.R.; Berger, P.; Vaartjes, I.; de Keizer, B.; Vonken, E.J.; Slart, R.H.; de Borst, G.J.; Zeebregts, C.J. Modest utility of quantitative measures in 18F-fluorodeoxyglucose positron emission tomography scanning for the diagnosis of aortic prosthetic graft infection. *J. Vasc. Surg.* **2015**, *61*, 965–971. [CrossRef]
51. Bruggink, J.L.; Glaudemans, A.W.; Saleem, B.R.; Meerwaldt, R.; Alkefaji, H.; Prins, T.R.; Slart, R.H.; Zeebregts, C.J. Accuracy of FDG-PET-CT in the diagnostic work-up of vascular prosthetic graft infection. *Eur. J. Vasc. Endovasc. Surg.* **2010**, *40*, 348–354. [CrossRef]

52. Kagna, O.; Kurash, M.; Ghanem-Zoubi, N.; Keidar, Z.; Israel, O. Does Antibiotic Treatment Affect the Diagnostic Accuracy of 18F-FDG PET/CT Studies in Patients with Suspected Infectious Processes? *J. Nucl. Med.* **2017**, *58*, 1827–1830. [CrossRef] [PubMed]
53. Liberatore, M.; Misuraca, M.; Calandri, E.; Rizzo, L.; Speziale, F.; Iurilli, A.P.; Anagnostou, C. White blood cell scintigraphy in the diagnosis of infection of endovascular prostheses within the first month after implantation. *Med. Sci. Monit.* **2006**, *12*, MT5–MT9. [PubMed]

8

Comparison of the Diagnostic Value of MRI and Whole Body ^{18}F-FDG PET/CT in Diagnosis of Spondylodiscitis

Corinna Altini [1], Valentina Lavelli [1], Artor Niccoli-Asabella [2], Angela Sardaro [3], Alessia Branca [1], Giulia Santo [1], Cristina Ferrari [1,*] and Giuseppe Rubini [1]

[1] Nuclear Medicine Unit, Interdisciplinary Department of Medicine, University of Bari Aldo Moro, Piazza Giulio Cesare, 11–70124 Bari, Italy; corinna.altini@hotmail.it (C.A.); valentina.lavelli@gmail.com (V.L.); alessia9130@gmail.com (A.B.); giuliasanto92@gmail.com (G.S.); giuseppe.rubini@uniba.it (G.R.)
[2] Nuclear Medicine Unit, AOU Policlinic "A. Perrino", 72100 Brindisi, Italy; artor.niccoliasabella@asl.brindisi.it
[3] Section of Radiology and Radiation Oncology, Interdisciplinary Department of Medicine, University of Bari Aldo Moro, Piazza Giulio Cesare, 11–70124 Bari, Italy; angela.sardaro@uniba.it
* Correspondence: ferrari_cristina@inwind.it

Abstract: Spondylodiscitis is a spine infection for which a diagnosis by a magnetic resonance imaging (MRI) is considered the most appropriate imaging technique. The aim of this study was to compare the role of an ^{18}F-fluorodeoxyglucose positron emission tomography/computed tomography (^{18}F-FDG PET/CT) and an MRI in this field. For 56 patients with suspected spondylodiscitis for whom MRI and ^{18}F-FDG PET/CT were performed, we retrospectively analyzed the results. Cohen's κ was applied to evaluate the agreement between the two techniques in all patients and in subgroups with a different number of spinal districts analyzed by the MRI. Sensitivity, specificity, and accuracy were also evaluated. The agreements of the ^{18}F-FDG PET/CT and MRI in the evaluation of the entire population, whole-spine MRI, and two-districts MRI were moderate ($\kappa = 0.456$, $\kappa = 0.432$, and $\kappa = 0.429$, respectively). In patients for whom one-district MRI was performed, ^{18}F-FDG PET/CT and MRI were both positive and completely concordant ($\kappa = 1$). We also separately evaluated patients with suspected spondylodiscitis caused by *Mycobacterium tuberculosis* for whom the MRI and ^{18}F-FDG PET/CT were always concordant excepting in 2 of the 18 (11%) patients. Sensitivity, specificity, and accuracy of the MRI and ^{18}F-FDG PET/CT were 100%, 60%, 97%, and 92%, 100%, and 94%, respectively. Our results confirmed the ^{18}F-FDG PET/CT diagnostic value in the diagnosis of spondylodiscitis is comparable to that of MRI for the entire spine evaluation. This could be considered a complementary technique or a valid alternative to MRI.

Keywords: spondylodiscitis; spine infection; MRI; ^{18}F-FDG PET/CT

---

1. Introduction

Spondylodiscitis is an infection of the vertebral body or disc that can extend to contiguous soft tissues [1]. Its incidence is rising due to increased life expectancy. It mainly affects men aged between 50 and 70 years [1,2]. It is often associated to the presence of debilitating conditions, such as endocarditis, diabetes mellitus, septic arthritis, urinary tract infections and indwelling catheter infections, malignancy, and spinal surgery [1,2]. The most frequent district involved is the lumbar spine, followed by the dorsal tract and the cervical tract [2]. The principal causes of spondylodiscitis are pyogenic agents, most commonly *Staphylococcus aureus*, followed by *Escherichia coli*. Less commonly, spondylodiscitis is caused by non-pyogenic agents, such as *Mycobacterium tuberculosis*, *Brucella*, *fungi*, and *parasites* [1,3].

The diagnosis of spondylodiscitis is based on a clinical suspect for the presence of symptoms, such as focal back pain, fever and/or neurological deficit associated with nonspecific laboratory findings [2,4,5]. Imaging findings are also fundamental for diagnosis and magnetic resonance imaging (MRI) is considered the most accurate technique for the early detection of spondylodiscitis [4,6,7].

More recently, ^{18}F-fluorodeoxyglucose positron emission tomography/computed tomography (^{18}F-FDG PET/CT) was proven to be a useful multimodality imaging method to study infectious and other benign disease, including spondylodiscitis [8,9].

The aim of this study was to compare the role of an ^{18}F-FDG PET/CT and MRI in the diagnosis of spondylodiscitis.

2. Experimental Section

We retrospectively analyzed patients who underwent a whole-body ^{18}F-FDG PET/CT for the suspicion of spondylodiscitis, performed from April 2013 to October 2018. There were 105 patients (74 men, 31 women; mean age 63 years; range: 18–90 years) for whom ^{18}F-FDG PET/CT was performed. Only 56/105 patients for whom MRI was performed before ^{18}F-FDG PET/CT were included in the analysis, whereas the other 49/105 were excluded. All the MRIs were performed in an average of 8 days before the ^{18}F-FDG PET/CT (range: 3–15 days) and included at least one spinal district.

All patients had already given their consent for the use of their data for clinical research. Our Institutional Review Board does not require the Ethical Committee's approval for the review of the patients' files.

The MRI examinations of the spine were acquired on a 1.5 T scanner (ACHIEVA, Philips Healthcare, Amsterdam, Netherlands). The choice of which and how many spinal districts to scan was driven by clinical suspicion. The MRI scan protocol consisted of a T1-weighted (T1-W), Turbo Spine Echo (TSE), T2-Weighted (T2-W), and Short Time Inversion Recovery-Weighted (STIR-W). The T1-W sagittal, axial, and coronal scans were performed after the contrast agent was administered to all patients. The total duration of the examination was 20–25 minutes without considering post-processing. The MRI findings indicative of spondylodiscitis were decrease signal intensity from the disc and adjacent vertebral bodies on T1-W images, increase signal intensity from the disc and adjacent vertebral bodies on T1-W, increase signal intensity on T2-W images (due to edema), and loss of endplate definition on T1-W. The gadolinium enhancement of the discs, vertebrae, and surrounding soft tissue helped to differentiate the infective lesions from degenerative changes (Modic type 1 abnormalities) or neoplasm [10].

An integrated PET/CT scanner Discovery IQ (GE, Healthcare Technologies, Milwaukee, WI, USA) was used for obtaining results. Patients were recommended to fast for six hours before the acquisition of the PET/CT. Before the ^{18}F-FDG injection, the blood sugar levels were measured and the optimal value was <140 mg/dL. We proceeded with the intravenous injection of 2.5–3 MBq/kg of ^{18}F-FDG using a venous line and the patients were allowed to stay in the room for approximately 60 minutes. Whole-body PET/CT acquisitions were performed by placing patients in a supine position with their arms raised above their heads. PET images were obtained in a three-dimensional mode and were analyzed qualitatively and semi-quantitatively with a Multivol PET/CT program of Advantage™ workstation (GE, Healthcare Technologies, Milwaukee, WI, USA). PET findings were analyzed by evaluating the different ^{18}F-FDG uptakes between the soft tissue infection and the bone marrow.

In all patients, the final diagnosis of spondylodiscitis was confirmed or excluded on the basis of resolution or significant improvement of constitutional symptoms (back pain and/or fever), laboratory, such as C-reactive protein (CRP), erythrocyte sedimentation rate (ESR), and white blood cells (WBCs), and instrumental (e.g., MRI and biopsy) follow-ups were performed for at least 6 months.

Sensitivity, specificity, and accuracy of the MRI and ^{18}F-FDG PET/CT were calculated. Cohen's κ was also applied to evaluate the agreement between the MRI and ^{18}F-FDG PET/CT in the entire population analyzed and in subgroups who performed whole-spine, two-districts and one-district MRI. Analyses were performed by MedCalc®statistical software version 2020 (MedCalc Software Ltd., Ostend, Belgium).

3. Results

The demographic and clinical characteristics of the 56 patients are shown in Table 1.

Table 1. Baseline characteristics.

Variable	Number (Percentage)
Total Number of Patients	**56**
Sex	
Male	39 (70%)
Female	17 (30%)
Median age (years)	63 (18–90)
Symptoms	
Fever	35 (62%)
Back pain	38 (69%)
None	18 (32%)
Etiological agent	52 (93%)
Mycobacterium tuberculosis	18 (35%)
Staphilococcus aureus	14 (27%)
Escherichia coli	4 (8%)
Haemophilus influenzae	4 (8%)
Brucella	3 (6%)
Propionibacterium acnes	2 (3%)
Streptococcus epidermidis	2 (3%)
Pseudomonas aeruginosa	1 (2%)
Candida albicans	1 (2%)
Aspergillus	1 (2%)
Staphilococcus capitis	1 (2%)
Granulicatella elegans	1 (2%)
Not found	4 (7%)
MRI district study	
One	19 (34%)
Cervical	1 (5%)
Dorsal	5 (26%)
Lumbar	13 (69%)
Two	12 (21%)
Cervical/dorsal	1 (8%)
Dorsal/lumbar	5 (42%)
Cervical/lumbar	1 (8%)
Lumbar/sacral	5 (42%)
Whole-spine	25 (45%)

None of patients were started on any antibiotic therapies before the imaging techniques performance.

The sensitivity, specificity, and accuracy for ^{18}F-FDG PET/CT were 92%, 100%, and 94%, and for MRI were 100%, 60%, and 97%, respectively.

In agreement with clinical and instrumental findings, final diagnosis of spondylodiscitis in 51/56 (91%) patients was confirmed, whereas in 5/56 (9%) patients, it was ruled out.

^{18}F-FDG PET/CT showed pathological uptake in the spine and correctly identified 44/56 (79%) patients with spondylodiscitis. Equally, ^{18}F-FDG PET/CT showed no significant uptake in the spine and therefore, correctly ruling out spondylodiscitis in 12/56 patients (21%). The MRI identified 53/56 patients (95%) with spinal infection and ruled out infection in 3/56 patients (5%). ^{18}F-FDG PET/CT had a false-negative in 4/56 patients (7%). MRI had a false-positive in 2/56 patients (4%) with a final diagnosis of severe degenerative disc disease.

Table 2 reports the κ values for the agreement results.

Table 2. Agreement results in all patients and MRI subgroups.

		κ	95% Confidence Interval
All patients	56	0.456	0.11–0.80
Subgroup I (whole-spine MRI)	25/56 (45%)	0.432	0.01–0.85
Subgroup II (two-district MRI)	12/56 (21%)	0.429	0–1.00
Subgroup III (one-district MRI)	19/56 (34%)	1	0.79–1.00

Table 3 reports the MRI and ^{18}F-FDG PET/CT results for all patients and subgroups.

Table 3. Results in all patients and in MRI subgroups.

	MRI (+)	MRI (+)	MRI (−)	MRI (−)
	^{18}F-FDG PET/CT (+)	^{18}F-FDG PET/CT (−)	^{18}F-FDG PET/CT (+)	^{18}F-FDG PET/CT (−)
All patients (n = 56)	47	6	0	3
Subgroup I (whole-spine MRI)	19	4	0	2
Subgroup II (two-districts MRI)	9	2	0	1
Subgroup III (one-district MRI)	19	0	0	0

Note: MRI (+), ^{18}F-FDG PET/CT (+), positive concordance; MRI (+/−), ^{18}F-FDG PET/CT (− /+), discordance; MRI (−), ^{18}F-FDG PET/CT (−), negative concordance.

Figure 1 reports an example case of spine infection detected by both MRI and ^{18}F-FDG PET/CT. Figure 2 reports a case of discordance between the MRI and ^{18}F-FDG PET/CT.

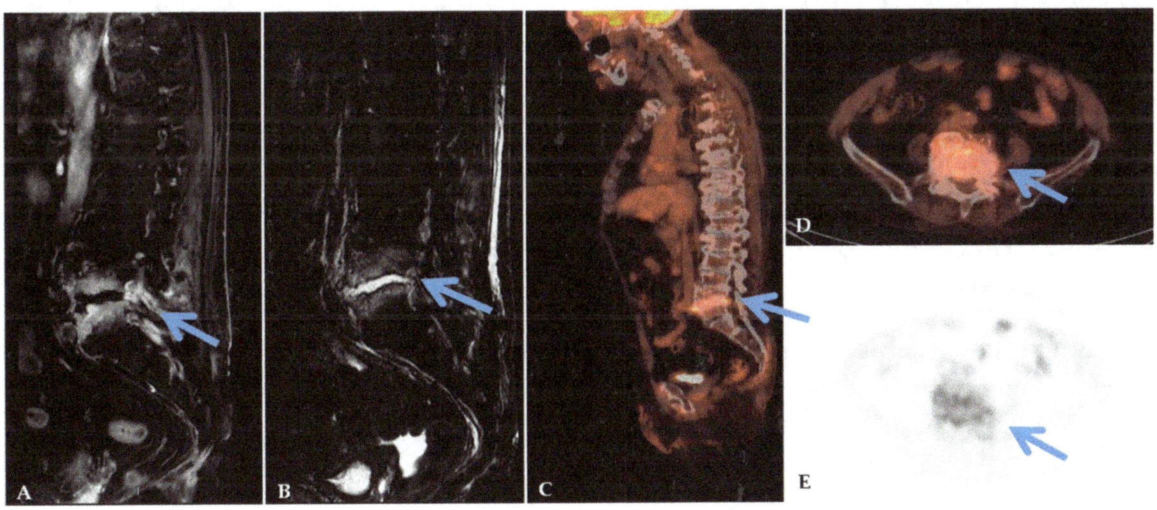

Figure 1. MRI and ^{18}F-FDG PET/CT in a 55-year-old man with back pain, fever, and with positive microbiology culture (*Staphilococcus aureus*). Sagittal MRI images showed in T1-Weighted (**A**) and Short Time Inversion Recovery (**B**) sequences pathological signal in the L4-L5 intervertebral disc and bone marrow edema (arrows). ^{18}F-FDG PET/CT images (**C**–**E**) showed pathological uptake in L4–L5 (Standardized Uptake Value 6.7) (arrows). The final diagnosis of spondylodiscitis was confirmed.

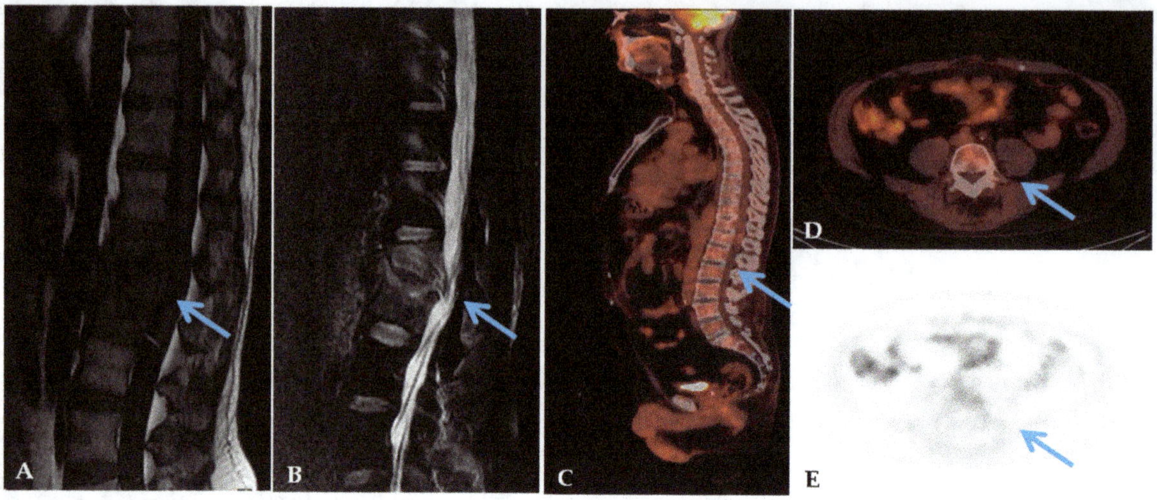

Figure 2. MRI and ^{18}F-FDG PET/CT in a 62-year-old man with back pain and low-grade fever. Sagittal MRI T1-Weighted (**A**) and T2-Weighted (**B**) images showed low T1 and high T2 signal at the L1–L2 end plates (arrows). ^{18}F-FDG PET/CT images (**C–E**) showed no significant FDG uptake in the spine (arrows). These findings confirmed severe degenerative disc disease.

In the subgroup of patients for whom whole-spine MRI was performed, 14/19 patients (74%), had the same lesions where the two techniques were identified. In 4/19 patients (21%), the MRI identified lesions in two districts, whereas the ^{18}F-FDG PET/CT only in one. In 1/19 patients (5%), the ^{18}F-FDG PET/CT identified one lesion more than MRI.

In the subgroup of patients for whom two-districts MRI was performed, seven of nine patients (78%) had the same lesions which the two techniques identified. In one of nine patients (11%), MRI identified lesions in two districts whereas the ^{18}F-FDG PET/CT in only one. In one of nine patients (11%), the ^{18}F-FDG PET/CT identified one lesion more than the MRI.

In the subgroup of 19 patients for whom the one-district MRI was performed, the ^{18}F-FDG PET/CT and the MRI were both positive and completely concordant for lesions identified that were: cervical in 1/19 (5%), dorsal in 5/19 (26%), and lumbar in 13/19 (69%).

The average value of Standardized Uptake Value (SUVmax) was 6.7 (SD ± 3.2).

The results concerning patients with *Mycobacterium tuberculosis* (TBC) etiology are reported separately in Table 4.

Table 4. Results in all patients affected by *Mycobacterium tuberculosis* and MRI subgroups.

	MRI (+)	MRI (+)	MRI (−)	MRI (−)
	^{18}F-FDG PET/CT (+)	^{18}F-FDG PET/CT (−)	^{18}F-FDG PET/CT (+)	^{18}F-FDG PET/CT (−)
All patients (*n* = 18)	16	2	0	0
Subgroup I (whole-spine MRI)	5	2	0	0
Subgroup II (two-districts MRI)	3	0	0	0
Subgroup III (one-district MRI)	8	0	0	0

Note: MRI (+); ^{18}F-FDG PET/CT (+): positive concordance. MRI (+/−); ^{18}F-FDG PET/CT (− /+): discordance. MRI (−); ^{18}F-FDG PET/CT (−): negative concordance.

4. Discussion

Diagnosis of spondylodiscitis is a combination of clinical, laboratory, and radiological findings. Symptoms and clinical signs of spondylodiscitis are non-specific and include severe back pain, fever and, in one-third of cases, neurological deficit such as leg weakness, paralysis, sensory deficit, radiculopathy, and loss of sphincter control [2,11]. For this reason, spondylodiscitis is difficult to diagnose because laboratory results are also nonspecific and not always present; they could include elevated levels of CRP, increased ESR, and elevated WBC [1].

Diagnosis of certainty associated with the detection of the etiological agent can be obtained by invasive investigations, such as biopsy, but this is associated with significant risks and side effects. For this reason, it is necessary to be able to have non-invasive diagnostic methods with repeatable and high performance value [2,12].

Generally, the first imaging modality required for suspected spinal infection, despite its low sensitivity and specificity, are plain radiographs [2,13–16]. Usually, the signs are not present on radiographs until two to eight weeks after the onset of symptoms and may not be evident in patients with severe degenerative disc disease [2,15,16]. Nowadays, MRI is the imaging procedure most used due to its high sensitivity in the diagnosis of infection and in assessing the extent of disease [4,17]. The main MRI findings for spondylodiscitis are impairment of the intervertebral discs associated with disc space narrowing or possible epidural involvement and increased contrast enhancement in the spine [4,6]. Contrast-enhanced MRI is the method of choice in clinical practice due to its advantages including high contrast resolution, high sensitivity for soft tissue, absence of ionizing radiation exposure, and the possibility to show evidence of bone marrow abnormalities [2,5]. MRI cannot be performed in patients with cardiac implantable electronic devices, cardioverter defibrillators, or cardiac resynchronization devices; even patients with metallic implants cannot undergo the process. The high costs and long run times for whole-spine examination do not make it a suitable examination for all patients. MRI diagnostic performance decreases in follow-up evaluation and in post-operative infection of the spine [2,17–23]. These drawbacks, over time, lead many to look for other methods that could replace an MRI, mostly when it is contraindicated, not available, or doubtful [2,24,25].

Over the years, ^{18}F-FDG PET/CT, a whole-body technique, has shown advantages in the clinical and therapeutic management of oncological disease and, simultaneously, its usefulness in the management of several non-oncological disease has been proven [26]. However, different from MRI, ^{18}F-FDG PET/CT exposes patients to ionizing radiation even if updated protocols minimize radio exposure. In patients with spondylodiscitis, ^{18}F-FDG PET/CT allows for differentiation of degenerative and infectious abnormalities found on an MRI [4,27]. It is considered positive when ^{18}F-FDG uptake is higher than bone marrow uptake in adjacent vertebrae or soft tissue around the spine. Therefore, unlike morphological imaging, ^{18}F-FDG PET/CT highlights glycidic metabolism, which may already be increased in the early stages of infection [4,5].

The diagnostic value of an MRI and ^{18}F-FDG PET/CT in our study is in line with current literature and confirm the higher sensitivity of an MRI and its relatively lower specificity than ^{18}F-FDG PET/CT (100% vs. 92% and 60% vs. 100%, respectively). The two techniques showed similar accuracy (94% and 97%). The high sensitivity of an MRI allows the identification of almost all spondylodiscitis lesions, but the lower specificity is indicative of the possibility of misunderstanding lesions due to inflammatory or degenerative spondyloarthropathy, recent vertebral fractures, postoperative inflammation, or bone tumors. The high specificity of ^{18}F-FDG PET/CT improves the interpretation of ambiguous MRI images [9].

Previous studies that investigated the value of an MRI in diagnosing spondylodiscitis showed results similar to our study, such as sensitivity of 82–96%, specificity of 85–93%, and accuracy of 81–94% [5,28–30].

Even though this imaging modality is considered the gold standard for spinal infection diagnoses, in 2015, a prospective study of 26 patients who underwent an MRI and ^{18}F-FDG PET/CT reported encouraging results for the use of an ^{18}F-FDG PET/CT as a valid alternative in the evaluation of patients with suspected spondylodiscitis that could not perform an MRI. In particular, Fauster et al. found sensitivity and specificity of 83% and 88% for ^{18}F-FDG PET/CT and 94% and 38% for MRI, respectively [4]. Similar results were reported in a recent meta-analysis that ^{18}F-FDG PET/CT has a superior accuracy than MRI (97% vs. 81%) in detecting spondylodiscitis, as well as high sensitivity (95% vs. 85%) and specificity (88% vs. 66%) [31]. Smids et al. analyzed a group of 75 patients with clinical suspicion of spondylodiscitis and found that ^{18}F-FDG PET/CT had higher sensitivity and accuracy in the early diagnosis of spondylodiscitis than MRI, especially when performed in the first two weeks of the onset of symptoms [5].

Our study included a homogeneous group of 56 patients with suspected spondylodiscitis, even though the comparison for the entire spine was not performed for all patients. For this reason, we also evaluated the agreement of the two techniques for all of the lesions and it always resulted moderately except for patients with a single-spine district MRI, for whom the agreement was complete and absolute. The differentiation in groups, based on the district studied from the MRI, was necessary to compare overlapping data and therefore to identify differences in numbers and locations of the infection, which can involve multiple spine sites.

Discordant results were found in 6 of 56 patients for whom the MRI was positive, but the ^{18}F-FDG PET/CT did not reveal any lesions. In four of them, the diagnosis of spondylodiscitis was confirmed and false-negative ^{18}F-FDG PET/CT results were probably due to a weak infection characterized only by epidural involvement, whereas the low ^{18}F-FDG uptake may have been related to the different immune reaction caused by the various etiological agents [22,32,33]. In the remaining two patients, spondylodiscitis was finally not confirmed by follow-up and the false-positive MRI results were due to the presence of severe degenerative disc disease [22].

Differences among patients in whom the MRI and ^{18}F-FDG PET/CT were concordant in the identification of the suspected lesions were observed. In patients for whom the whole-body MRI was performed, MRI identified one lesion more than the ^{18}F-FDG PET/CT in four patients, whereas the ^{18}F-FDG PET/CT detected one lesion more than the MRI in only one patient. Similarly, in the subgroup for whom two-districts MRI was performed, it identified one lesion more than the ^{18}F-FDG PET/CT in one patient, whereas the ^{18}F-FDG PET/CT detected one lesion more than the MRI in only one patient. The higher number of lesions identified by the MRI was related to the presence of edema-like changes in the end plates and to epidural abscesses. The patients in whom additional ^{18}F-FDG PET/CT lesions were found, psoas abscesses were detected. For all the additional lesions found by the two techniques, the final diagnosis of spondylodiscitis was confirmed.

Mycobacterium tuberculosis is one of the etiological agents of spondylodiscitis, but it can differ from bacterial disease for clinical and imaging. In these patients, the back pain and neurological deficit onset occurred only later in chronic forms [34]. Imaging-guide vertebral biopsy is a gold standard for differentiating tubercular and pyogenic spondylodiscitis. MRI and ^{18}F-FDG PET/CT were helpful for evaluating the extension of the infection [35]. The main MRI findings, suggestive for tubercular spondylodiscitis, indicated sparing of the intervertebral disc in the early stages of infection, loss of vertebral body cortical definition, multiple vertebral involvement, and the presence of muscular (paraspinal, psoas) abscesses [34,35]. Tuberculous spondylodiscitis ^{18}F-FDG PET/CT commonly presents as ^{18}F-FDG uptake lesions. However, in some cases, a cold abscess is characterized by moderate ^{18}F-FDG uptake in the cortex and low uptake in the center [36].

In our study, we described separate patients with tuberculous spondylodiscitis. In most of them, the MRI and ^{18}F-FDG PET/CT results were both of positive and in concordance in identifying lesions due to their typical imaging presentation at two techniques. The remaining two patients' results were discordant. The false-positive MRI result was the same as described in the entire population and therefore was due to degenerative end-plate abnormalities. Similarly, the false-negative ^{18}F-FDG PET/CT result was previously described and may be related to low-virulence bacteria.

Despite the encouraging results, some limitations of our study should be reported. First of all, we analyzed a small sample size in line with the literature. Other limitations were the heterogeneous groups of pathogens and the difference in the numbers of spine districts examined by the MRI.

Our results show the complementary role of ^{18}F-FDG PET/CT and MRI in a spondylodiscitis diagnosis. The combination of ^{18}F-FDG PET/CT and MRI detected lesions in 100% of patients with spondylodiscitis, identifying the site and the extent of the disease and correctly guiding the therapeutic choice [2,4,37,38].

5. Conclusions

Our results confirmed the high diagnostic value of ^{18}F-FDG PET/CT in the diagnosis of spondylodiscitis in comparison with MRI. Given the increasing evidence of the diagnostic value of ^{18}F-FDG PET/CT, it could be proposed as a possible alternative to MRI, especially when MRI is contraindicated, non-diagnostic, or inconclusive. The agreement between these two techniques suggests their complementary role in selected and more complicated patients.

Author Contributions: Conceptualization, C.A.; methodology, V.L.; data curation, G.S.; writing—original draft preparation, A.B.; writing—review and editing, A.S.; visualization, A.N.-A.; supervision, C.F.; project administration, G.R. All authors have read and agreed to the published version of the manuscript.

References

1. Raghavan, M.; Lazzeri, E.; Palestro, C.J. Imaging of Spondylodiscitis. *Semin. Nucl. Med.* **2018**, *48*, 131–147. [CrossRef] [PubMed]
2. Lazzeri, E.; Bozzao, A.; Cataldo, M.A.; Petrosillo, N.; Manfrè, L.; Trampuz, A.; Signore, A.; Muto, M. Joint EANM/ESNR and ESCMID-endorsed consensus document for the diagnosis of spine infection (spondylodiscitis) in adults. *Eur. J. Nucl. Med. Mol. Imaging* **2019**, *46*, 2464–2487. [CrossRef] [PubMed]
3. Prodi, E.; Grassi, R.; Iacobellis, F.; Cianfoni, A. Imaging in Spondylodiskitis. *Magn. Reson. Imaging Clin. North Am.* **2016**, *24*, 581–600. [CrossRef] [PubMed]
4. Fuster, D.; Tomás, X.; Mayoral, M.; Soriano, A.; Manchón, F.; Cardenal, C.; Monegal, A.; Granados, U.; Garcia, S.; Pons, F. Prospective comparison of whole-body 18F-FDG PET/CT and MRI of the spine in the diagnosis of haematogenous spondylodiscitis. *Eur. J. Nucl. Med. Mol. Imaging* **2014**, *42*, 264–271. [CrossRef] [PubMed]
5. Smids, C.; Kouijzer, I.J.E.; Vos, F.J.; Sprong, T.; Hosman, A.J.F.; de Rooy, J.W.J.; Aarntzen, E.H.J.G.; de Geus-Oei, L.F.; Oyen, W.J.G.; Bleeker-Rovers, C.P. A comparison of the diagnostic value of MRI and 18F-FDG-PET/CT in suspected spondylodiscitis. *Infection* **2016**, *45*, 41–49. [CrossRef]
6. Cottle, L.; Riordan, T. Infectious spondylodiscitis. *J. Infect.* **2008**, *56*, 401–412. [CrossRef]
7. Gaudio, F.; Pedote, P.; Niccoli Asabella, A.; Ingravallo, G.; Sindaco, P.; Alberotanza, V.; Perrone, T.; Laddaga, F.E.; Rubini, G.; Stabile Ianora, A.A.; et al. Bone involvement in hodgkin's lymphoma: Clinical features and outcome. *Acta Haematol.* **2018**, *140*, 178–182. [CrossRef]
8. Inanami, H.; Oshima, Y.; Iwahori, T.; Takano, Y.; Koga, H.; Iwai, H. Role of 18F-fluoro-d-deoxyglucose PET/CT in diagnosing surgical site infection after spine surgery with instrumentation. *Spine* **2015**, *40*, 109–113. [CrossRef]
9. Treglia, G.; Pascale, M.; Lazzeri, E.; van der Bruggen, W.; Delgado Bolton, R.C.; Glaudemans, A.W.J.M. Diagnostic performance of 18F-FDG PET/CT in patients with spinal infection: A systematic review and a bivariate meta-analysis. *Eur. J. Nucl. Med. Mol. Imaging* **2020**, *47*, 1287–1301. [CrossRef]
10. Niccoli Asabella, A.; Iuele, F.; Simone, F.; Fanelli, M.; Lavelli, V.; Ferrari, C.; Di Palo, A.; Notaristefano, A.; Merenda, N.C.; Rubini, G. Role of (18)F-FDG PET/CT in the evaluation of response to antibiotic therapy in patients affected by infectious spondylodiscitis. *Hell. J. Nucl. Med.* **2015**, *18* (Suppl. 1), 17–22.
11. Mylona, E.; Samarkos, M.; Kakalou, E.; Fanourgiakis, P.; Skoutelis, A. Pyogenic Vertebral Osteomyelitis: A Systematic Review of Clinical Characteristics. *Semin. Arthritis Rheum.* **2009**, *39*, 10–17. [CrossRef] [PubMed]
12. Chaudhary, S.B.; Vives, M.J.; Basra, S.K.; Reiter, M.F. Postoperative spinal wound infections and postprocedural diskitis. *J. Spinal Cord Med.* **2007**, *30*, 441–451. [CrossRef] [PubMed]
13. Duarte, R.M.; Vaccaro, A.R. Spinal infection: State of the art and management algorithm. *Eur. Spine J.* **2013**, *22*, 2787–2799. [CrossRef]
14. Jevtic, V. Vertebral infection. *Eur. Radiol. Suppl.* **2004**, *14*, 1. [CrossRef] [PubMed]
15. Khoo, L.A.L.; Heron, C.; Patel, U.; Given-Wilson, R.; Grundy, A.; Khaw, K.T.; Dundas, D. The diagnostic contribution of the frontal lumbar spine radiograph in community referred low back pain—A prospective study of 1030 patients. *Clin. Radiol.* **2003**, *58*, 606–609. [CrossRef]

16. Leone, A.; Dell'atti, C.; Magarelli, N.; Colelli, P.; Balanika, A.; Casale, R.; Bonomo, L. Imaging of spondylodiscitis. *Eur. Rev. Med. Pharmacol. Sci.* **2012**, *16*, 8–19. [PubMed]
17. Desanto, J.; Ross, J.S. Spine infection/inflammation. *Radiol. Clin. North Am.* **2011**, *49*, 105–127. [CrossRef]
18. Tins, B.J.; Cassar-Pullicino, V.N. MR imaging of spinal infection. *Semin. Musculoskelet. Radiol.* **2004**, *8*, 215–229. [CrossRef]
19. Grane, P.; Josephsson, A.; Seferlis, A.; Tullberg, T. Septic and aseptic post-operative discitis in the lumbar spine—Evaluation by MR imaging. *Acta Radiol.* **1998**, *39*, 108–115. [CrossRef]
20. Kawakyu-O'Connor, D.; Bordia, R.; Nicola, R. Magnetic Resonance Imaging of Spinal Emergencies. *Magn. Reson. Imaging Clin. North Am.* **2016**, *24*, 325–344. [CrossRef]
21. Danchaivijitr, N.; Temram, S.; Thepmongkhol, K.; Chiewvit, P. Diagnostic accuracy of MR imaging in tuberculous spondylitis. *J. Med. Assoc. Thail.* **2007**, *90*, 1581–1589.
22. Rosen, R.S.; Fayad, L.; Wahl, R.L. Increased 18F-FDG uptake in degenerative disease of the spine: Characterization with 18F-FDG PET/CT. *J. Nucl. Med.* **2006**, *47*, 1274–1280.
23. Hong, S.H.; Choi, J.Y.; Lee, J.W.; Kim, N.R.; Choi, J.A.; Kang, H.S. MR imaging assessment of the spine: Infection or an imitation? *Radiographics* **2009**, *29*, 599–612. [CrossRef] [PubMed]
24. Di Martino, A.; Papapietro, N.; Lanotte, A.; Russo, F.; Vadalà, G.; Denaro, V. Spondylodiscitis: Standards of current treatment. *Curr. Med. Res. Opin.* **2012**, *28*, 689–699. [CrossRef] [PubMed]
25. Diehn, F.E. Imaging of Spine Infection. *Radiol. Clin. North Am.* **2012**, *50*, 777–798. [CrossRef]
26. Niccoli Asabella, A.; Di Palo, A.; Altini, C.; Ferrari, C.; Rubini, G. Multimodality Imaging in Tumor Angiogenesis: Present Status and Perspectives. *Int. J. Mol. Sci.* **2017**, *18*, 1864. [CrossRef]
27. Stumpe, K.D.M.; Zanetti, M.; Weishaupt, D.; Hodler, J.; Boos, N.; Von Schulthess, G.K. FDG positron emission tomography for differentiation of degenerative and infectious endplate abnormalities in the lumbar spine detected on MR imaging. *Am. J. Roentgenol.* **2002**, *179*, 1151–1157. [CrossRef]
28. Gratz, S.; Dörner, J.; Fischer, U.; Behr, T.M.; Béhé, M.; Altenvoerde, G.; Meller, J.; Grabbe, E.; Becker, W. 18F-FDG hybrid PET in patients with suspected spondylitis. *Eur. J. Nucl. Med. Mol. Imaging* **2002**, *29*, 516–524. [CrossRef]
29. Modic, M.T.; Feiglin, D.H.; Piraino, D.W.; Boumphrey, F.; Weinstein, M.A.; Duchesneau, P.M.; Rehm, S. Vertebral osteomyelitis: Assessment using MR. *Radiology* **1985**, *157*, 157–166. [CrossRef]
30. Ledermann, H.P.; Schweitzer, M.E.; Morrison, W.B.; Carrino, J.A. MR imaging findings in spinal infections: Rules or myths? *Radiology* **2003**, *228*, 506–514. [CrossRef]
31. Kim, S.J.; Pak, K.; Kim, K.; Lee, J.S. Comparing the Diagnostic Accuracies of F-18 Fluorodeoxyglucose Positron Emission Tomography and Magnetic Resonance Imaging for the Detection of Spondylodiscitis: A Meta-analysis. *Spine* **2019**, *44*, E414–E422. [CrossRef] [PubMed]
32. Dauchy, F.A.; Dutertre, A.; Lawson-Ayayi, S.; de Clermont-Gallerande, H.; Fournier, C.; Zanotti-Fregonara, P.; Dutronc, H.; Vital, J.M.; Dupon, M.; Fernandez, P. Interest of [18F] fluorodeoxyglucose positron emission tomography/computed tomography for the diagnosis of relapse in patients with spinal infection: A prospective study. *Clin. Microbiol. Infect.* **2016**, *22*, 438–443. [CrossRef] [PubMed]
33. Squaiella, C.C.; Ananias, R.Z.; Mussalem, J.S.; Braga, E.G.; Rodrigues, E.G.; Travassos, L.R.; Lopes, J.D.; Longo-Maugéri, I.M. In vivo and in vitro effect of killed Propionibacterium acnes and its purified soluble polysaccharide on mouse bone marrow stem cells and dendritic cell differentiation. *Immunobiology* **2006**, *211*, 105–116. [CrossRef] [PubMed]
34. Kumar, Y.; Gupta, N.; Chhabra, A.; Fukuda, T.; Soni, N.; Hayashi, D. Magnetic resonance imaging of bacterial and tuberculous spondylodiscitis with associated complications and non-infectious spinal pathology mimicking infections: A pictorial review. *BMC Musculoskelet. Disord.* **2017**, *18*, 244. [CrossRef]
35. Bassetti, M.; Merelli, M.; Di Gregorio, F.; Della Siega, P.; Screm, M.; Scarparo, C.; Righi, E. Higher fluorine-18 fluorodeoxyglucose positron emission tomography (FDG-PET) uptake in tuberculous compared to bacterial spondylodiscitis. *Skelet. Radiol.* **2017**, *46*, 777–783. [CrossRef]
36. Yago, Y.; Yukihiro, M.; Kuroki, H.; Katsuragawa, Y.; Kubota, K. Cold tuberculous abscess identified by FDG PET. *Ann. Nucl. Med.* **2005**, *19*, 515–518. [CrossRef]
37. Mazzie, J.P.; Brooks, M.K.; Gnerre, J. Imaging and Management of Postoperative Spine Infection. *Neuroimaging Clin. North Am.* **2014**, *24*, 365–374. [CrossRef]
38. Skanjeti, A.; Penna, D.; Douroukas, A.; Cistaro, A.; Arena, V.; Leo, G.; Longo, G.; Traverso, A.; Belloro, S.; Pelosi, E. PET in the clinical work-up of patients with spondylodiscitis: A new tool for the clinician? *Q. J. Nucl. Med. Mol. Imaging* **2012**, *56*, 569.

9

Theranostic Designed Near-Infrared Fluorescent Poly (Lactic-co-Glycolic Acid) Nanoparticles and Preliminary Studies with Functionalized VEGF-Nanoparticles

Michela Varani [1], Filippo Galli [1], Gabriela Capriotti [1], Maurizio Mattei [2], Rosella Cicconi [2], Giuseppe Campagna [1], Francesco Panzuto [3] and Alberto Signore [1,*]

1 Nuclear Medicine Unit, Department of Medical-Surgical Sciences and of Translational Medicine, Faculty of Medicine and Psychology, "Sapienza" University of Rome, 00189 Roma, Italy; varanimichela@gmail.com (M.V.); filippo.galli@uniroma1.it (F.G.); gabriela.capriotti@uniroma1.it (G.C.); gius.campagna@gmail.com (G.C.)

2 Department of Biology and Centro di Servizi Interdipartimentale-Stazione per la Tecnologia Animale, "Tor Vergata" University of Rome, 00189 Roma, Italy; mattei@uniroma2.it (M.M.); rosella.cicconi@uniroma2.it (R.C.)

3 Digestive Disease Unit, Sant'Andrea University Hospital, ENETS Center of Excellence Rome, 00189 Roma, Italy; fpanzuto@ospedalesantandrea.it

* Correspondence: alberto.signore@uniroma1.it

Abstract: Poly-lactic-co-glycolic acid nanoparticles (PLGA-NPs) were approved by the Food and Drug Administration (FDA) for drug delivery in cancer. The enhanced permeability and retention (EPR) effect drives their accumulation minimizing the side effects of chemotherapeutics. Our aim was to develop a new theranostic tool for cancer diagnosis and therapy based on PLGA-NPs and to evaluate the added value of vascular endothelial growth factor (VEGF) for enhanced tumor targeting. In vitro and in vivo properties of PLGA-NPs were tested and compared with VEGF-PLGA-NPs. Dynamic light scattering (DLS) was performed to evaluate the particle size, polydispersity index (PDI), and zeta potential of both preparations. Spectroscopy was used to confirm the absorption spectra in the near-infrared (NIR). In vivo, in BALB/c mice bearing a syngeneic tumor in the right thigh, intravenously injected PLGA-NPs showed a high target-to-muscle ratio (4.2 T/M at 24 h post-injection) that increased over time, with a maximum uptake at 72 h and a retention of the NPs up to 240 h. VEGF-PLGA-NPs accumulated in tumors 1.75 times more than PLGA-NPs with a tumor-to-muscle ratio of 7.90 ± 1.61 (versus 4.49 ± 0.54 of PLGA-NPs). Our study highlights the tumor-targeting potential of PLGA-NPs for diagnostic and therapeutic applications. Such NPs can be conjugated with proteins such as VEGF to increase accumulation in tumor lesions.

Keywords: polymeric nanoparticles; PLGA; optical imaging; tumor targeting

---

1. Introduction

The latest advances in molecular imaging are closely related to the use of new tools, such as nano- or micro-particles that can be used for several applications, from detection and diagnosis to drug delivery and treatment [1]. Different nanomaterials are used to create particles with a range from 1 to 1000 nm, and so, are defined as nano-particles (NPs) [2]. They offer the advantage to deliver drugs to the target with high efficiency and low systemic toxicity [3,4]. The NPs formulated with organic polymers (polymeric NPs) are generally one of the best choices for clinical or pre-clinical use due to their favorable characteristics such as non-immunogenicity, non-toxicity, biodegradability, and biocompatibility [5].

Indeed, PLGA have been approved by the Food and Drug Administration (FDA) and the European Medicine Agency (EMA) as copolymers to deliver drugs, and today about 16 approved pharmaceuticals are based on the use of these NPs [6,7]. Their in vivo biodistribution is greatly influenced by different physical and chemical characteristics, among which size and glycolic:lactic acid ratio play a key role [8,9]. The NPs accumulate in target lesions with an active or passive mechanism. The passive mechanism is represented by the enhanced permeability and retention (EPR) effect, that allows NPs with a size in the 20–200 nm range to accumulate in cancer lesions with an impaired vasculature [10,11]. Therefore, this mechanism is of great importance when using nanotechnologies in oncology [12–14]. Moreover, the flexibility of PLGA-NPs offers the advantage to combine their ability to deliver drugs with the possibility to functionalize them with peptides, proteins, or imaging probes [15]. Since tumor and stromal cells produce several proangiogenic factors, such as proteins from the vascular endothelial growth factor (VEGF) family, they are usually characterized by high and irregular vascularization [16]. Therefore, targeting of either VEGF or VEGF receptor (VEGFR) can be achieved and exploited to increase PLGA accumulation in tumor lesions [17].

In the present study, we investigated the possibility of using specifically designed PLGA-NPs as a tool for future theranostic applications. We selected PLGA-NPs (lactic acid:glycolic acid ratio of 50:50, average size of 100–200 nm) conjugated with a near-infrared (NIR) fluorochrome with an excitation wavelength at 780 nm and emission wavelength at 825 nm, allowing a deeper tissue penetration of fluorescence [18]. The target capacity and the pharmacokinetic of native PLGA-NPs was investigated in vivo to evaluate the tumor detection and then the retention of PLGA-NPs up to 240 h.

To actively target tumor cells over-expressing VEGFR, the PLGA-NPs were loaded with a recombinant human VEGF-A165 (rhVEGF) analog by the 1-Ethyl-3-[3-dimethylaminopropyl] carbodiimide hydrochloride/N-hydroxysuccinimide (EDC/NHS) covalent coupling method. The successful functionalization of NPs was examined with an in vitro kinetic binding of VEGF-PLGA-NPs with the VEGF Receptor-2 (KDR)/Fc chimera human compared to native PLGA-NPs. Tumor targeting of VEGF-PLGA-NPs was examined in vivo 24 h post-injection (p.i.) and compared with native PLGA-NPs. The T/M showed an increasing of PLGA-NPs capability to target the tumor over-expressing VEGFR.

2. Materials and Methods

2.1. PLGA-NPs

PLGA (D, L-lactide-co-glycolide) nanoparticles with a lactic acid:glycolic acid ratio of 50:50, average size of 100–200 nm, conjugated with a NIR fluorochrome with an excitation/emission wavelength of 780/825 nm, were purchased from Degradex® (Phosphorex Inc., Hopkinton, MA, USA).

2.2. PLGA-NPs Functionalization with VEGF

The conjugation of VEGF was performed by using the 1-Ethyl-3-(3-dimethylaminopropyl) carbodiimide (EDC) and N-hydroxysuccinimide (NHS) coupling protocol. EDC and NHS were purchased from Thermo Scientific (ThermoFisher, Waltham, MA, USA). The recombinant human VEGF-A165 analog with a molecular weight of 38.2 kDa was purchased by Prospec-Tany Technogene Ltd. (Rehovot, Israel). This molecule shares 88% homology with murine VEGF and has been previously used in mice [19,20]. The carboxylate (-COOH) PLGA-NPs react with NHS in the presence of EDC to create a stable crosslinking with the primary amines (-NH_2) of the VEGF molecule. The conjugation condition was initially optimized with the use of bovine serum albumin (BSA), evaluating the protein-particle ratio, pH, the choice of buffer, the reaction time, and the purification method. A suspension of 6 mL MES buffer (pH 6.0) containing a concentration of PLGA-NPs (5 mg/mL) were first reacted with 30 mg of EDC (5 mg/mL in phosphate-buffered saline (PBS) pH 7.4). Then, 30 mg of NHS (5 mg/mL in PBS, pH 7.4) were added to the solution and incubated at room temperature with agitation for 15 min. To separate the activated PLGA-NPs from an excess of EDC, EDC-by-products, and NHS, the sample was centrifuged with a high-speed micro-centrifuge (ThermoFisher, Waltham, MA, USA) at 12,000 rpm (9500× *g*) 4 °C for 20 min and washing 3 times with 1 mL PBS (pH 7.4). The EDC coupling creates an unstable reactive o-acylisourea ester group that is easily substituted by an amine-reactive ester in the presence of NHS. The resulting NHS ester is semi-stable but very reactive towards the amino groups on the VEGF molecule. The carboxyl-amine reaction allows the conjugation of the VEGF onto the PLGA-NPs. RhVEGF (2 mg) was added to the PLGA-NPs suspension and the conjugation proceeded for 2 h at room temperature. The resulting VEGF-PLGA-NPs were collected by 3 times ultracentrifugation at 12,000 rpm (9500× *g*), 4 °C for 20 min, and was washed with 1 mL of PBS (pH 7.4) to remove unconjugated VEGF.

2.3. *Calculation of Average Size and Zeta Potential*

The mean size, the polydispersity index (PDI), and the net surface charges (zeta potential) of native and functionalized PLGA-NPs were measured by dynamic light scattering (DLS), using photon correction spectroscopy, electrophoretic mobility analysis, and potential distribution at 25 °C with water as suspension medium. Reading was performed with a NanoZetaSizer analyzer (Malvern Instruments Ltd., Malvern, UK) equipped with a 5 mW HeNe laser (wavelength λ = 632.8 nm), a digital logarithmic correlator and a non-invasive backscattering (NIBS) optical system. Briefly, 10 μL (100 μg) PLGA-NPs were suspended with 90 μL H_2O and loaded in Sarstedt polystyrol/polystyrene cuvettes (10 × 10 × 45 mm) for size and PDI measurements. For zeta potential analysis, 20 μL (200 μg) PLGA-NPs and VEGF-PLGA-NPs were suspended with 980 μL H_2O, sonicated to reduce the aggregation and loaded in Malvern folded capillary cells for zeta potential measurements. Absorption spectra were acquired by a Jasco V-630 spectrophotometer. Briefly, 50 μL (500 μg) PLGA-NPs and VEGF-PLGA-NPs were diluted with 400 μL H_2O and loaded in J18 Jasco quartz cells (path length = 10 mm). Water solution was measured separately as a blank solution and subtracted by sample spectra. All experiments were performed in triplicate.

2.4. *In Vitro Binding of VEGF-PLGA-NPs and PLGA-NPs to KDR-Fc*

In vitro binding of native or VEGF-functionalized PLGA-NPs was performed with Nunc MaxiSorp™ 96 well plates (ThermoFisher, Waltham, MA, USA). The binding properties due to the hydrophilic surface of the wells allowed the coating of the VEGF Receptor-2 (KDR)/Fc chimera human (Sigma-Aldrich, St. Louis, MO, USA). Briefly, 50 μL of KDR-Fc in a final concentration of 0.002 μg/μL in bicarbonate/carbonate coating buffer (100 mM) was added to each well and the plate was covered and incubated 48 h at 4 °C. The coating solution was removed and the wells were rinsed two times with PBS (pH 7.4). Then, 150 μL of skimmed milk powder 2% (*w/v*) in PBS were added per well to block residual binding sites for 1 h at 37 °C. As a negative control, a blocking solution was added to each well that had not been coated with KDR-Fc. The blocking solution was removed by rinsing twice with 1 × PBS, pH 7.4. Then, 100 μL of two-fold dilution of VEGF-PLGA-NPs and native PLGA-NPs were added to each well followed by overnight incubation at 4 °C. KDR-Fc-uncoated wells were used to evaluate non-specific binding to the plastic. After incubation, the plate was washed two times with PBS and imaged with an in vivo FX station (Molecular Imaging Software, Kodak, Sevie County, TN, USA). Regions of interest (ROIs) were drawn for each well and the mean fluorescent intensity (mean IF) was calculated. The mean IF from wells without KDR-Fc (−KDR) was subtracted to the mean IF calculated in well coated with KDR-Fc (+KDR) to obtain PLGA-NPs and VEGF-PLGA-NPs net binding to KDR-Fc. Experiments were performed in triplicate.

2.5. *In Vivo Studies*

2.5.1. Mouse Model

All animal experiments were carried out in compliance with the local ethics committee and in agreement with the National rules and the EU regulation (Study 204/2018-PR). A syngeneic murine tumor model was used for in vivo studies. The model was obtained by subcutaneous injection in the right thigh of 10^6 J774a.1 cells (reticulum cell sarcoma) in a medium: Matrigel® (BD-Biosciences, Bergen, NJ, USA) solution (200 μL, 50:50, v:v), in female BALB/c mice (8 weeks). Cells were purchased from American Type Culture Collection (ATCC® TIB-67™, Milan, Italy) and grown in ATCC-formulated Dulbecco's Modified Eagle's Medium supplemented with 10% of fetal bovine serum at 37 °Cand in 5% CO_2. The 8-week-old female BALB/c mice were purchased from Harlan Laboratories. After about 20 days from the inoculation, the tumors became palpable and the targeting experiments were performed.

2.5.2. Pharmacokinetic of PLGA-NPs

To evaluate the kinetics and tumor targeting of native PLGA-NPs, 100 μL of NPs (500 μg) diluted with 50 μL NaCl were injected in the tail vein of 22 BALB/c mice, bearing a subcutaneous syngeneic tumor (reticulum cells sarcoma). At 2, 24, 48, and 72 h p.i. 5 mice per time point were anesthetized to acquire whole-body images with a Kodak in vivo FX station. Then, mice were sacrificed to excise major organs (liver, spleen, lungs, kidneys, muscle, tumor) to perform ex vivo optical imaging and quantify the uptake of PLGA-NPs in selected organs. ROIs were drawn over each organ, and the fluorescence signal was calculated as net fluorescence/area of the organ. Whole-body optical imaging only was performed in the last two mice up to 240 h.

2.5.3. Tumor Targeting of VEGF-PLGA-NPs and of PLGA-NPs

For tumor targeting experiments, fluorescent PLGA-NPs and VEGF-PLGA-NPs (500 μg in 150 μL 0.9% NaCl solution) were injected in the tail vein of 10 BALB/c mice (5 mice for each compound), bearing a subcutaneous syngeneic tumor (reticulum cells sarcoma). After 24 h, whole-body images were acquired and then mice were sacrificed. Liver, spleen, lungs, kidney, muscle, and tumor were excised for ex vivo optical imaging. On ex vivo images, ROIs were drawn to quantify the uptake of PLGA-NPs and VEGF-PLGA-NPs in selected organs and to calculate the tumor-to-muscle ratio (T/M). The fluorescence signal was calculated as net fluorescence/area.

2.6. Statistical Analysis

Statistical analysis was performed using SAS v. 9.4 (SAS Institute Inc., Cary, NC, USA).

Variables continuous was showed as mean ± standard deviation (SD). Shapiro-Wilk test was used to verify the normality of distribution of continuous variables. We applied the Box-Cox procedure which allowed to identify suitable mathematical functions (log10, quadratic, and inverse) which make the non-normal continuous variables/residuals subsequently distributed according to the Gauss condition. Comparisons between "PLGA-NPs" vs. "VEGF-PLGA-NPs" and continuous variables were analyzed by t-test. We used the Satterthwaite formula when the variances were unequal. Differences between time (2 h, 24 h, 48 h, and 72 h) and the continuous variables were tested by GLM (General Liner Model) test. Homoscedasticity was verified by Levene and Brown-Forsythe tests. Post-hoc analysis was performed by the Tukey test. Mann-Whitney test was used comparing data of net binding of PLGA-NPs and VEGF-PLGA-NPs to KDR. A $p < 0.05$ was considered statistically significant.

3. Results

3.1. Characterization of Native and VEGF Functionalized PLGA-NPs

Preliminary characterization showed that native PLGA-NPs have a zeta average of 180 ± 17.08 nm with a PDI of 0.25 ± 0.02. The VEGF-PLGA-NPs have a zeta average of 173 ± 7.39 nm with a PDI of 0.17 ± 0.01. The zeta average and the PDI were reported as mean ± standard deviation (SD) of three measurements performed on the same sample (Table 1). Native PLGA-NPs showed a negative zeta potential value of −37.60 ± 0.67 mV, that excludes the presence of aggregates due to the Van der Waal interactions. The VEGF-PLGA-NPs have a zeta potential value of −9.43 mV that indicated a change in the potential difference across the boundaries between liquid and the NPs surface, revealing that the conjugation was successful (Figure 1).

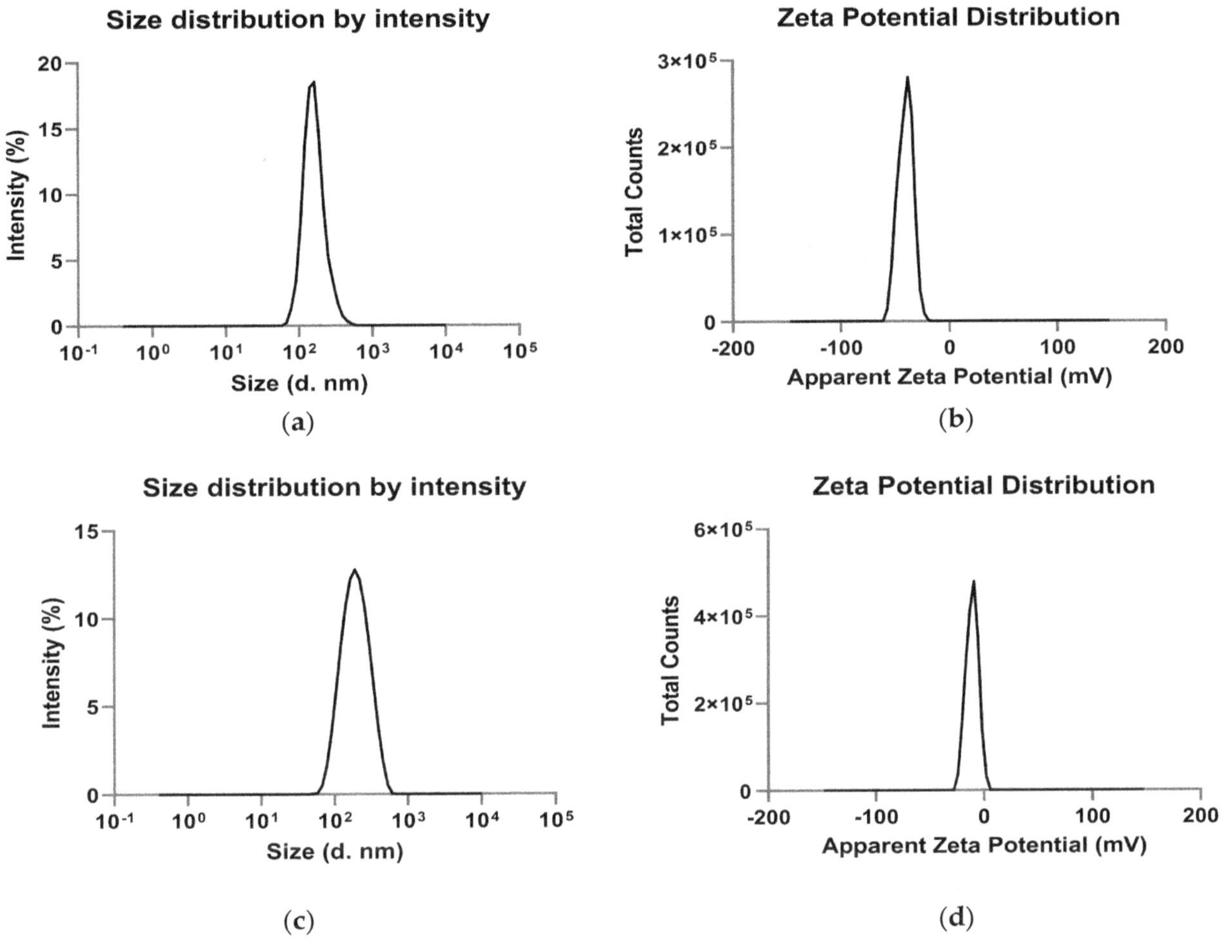

Figure 1. Particle size distribution and zeta measurement profile of native (**a**,**b**) and vascular endothelial growth factor-conjugated poly-lactic-co-glycolic acid nanoparticles (VEGF-PLGA-NPs) (**c**,**d**). Data are three different measurements made by the instrument on the same sample. (**a**) Size distribution of PLGA-NPs; (**b**) zeta potential distribution of PLGA-NPs; (**c**) size distribution of VEGF-PLGA-NPs; (**d**) zeta potential distribution of VEGF-PLGA-NPs.

Table 1. Characterization of PLGA-NPs and VEGF-PLGA-NPs to the DLS. Data are expressed as mean ± SD of three measurements.

	PLGA-NPs Mean ± SD	VEGF-PLGA-NPs Mean ± SD	*t* Test (*p*)
Zeta average (nm)	180.2 ± 17.08	173.03 ± 7.39	n.s.
Polydispersity index	0.25 ± 0.02	0.17 ± 0.01	**0.01**
Mean intensity (nm)	169.73 ± 15.10	208.60 ± 4.97	**0.03**
Zeta potential (mV)	−37.6 ± 0.67	−9.43 ± 0.25	**0.0001**

Bold: statistically significant ($p < 0.05$).

The spectroscopy was performed to confirm the absorbance of the sample. The results confirmed the absorbance of the fluorochrome conjugated with PLGA in the near-infrared region, generating an emission peak >700 nm (Figure 2).

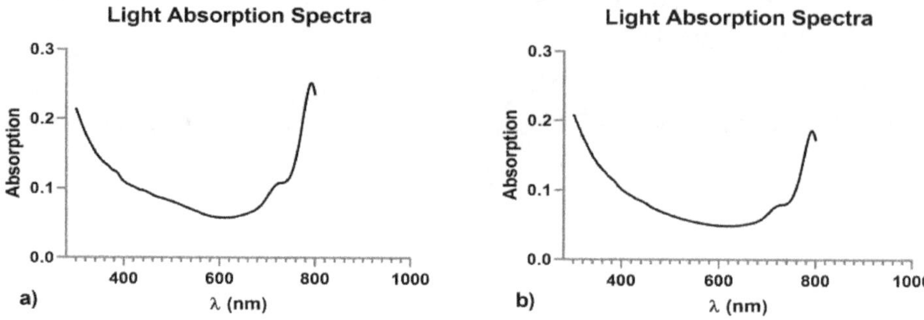

Figure 2. Light absorption spectra of poly-lactic-co-glycolic acid nanoparticles (PLGA-NPs) (**a**), and vascular endothelial growth factor-conjugated poly-lactic-co-glycolic acid nanoparticles (VEGF-PLGA-NPs) (**b**). Both the nano-formulations generated an emission peak >700 nm. Solvent was bidistilled water, pH 5.0.

3.2. In Vitro Binding of PLGA-NPs and VEGF-PLGA-NPs to KDR-Fc

In vitro binding studies with PLGA-NPs and VEGF-PLGA-NPs are summarized in Figure 3.

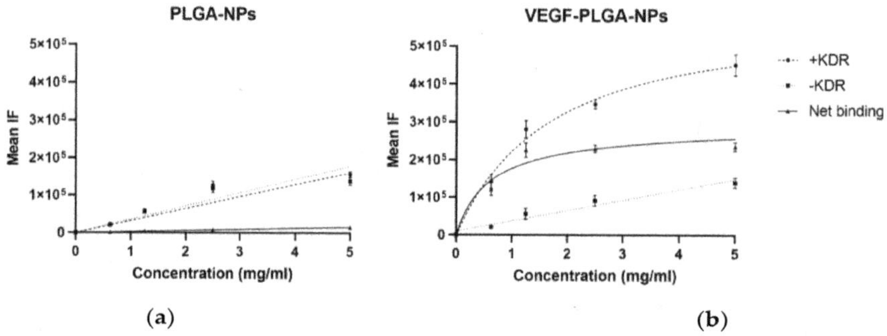

Figure 3. In vitro binding assay of PLGA-NPs (**a**) and VEGF-PLGA-NPs (**b**) to VEGF Receptor-2 (KDR)/Fc chimera human (KDR-Fc). KDR-Fc at concentration of 0.002 μg/μL was coated on the surface of 96-well plates. Two-fold dilutions of PLGA-NPs and VEGF-PLGA-NPs were incubated overnight at 4 °C. The mean fluorescent intensity (IF) was calculated for each well using in vivo FX station Kodak. Net binding was calculated by subtracting the mean IF in - KDR wells (negative control) to the mean IF calculated in +KDR well. One well for each dilution has not been coated with KDR-Fc and it was used as a negative control (-KDR). Results are presented as the means ± S.D (bars) of three separate experiments. Statistical analysis by Mann–Witney test showed significant difference between the two binding curves ($p < 0.0001$).

PLGA-NPs showed low NET binding to KDR-Fc that increased linearly with the concentration, properly due to non-specific interactions.

On the other hand, NET binding of VEGF-PLGA-NPs reached a plateau at 1.2 mg/mL due to a VEGFR saturation, demonstrating the specific interaction between VEGF and KDR-Fc.

The results indicated the binding specificity of VEGF functionalized PLGA-NPs with the KDR-Fc.

3.3. In Vivo Studies

Pharmacokinetic and Tumor Targeting of PLGA-NPs

In vivo pharmacokinetic studies of PLGA-NPs showed maximum tumor uptake at 72 h p.i., as shown in Figure 4. This result was confirmed by ex vivo imaging of the collected organs and a semi-quantitative analysis of the ROIs (Figure 5, Table 2). After PLGA-NPs injection, the tumor was clearly visible in planar whole body images, with a signal that increased up to 24 h with a high contrast to noise ratio. Tumor accumulation of PLGA-NPs gradually decreased with time over 240 h p.i.

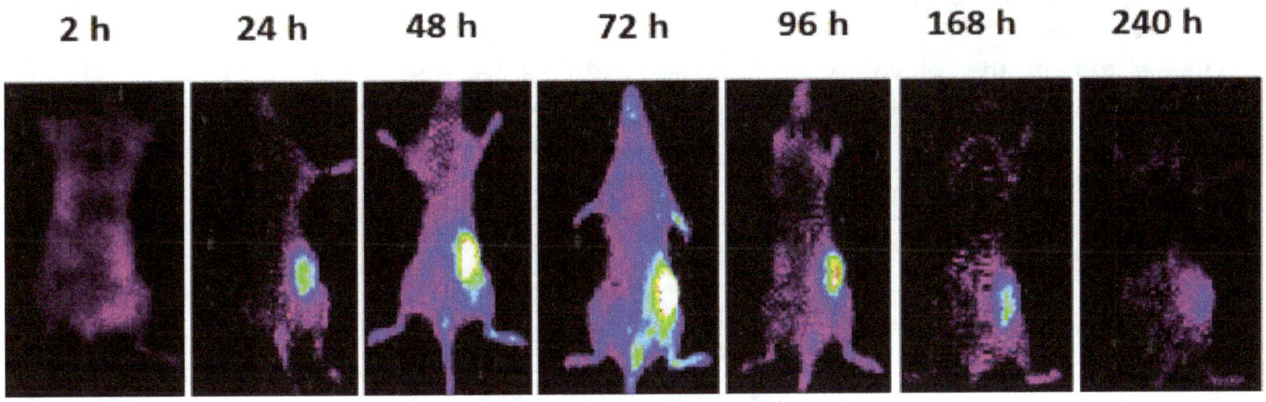

Figure 4. Whole body optical images of the same mouse bearing a subcutaneous syngeneic tumor at 2, 24, 48, 72, 96, 168, 240 h post-injection of 500 μg of fluorescent PLGA-NPs subcutaneously in the right flank.

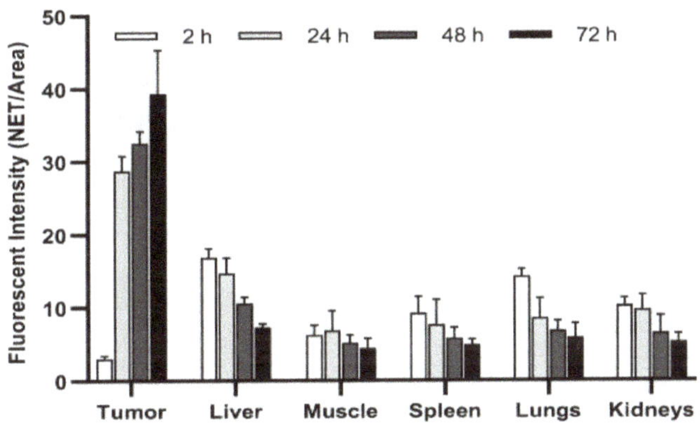

Figure 5. Biodistribution of PLGA-NPs in BALB/c mice. Data are expressed as average fluorescence (NET/Area) ± SD of five different mice per time point.

Table 2. Ex vivo fluorescence (NET/Area) of organs at different time points.

Parameter	2 h	24 h	48 h	72 h	*p*
	Mean ± SD (95% CI)	**Mean ± SD (95% CI)**	**Mean ± SD (95% CI)**	**Mean ± SD (95% CI)**	
Tumor *	3.03 ± 0.37 (2.58 to 3.49)	28.75 ± 2.02 (26.23 to 31.26)	32.58 ± 1.62 (30.57 to 34.59)	39.32 ± 5.95 (31.92 to 46.71)	**<0.0001**
Liver **	16.94 ± 1.19 (15.47 to 18.41)	14.67 ± 2.19 (11.94 to 17.39)	10.56 ± 0.85 (9.50 to 11.61)	7.26 ± 0.51 (6.62 to 7.89)	**<0.0001**
Muscle **	6.23 ± 1.34 (4.57 to 7.89)	6.83 ± 2.72 (3.46 to 10.21)	5.16 ± 1.05 (3.86 to 6.46)	4.39 ± 1.34 (2.73 to 6.05)	n.s.
Spleen	9.25 ± 2.19 (6.53 to 11.96)	7.64 ± 3.38 (3.44 to 11.84)	5.73 ± 1.52 (3.84 to 7.62)	4.84 ± 0.75 (3.90 to 5.77)	**0.02**
Lungs	14.22 ± 1.01 (12.96 to 15.48)	8.56 ± 2.64 (5.28 to 11.85)	6.83 ± 1.29 (5.22 to 8.44)	5.86 ± 1.92 (3.47 to 8.25)	**<0.0001**
Kidneys	10.21 ± 1.01 (8.96 to 11.46)	9.70 ± 1.96 (7.26 to 12.14)	6.49 ± 2.35 (3.58 to 9.40)	5.28 ± 1.08 (3.93 to 6.62)	**0.0006**

* $\log_{10}$ transformed; ** quadratic transformed; Tumor: post-hoc analysis: p (2 h vs. 24 h) **< 0.0001;** p (2 h vs. 48 h) **< 0.0001;** p (2 h vs. 72 h) **< 0.0001;** p (24 h vs. 72 h) = **0.0023;** Liver: post-hoc analysis: p (2 h vs. 24 h) = **0.042;** p (2 h vs. 48 h) **< 0.0001;** p (2 h vs. 72 h) **< 0.0001;** p (24 h vs. 48 h) = **0.0016;** p (24 h vs. 72 h) **< 0.0001;** Spleen: post-hoc analysis: p (2 h vs. 72 h) = **0.026;** Lungs: post-hoc analysis: p (2 h vs. 24 h) = **0.0008;** p (2 h vs. 48 h) **< 0.0001;** p (2 h vs. 72 h) **< 0.0001;** Kidneys: post-hoc analysis: p (2 h vs. 48 h) = **0.015;** p (2 h vs. 72 h) = **0.0015;** p (24 h vs. 48 h) = **0.039;** p (24 h vs. 72 h) = **0.004.** Bold: statistically significant ($p < 0.05$).

Ex vivo studies (Table 2) revealed that the main route of excretion is the liver due to the size of PLGA-NPs that exceed the glomerular filtration cut-off. However, fluorescence from the kidneys was also observed, probably due to the elimination of PLGA metabolites. In the blood circulation,

PLGA are cleared by the cells of the mononuclear phagocytic system (MPS), that are also present in lungs, thus explaining their mean IF.

The signal from the spleen, lungs, liver, and kidneys decreases from 2 h to 24 h, whereas the signal from the tumor increases with time. Imaging studies with PLGA-NPs and VEGF-PLGA-NPs are reported in Figure 6. Mice injected with VEGF-PLGA-NPs showed increased tumor uptake and higher T/M ratio if compared to PLGA-NPs (Figure 7, Table 3).

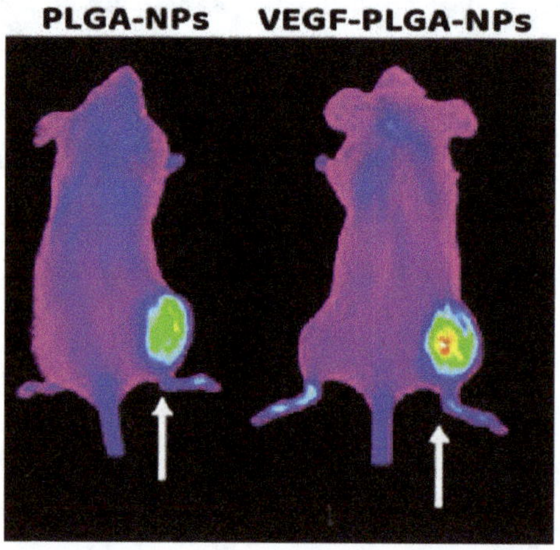

Figure 6. Whole body images of two mice bearing a syngeneic J744a.1 tumor in the right thigh and acquired 24 h post-injection (p.i.) of native PLGA-NPs (left) and VEGF-PLGA-NPs (right).

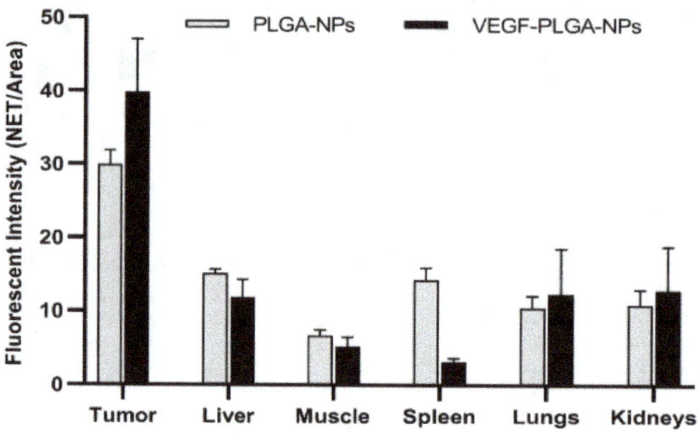

Figure 7. Comparative distribution of PLGA-NPs and VEGF-PLGA-NPs at 24 h post-injection (p.i.) in collected organs. Data are expressed as average fluorescence (NET/Area) ± SD of five different mice per group.

Table 3. fluorescence (NET/Area) of different organs at 24 h p.i. of PLGA-NPs and VEGF-PLGA-NPs.

Parameter	**PLGA-NPs**	**VEGF-PLGA-NPs**	***t* Test**
	Mean ± SD (95% CI)	**Mean ± SD (95% CI)**	**(*p*)**
Tumor °	29.95 ± 1.92 (27.56 to 32.33)	39.83 ± 7.17 (30.92 to 48.74)	**0.03**
Liver °	15.17 ± 0.55 (14.48 to 15.85)	11.86 ± 2.42 (5.84 to 17.88)	n.s.
Muscle	6.73 ± 0.73 (5.82 to 7.65)	5.18 ± 1.31 (3.56 to 6.80)	n.s.
Spleen °	14.29 ± 1.71 (12.18 to 16.41)	3.20 ± 0.44 (2.50 to 3.89)	**<0.0001**
Lungs °	10.53 ± 1.59 (8.55 to 12.50)	12.37 ± 6.24 (4.62 to 20.12)	n.s.
Kidneys	10.96 ± 2.03 (8.43 to 13.49)	12.92 ± 5.99 (5.48 to 20.36)	n.s.
T/M *	4.49 ± 0.54 (3.81 to 5.17)	7.90 ± 1.61 (5.90 to 9.90)	**0.0003**

* Inverse transformed; ° Satterthwaite correction. Bold: statistically significant ($p < 0.05$).

4. Discussion

Recently, biodegradable PLGA-NPs have been intensively investigated as carriers for drugs, peptides, and other molecules to treat cancer with low systemic toxicity [21,22]. However, nanoparticles are versatile molecules that could be also used for diagnostic imaging [23].

PLGA-NPs characteristics such as size, surface charge, and polymer composition, can be tuned to modify their in vivo biodistribution and make them suitable tools for different purposes [24,25].

For example, they could be even modified to enhance binding and active targeting to specific tumor antigens [26,27]. Given the many reports on the use of PLGA-NPs as a delivery system, we wanted to test the potential of specifically designed (lactic acid:glycolic acid ratio of 50:50, average size of 100–200 nm) NIR-fluorescent PLGA-NPs as theranostic tools for diagnosis and therapy of cancer. Preliminary results obtained by our group and confirmed by this study, showed that PLGA-NPs have suitable characteristics to be used as an in vivo targeting tool due to high accumulation in tumors thanks to the EPR effect. Indeed, high T/B ratios in tumors are achieved within 24 h p.i. of NIR-PLGA-NPs and reach their maximum at 72 h. To increase their accumulation in tumor lesions and reduce uptake in the liver and kidneys, we also developed fluorescent VEGF-conjugated NPs. Indeed, pathological neo-angiogenesis is involved in tumor growth and distant metastatization [28]. The angiogenic cytokines, as the vascular endothelial growth factor A (VEGF-A), are involved in the growth and remodeling of vessels in the tumor microenvironment [29–31]. Several targeted therapies based on VEGF/VEGFR signaling have been developed in different oncological diseases [32]. For example, the clinically approved anti-VEGF monoclonal antibody (mAb), bevacizumab, recognizes the free VEGF isoforms blocking their binding with VEGFR [33]. The anti-angiogenic tyrosine kinase inhibitors (TKIs), sorafenib, and sunitinib, were approved to target the VEGFR2, blocking the signaling cascade [34].

The clinical implications of VEGF-targeted therapies caused several benefits for the majority of patients, with the exception of a small fraction [35]. This highlighted the importance of angiogenic markers when it comes to theranostic. In literature PLGA-NPs are widely described as a delivery system, encapsulating inside the polymers drugs or molecules usually with the double emulsion-solvent evaporation technique or nanoprecipitation method [36–38]. VEGF molecules are usually encapsulated inside the PLGA-NPs for therapeutic purposes as therapeutic angiogenesis or tissue regeneration [39,40]. In the present study, we functionalized the surface of NIR-fluorescent PLGA-NPs with the rhVEGF-A165 analog to enhance their accumulation in tumors.

A similar approach has been described by Shi et al. that used recombinant human VEGF-C and achieved successful conjugation of the protein with NPs. However, their particle size was bigger than our (400 nm vs. 150 nm) and no biodistribution in vivo was shown [41].

Our results from DLS analysis showed a significant drop in the zeta potential from −37.6 mV (of PLGA-NPs) to −9.4 mV (of VEGF-PLGA-NPs). However, the zeta potential indicates the potential difference across the boundaries between liquid and solid phases. This value should be higher than +25 mV or lower than −25 mV to indicate good stability. In the range between +25mV and −25 mV it indicates poor or no stability. The zeta potential should be evaluated together with the PDI that shows the dispersity of NPs in the liquid suspension and should be closer to 0. This index reveals the degree of dispersion of NPs in suspension (PDI higher than 0.7 indicates polydisperse NPs and aggregates; PDI less than 0.5 indicates monodisperse NPs without aggregates) [42]. Our results showed that VEGF-NPs, despite a suboptimal zeta potential (−9.4 mV), have an excellent value of PDI (0.17) and therefore reasonably stable to be used for in vitro or in vivo studies.

In vitro binding studies to KDR-Fc, showed that, despite some non-specific interactions with the plastic surface, the binding of VEGF-PLGA-NPs to VEGF receptors (KDR-Fc) is specific. This result supports the finding of an increased T/M ratio of VEGF-PLGA-NPs if compared to PLGA-NPs. We also observed in vivo a lower uptake in other major organs (e.g., liver and spleen) and higher accumulation in kidneys. From a translational point of view, it would be very useful to have a diagnostic imaging probe that allows us to evaluate the degree of accumulation in tumors prior to administer the same NPs containing an anticancer drug. Fluorescent probes, despite their usefulness in pre-clinical applications, have limited penetration in tissues and are not suitable for human studies [43]. The limited penetration of light can be overcome by the use of radioactive isotopes, such as Copper-64 ($T_{1/2}$ = 12.7 h) for positron emission tomography (PET) or Technetium-99 m ($T_{1/2}$ = 6 h) for gamma-camera imaging [44]. Our study, showing high tumor accumulation of PLGA-NPs (with or without VEGF) within 24 h from injection, is preparatory for the development of radiolabeled NPs with diagnostic and/or therapeutic purposes, replacing the NIR-fluorescent probe. The use of radioisotopes, especially alfa or beta-emitters, poses a serious problem of liver and kidneys radiotoxicity and we believe that the added value of VEGF (or other targeting molecules) functionalization might mitigate this issue [45,46]. In this perspective, we selected for targeting studies the time point of 24 h p.i., as it matches with the half-life of most common diagnostic isotopes. Indeed, it would be of great interest to investigate later time points with VEGF-NPs, especially if radiolabeled with a therapeutic isotope, but priority should be given to test NPs radiolabeled with diagnostic isotopes to confirm the results obtained with optical imaging.

5. Conclusions

The use of PLGA as a delivery system for several drugs has already been approved by the FDA and several studies have focused on their design for this purpose. Despite the extensive work with the PLGA in the therapeutic field, they have not been extensively explored as an imaging tool in humans [47,48]. Despite the recent progress in nanomedicine, the imaging depth-limit of fluorescence does not allow the application of these NPs for human diagnostic purposes [49]. For this reason, our strategy was to use fluorescent-PLGA-NPs as screening probes to assess pharmacokinetic, tumor targeting, and T/M ratio of native and functionalized PLGA-NPs. Second step will be to develop radiolabeled NPs with translational potential.

In summary, our study confirms the potential of 50:50 100–200 nm PLGA-NPs as a theranostic tool in oncology. Functionalization with targeting molecules, such as VEGF, can increase their T/M ratio in vivo, but the replacement of fluorescent probes is mandatory to translate results in humans.

Author Contributions: Conceptualization—A.S., G.C. (Gabriela Capriotti), F.P., and M.V. Methodology—M.V., M.M., R.C., and F.G. Writing first draft—M.V., M.M., G.C. (Giuseppe Campagna), R.C., F.G. Final writing, review and editing of paper—A.S., F.P., and G.C. (Gabirela Capriotti). All authors have read and agreed to the published version of the manuscript.

References

1. Yohan, D.; Chithrani, B.D. Applications of nanoparticles in nanomedicine. *J. Biomed. Nanotechnol.* **2014**, *10*, 2371–2392. [CrossRef] [PubMed]
2. ASTM E2456-06 (2012), Standard Terminology Relating to Nanotechnology. ASTM International. Available online: www.astm.org (accessed on 1 May 2012).
3. Chu, K.S.; Hasan, W.; Rawal, S.; Walsh, M.D.; Enlow, E.M.; Luft, J.C.; Bridges, A.S.; Kuijer, J.L.; Napier, M.E.; Zamboni, W.C.; et al. Plasma, tumor and tissue pharmacokinetics of Docetaxel delivered via nanoparticles of different sizes and shapes in mice bearing SKOV-3 human ovarian carcinoma xenograft. *Nanomedicine* **2013**, *9*, 686–693. [CrossRef] [PubMed]
4. Tao, W.; Zeng, X.; Liu, T.; Wang, Z.; Xiong, Q.; Ouyang, C.; Huang, L.; Mei, L. Docetaxel-loaded nanoparticles based on star-shaped mannitol-core PLGA-TPCS diblock copolymer for breast cancer therapy. *Acta Biomater.* **2013**, *9*, 8910–8920. [CrossRef] [PubMed]
5. Chan, J.M.; Valencia, P.M.; Zhang, L.; Langer, R.; Farokhzad, O.C. Polymeric nanoparticles for drug delivery. *Methods Mol. Biol.* **2010**, *624*, 163–175. [PubMed]
6. Dinarvand, R.; Sepehri, N.; Manoochehri, S.; Rouhani, H.; Atyabi, F. Polylactide-co-glycolide nanoparticles for controlled delivery of anticancer agents. *Int. J. Nanomed.* **2011**, *6*, 877–895. [CrossRef]

7. Bobo, D.; Robinson, K.; Islam, J.; Thurecht, J.K.; Corrie, S.R. Nanoparticle-based medicines: A review of FDA-approved materials and clinical trials to date. *Pharm. Res.* **2016**, *33*, 2373–2387. [CrossRef]
8. Ernsting, M.J.; Murakami, M.; Roy, A.; Li, S.D. Factors controlling the pharmacokinetics, biodistribution and intratumoral penetration of nanoparticles. *J. Control. Release* **2013**, *172*, 782–794. [CrossRef]
9. Kulkarni, S.A.; Feng, S.S. Effects of particle size and surface modification on cellular uptake and biodistribution of polymeric nanoparticles for drug delivery. *Pharm. Res.* **2013**, *30*, 2512–2522. [CrossRef]
10. Greish, K. Enhanced permeability and retention (EPR) effect for anticancer nanomedicine drug targeting. *Methods Mol. Biol.* **2010**, *624*, 25–37.
11. Maeda, H.; Nakamura, H.; Fang, J. The EPR effect for macromolecular drug delivery to solid tumors: Improvement of tumor uptake, lowering of systemic toxicity, and distinct tumor imaging in vivo. *Adv. Drug Deliv. Rev.* **2013**, *65*, 71–79. [CrossRef]
12. Golombek, S.K.; May, J.N.; Theek, B.; Appold, L.; Drude, N.; Kiessling, F.; Lammers, T. Tumor targeting via EPR: Strategies to enhance patient responses. *Adv. Drug Deliv. Rev.* **2018**, *130*, 17–38. [CrossRef] [PubMed]
13. Lee, H.; Shields, A.F.; Siegel, B.A.; Miller, K.D.; Krop, I.; Ma, C.X.; LoRusso, P.M.; Munster, P.N.; Campbell, K.; Gaddy, D.F.; et al. 64Cu-MM-302 Positron Emission Tomography Quantifies Variability of Enhanced Permeability and Retention of Nanoparticles in Relation to Treatment Response in Patients with Metastatic Breast Cancer. *Clin. Cancer Res.* **2017**, *23*, 4190–4202. [CrossRef] [PubMed]
14. Baetke, S.C.; Lammers, T.; Kiessling, F. Applications of nanoparticles for diagnosis and therapy of cancer. *Br. J. Radiol.* **2015**, *88*, 20150207. [CrossRef]
15. Bi, Y.; Hao, F.; Yan, G.; Teng, L.; Lee, R.J.; Xie, J. Actively Targeted Nanoparticles for Drug Delivery to Tumor. *Curr. Drug Metab.* **2016**, *17*, 763–782. [CrossRef] [PubMed]
16. Carmeliet, P. VEGF as a key mediator of angiogenesis in cancer. *Oncology* **2005**, *69*, 4–10. [CrossRef] [PubMed]
17. Taurone, S.; Galli, F.; Signore, A.; Agostinelli, E.; Dierckx, R.A.J.O.; Minni, A.; Pucci, M.; Artico, M. VEGF in nuclear medicine: Clinical application in cancer and future perspectives. *Int. J. Oncol.* **2016**, *49*, 437–447. [CrossRef] [PubMed]
18. Ntziachristos, V.; Bremer, C.; Weissleder, R. Fluorescence imaging with near-infrared light: New technological advances that enable in vivo molecular imaging. *Eur. Radiol.* **2003**, *13*, 195–208. [CrossRef]
19. U.S. National Library of Medicine, Basic Local Alignment Search (BLAST®). Entrez Gene IDs: 7422 (Human); 22339 (Mouse). Available online: https://blast.ncbi.nlm.nih.gov/Blast.cgi (accessed on 3 April 2020).
20. Byrne, A.M.; Bouchier-Hayes, D.J.; Harmey, J.H. Angiogenic and cell survival functions of vascular endothelial growth factor (VEGF). *J. Cell Mol. Med.* **2005**, *9*, 777–794. [CrossRef]
21. Tian, J.; Min, Y.; Rodgers, Z.; Au, K.M.; Hagan, C.T.; Zhang, M.; Roche, K.; Yang, F.; Wagner, K.; Wang, A.Z. Co-delivery of paclitaxel and cisplatin with biocompatible PLGA-PEG nanoparticles enhances chemoradiotherapy in non-small cell lung cancer models. *J. Mater. Chem. B* **2017**, *5*, 6049–6057. [CrossRef]
22. Von Hoff, D.D.; Mita, M.M.; Ramanathan, R.K.; Weiss, G.J.; Mita, A.C.; Lo Russo, P.M.; Burris, H.A.; Hart, L.L.; Low, S.C.; Parsons, D.M.; et al. Phase I Study of PSMA-Targeted Docetaxel-Containing Nanoparticle BIND-014 in Patients with Advanced Solid Tumors. *Clin. Cancer Res.* **2016**, *22*, 3157–3163. [CrossRef]
23. Varani, M.; Galli, F.; Auletta, S.; Signore, A. Radiolabelled nanoparticles for cancer diagnosis. *Clin. Transl. Imaging* **2018**, *6*, 271–292. [CrossRef]
24. Pillai, G.J.; Greeshma, M.M.; Menon, D. Impact of poly(lactic-co-glycolic acid) nanoparticle surface charge on protein, cellular and haematological interactions. *Colloids Surf. B Biointerfaces* **2015**, *136*, 1058–1066. [CrossRef]
25. Fornaguera, C.; Calderó, G.; Mitjans, M.; Vinardell, M.P.; Solans, C.; Vauthier, C. Interactions of PLGA nanoparticles with blood components: Protein adsorption, coagulation, activation of the complement system and hemolysis studies. *Nanoscale* **2015**, *7*, 6045–6058. [CrossRef]
26. Karra, N.; Nassar, T.; Ripin, A.N.; Schwob, O.; Borlak, J.; Benita, S. Antibody conjugated PLGA nanoparticles for targeted delivery of paclitaxel palmitate: Efficacy and biofate in a lung cancer mouse model. *Small* **2013**, *9*, 4221–4236. [CrossRef] [PubMed]
27. Jahan, S.T.; Sadat, S.M.A.; Walliser, M.; Haddadi, A. Targeted Therapeutic Nanoparticles: An Immense Promise to Fight against Cancer. *J. Drug Deliv.* **2017**, *2017*, 9090325. [CrossRef] [PubMed]
28. Weidner, N.; Carroll, P.R.; Flax, J.; Blumenfeld, W.; Folkman, J. Tumor angiogenesis correlates with metastasis in invasive prostate carcinoma. *Am. J. Pathol.* **1993**, *143*, 401–409. [PubMed]

29. Fearnley, G.W.; Smith, G.A.; Abdul-Zani, I.; Yuldasheva, N.; Mughal, N.A.; Homer-Vanniasinkam, S.; Kearney, M.T.; Zachary, I.C.; Tomlinson, D.C.; Harrison, M.A.; et al. VEGF-A isoforms program differential VEGFR2 signal transduction, trafficking and proteolysis. *Biol. Open* **2016**, *5*, 571–583. [CrossRef] [PubMed]
30. Rydén, L.; Linderholm, B.; Nielsen, N.H.; Emdin, S.; Jönsson, P.E.; Landberg, G. Tumor specific VEGF-A and VEGFR2/KDR protein are co-expressed in breast cancer. *Breast Cancer Res. Treat.* **2003**, *82*, 147–154. [CrossRef]
31. Apte, R.S.; Chen, D.S.; Ferrara, N. VEGF in Signaling and Disease: Beyond Discovery and Development. *Cell* **2019**, *176*, 1248–1264. [CrossRef]
32. Ellis, L.M.; Hicklin, D.J. VEGF-targeted therapy: Mechanisms of anti-tumour activity. *Nat. Rev. Cancer* **2008**, *8*, 579–591. [CrossRef]
33. Ferrara, N.; Hillan, K.J.; Novotny, W. Bevacizumab (Avastin), a humanized anti-VEGF monoclonal antibody for cancer therapy. *Biochem. Biophys. Res. Commun.* **2005**, *333*, 328–335. [CrossRef] [PubMed]
34. Gotink, K.J.; Verheul, H.M. Anti-angiogenic tyrosine kinase inhibitors: What is their mechanism of action? *Angiogenesis* **2010**, *13*, 1–14. [CrossRef] [PubMed]
35. Lupo, G.; Caporarello, N.; Olivieri, M.; Cristaldi, M.; Motta, C.; Bramanti, V.; Avola, R.; Salmeri, M.; Nicoletti, F.; Anfuso, C.D. Anti-angiogenic Therapy in Cancer: Downsides and New Pivots for Precision Medicine. *Front Pharm.* **2017**, *7*, 519. [CrossRef] [PubMed]
36. Cohen-Sela, E.; Chorny, M.; Koroukhov, N.; Danenberg, H.D.; Golomb, G. A new double emulsion solvent diffusion technique for encapsulating hydrophilic molecules in PLGA nanoparticles. *J. Control. Release* **2009**, *133*, 90–95. [CrossRef]
37. Xie, H.; Smith, J.W. Fabrication of PLGA nanoparticles with a fluidic nanoprecipitation system. *J. Nanobiotechnol.* **2010**, *8*, 18. [CrossRef] [PubMed]
38. Karal-Yılmaz, O.; Serhatlı, M.; Baysal, K.; Baysal, B.M. Preparation and in vitro characterization of vascular endothelial growth factor (VEGF)-loaded poly (D,L-lactic-co-glycolic acid) microspheres using a double emulsion/solvent evaporation technique. *J. Microencapsul.* **2011**, *28*, 46–54. [CrossRef]
39. Rui, J.; Dadsetan, M.; Runge, M.B.; Spinner, R.J.; Yaszemski, M.J.; Windebank, A.J.; Wang, H. Controlled release of vascular endothelial growth factor using poly-lactic-co-glycolic acid microspheres: In vitro characterization and application in polycaprolactone fumarate nerve conduits. *Acta Biomater.* **2012**, *8*, 511–518. [CrossRef]
40. Jiang, X.; Lin, H.; Jiang, D.; Xu, G.; Fang, X.; He, L.; Xu, M.; Tang, B.; Wang, Z.; Cui, D.; et al. Co-delivery of VEGF and bFGF via a PLGA nanoparticle-modified BAM for effective contracture inhibition of regenerated bladder tissue in rabbits. *Sci. Rep.* **2016**, *6*, 20784. [CrossRef]
41. Shi, Y.; Zhou, M.; Zhang, J.; Lu, W. Preparation and cellular targeting study of VEGF-conjugated PLGA nanoparticles. *J. Microencapsul.* **2015**, *32*, 699–704. [CrossRef]
42. Kumar, A.; Dixit, C.K. *Methods for characterization of nanoparticles. Advances in Nanomedicine for the Delivery of Therapeutic Nucleic Acids*; Woodhead Publishing: Sawston, UK; Cambridge, UK, 2017; pp. 43–58.
43. Coll, J.L. Cancer optical imaging using fluorescent nanoparticles. *Nanomedicine* **2011**, *6*, 7–10. [CrossRef]
44. Weissleder, R.; Pittet, M.J. Imaging in the era of molecular oncology. *Nature* **2008**, *452*, 580–589. [CrossRef]
45. Raja, C.; Graham, P.; Rizvi, S.; Song, E.; Goldsmith, H.; Thompson, J.; Bosserhoff, A.; Morgenstern, A.; Apostolidis, C.; Kearsley, J.; et al. Interim analysis of toxicity and response in phase 1 trial of systemic targeted alpha therapy for metastatic melanoma. *Cancer Biol. Ther.* **2007**, *6*, 846–852. [CrossRef] [PubMed]
46. Galli, F.; Artico, M.; Taurone, S.; Manni, S.; Bianchi, E.; Piaggio, G.; Weintraub, B.D.; Szkudlinski, M.W.; Agostinelli, E.; Dierckx, R.A.J.O.; et al. Radiolabeling of VEGF165 with 99mTc to evaluate VEGFR expression in tumor angiogenesis. *Int. J. Oncol.* **2017**, *50*, 2171–2179. [CrossRef] [PubMed]
47. Jain, A.K.; Das, M.; Swarnakar, N.K.; Jain, S. Engineered PLGA nanoparticles: An emerging delivery tool in cancer therapeutics. *Crit. Rev. Ther. Drug Carrier Syst.* **2011**, *28*, 1–45. [CrossRef] [PubMed]
48. Lü, J.M.; Wang, X.; Marin-Muller, C.; Wang, H.; Lin, P.H.; Yao, Q.; Chen, C. Current advances in research and clinical applications of PLGA-based nanotechnology. *Expert Rev. Mol. Diagn.* **2009**, *9*, 325–341. [CrossRef] [PubMed]
49. Pratiwi, F.W.; Kuo, C.W.; Chen, B.C.; Chen, P. Recent advances in the use of fluorescent nanoparticles for bioimaging. *Nanomedicine* **2019**, *14*, 1759–1769. [CrossRef] [PubMed]

10

Comparison of White Blood Cell Scintigraphy, FDG PET/CT and MRI in Suspected Diabetic Foot Infection: Results of a Large Retrospective Multicenter Study

Chiara Lauri [1,2], Andor W.J.M. Glaudemans [2], Giuseppe Campagna [1], Zohar Keidar [3], Marina Muchnik Kurash [3], Stamata Georga [4], Georgios Arsos [4], Edel Noriega-Álvarez [5], Giuseppe Argento [6], Thomas C. Kwee [2], Riemer H.J.A. Slart [2,7] and Alberto Signore [1,2,*]

1 Nuclear Medicine Unit, Department of Medical-Surgical Sciences and of Translational Medicine, "Sapienza" University of Rome, 00161 Rome, Italy; chialau84@hotmail.it (C.L.); gius.campagna@gmail.com (G.C.)
2 Department of Nuclear Medicine and Molecular Imaging, University of Groningen, University Medical Center Groningen, 9700 Groningen, The Netherlands; a.w.j.m.glaudemans@umcg.nl (A.W.J.M.G.); t.c.kwee@umcg.nl (T.C.K.); r.h.j.a.slart@umcg.nl (R.H.J.A.S.)
3 Department of Nuclear Medicine, Rambam Health Care Campus, 3109601 Haifa, Israel; z_keidar@rambam.health.gov.il (Z.K.); kurash.marina@gmail.com (M.M.K.)
4 3rd Department of Nuclear Medicine, Aristotle University Medical School, Papageorgiou General Hospital, 56403 Thessaloniki, Greece; matageorga@gmail.com (S.G.); garsos@auth.gr (G.A.)
5 Department of Nuclear Medicine, University Hospital of Ciudad Real, 13005 Ciudad Real, Spain; edelnoriega@gmail.com
6 Radiology Unit, Sant'Andrea University Hospital, 00189 Rome, Italy; giuseppe.argento@uniroma1.it
7 Department of Biomedical Photonic Imaging, Faculty of Science and Technology, University of Twente, 7500 Enschede, The Netherlands
* Correspondence: alberto.signore@uniroma1.it

Abstract: Diabetic foot infections (DFIs) represent one of the most frequent and disabling morbidities of longstanding diabetes; therefore, early diagnosis is mandatory. The aim of this multicenter retrospective study was to compare the diagnostic accuracy of white blood cell scintigraphy (WBC), ^{18}F-fluorodeoxyglucose positron emission tomography/computed tomography ((^{18}F) FDG PET/CT), and Magnetic Resonance Imaging (MRI) in patients with suspected DFI. Images and clinical data from 251 patients enrolled by five centers were collected in order to calculate the sensitivity, specificity, and accuracy of WBC, FDG, and MRI in diagnosing osteomyelitis (OM), soft-tissue infection (STI), and Charcot osteoarthropathy. In OM, WBC acquired following the European Society of Nuclear Medicine (EANM) guidelines was more specific and accurate than MRI (91.9% vs. 70.7%, $p < 0.0001$ and 86.2% vs. 67.1%, $p = 0.003$, respectively). In STI, both FDG and WBC achieved a significantly higher specificity than MRI (97.9% and 95.7% vs. 83.6%, $p = 0.04$ and $p = 0.018$, respectively). In Charcot, both MRI and WBC demonstrated a significantly higher specificity and accuracy than FDG (88.2% and 89.3% vs. 62.5%, $p = 0.0009$; 80.3% and 87.9% vs. 62.1%, $p < 0.02$, respectively). Moreover, in Charcot, WBC was more specific than MRI (89.3% vs. 88.2% $p < 0.0001$). Given the limitations of a retrospective study, WBC using EANM guidelines was shown to be the most reliable imaging modality to differentiate between OM, STI, and Charcot in patients with suspected DFI.

Keywords: diabetic foot; infection; diagnosis; WBC scintigraphy; FDG PET/CT; MRI

1. Introduction

Diabetes-related foot complications represent some of the most frequent and disabling morbidities of longstanding diabetes and are associated with prolonged hospitalization and high social costs [1–5]. Patients with peripheral neuropathy and microvascular impairment have an increased risk of developing an ulcer that could represent a breach for the entry of bacteria, thus potentially causing an infection. The process initially involves the soft tissues (STs) of the foot, and later it could spread in depth for contiguity and reach the bone, leading to diabetic foot osteomyelitis (DFO). Osteomyelitis (OM) is a severe complication for the diabetic patient, with a high risk of amputation and mortality rates [6–8]. Considering that more than 50% of wounds are infected at their presentation [2], the prevention of foot ulcers, early diagnosis, and appropriate and prompt treatment are mandatory in order to avoid such a complication and amputation [9,10]. Moreover, about 2.5% of diabetic patients have a Charcot foot, a progressive degenerative disease of the musculoskeletal system characterized by destruction of the bony architecture, which usually involves tarsal and metatarsal joints [11]. The presence of this neuro-ostearthropathy further complicates the diagnostic approach to diabetic foot infection (DFI) since this condition may coexist with the presence of ulcers, thus making the correct diagnosis difficult to achieve. Nevertheless, a differential diagnosis between Charcot, OM, and soft tissue infection (STI) is crucial for the correct management in patients suspected of DFI.

The gold standard examination for the diagnosis of OM is represented by the isolation of the pathogen using microbiological assays. Bone biopsy, however, is an invasive procedure and its reliability strongly depends on the quality of the specimen obtained in the aseptic procedure. Moreover, clinical examination and biochemical inflammatory markers are often non-specific and do not allow a differentiation between infection and inflammation [12,13]. Several diagnostic imaging tests are currently available, including both radiological and nuclear medicine (NM) non-invasive imaging modalities. Despite a consensus document for the diagnosis of peripheral bone infections being recently published, it does not specifically address DFI [14]. Therefore, at present, no clear consensus on the most appropriate imaging technique in suspected DFI exists [7,15,16]. Magnetic resonance imaging (MRI) is the best radiological modality for the assessment of soft tissue abnormalities and may be able to differentiate between STI and OM. However, its specificity can be reduced in the presence of bone marrow edema, synovial effusion, dislocation, bony destruction, and loss of discernible bone and joint margins since they may characterize neuropathic joint disease as well as OM [17]. The NM gold standard in this field is represented by white blood cell scintigraphy (WBC), which provides an in vivo demonstration of the presence of the infective focus. The European Society of Nuclear Medicine (EANM) has previously published guidelines [14,18–22], aiming to define the correct labelling procedure, acquisition, and interpretation criteria for WBC. However, currently, not all institutes follow these recommended standards. The use of ^{18}F-fluorodeoxyglucose ((^{18}F) FDG) positron emission tomography combined with computed tomography (PET/CT) has gained a role in several indications in the field of infection and inflammation [21]. This technique is widely available and has the advantages of a short acquisition time, high image resolution, and no need of blood handling and manipulation. FDG, however, accumulates in both infection and sterile inflammation since all the involved cells use glucose as a source of energy [21]. Therefore, it is not clear if FDG PET/CT is adequate enough to discriminate among the different foot complications in diabetic patients [15]. In a recently published systematic review and meta-analysis comparing WBC, FDG PET/CT, and MRI in DFO, it emerged that the sensitivity is approximately 90% for all imaging modalities, with ^{99m}Technetium-hexamethylpropyleneamine oxime (^{99m}Tc-HMPAO)-labelled WBC scintigraphy demonstrating the highest specificity, followed by FDG PET/CT, MRI, and ^{111}Indium (^{111}In) oxine-labelled WBC [23].

To the best of our knowledge, no multicenter studies are available in the literature comparing these imaging modalities. Therefore, the aim of this retrospective study was to compare the accuracy of WBC scintigraphy, FDG PET/CT, and MRI in differentiating OM, STI, and Charcot in patients with suspected DFI. In particular, our primary end point was to evaluate the diagnostic approaches adopted among different centers in daily practice, aiming to provide a panoramic view on the diagnostic management in different countries. Moreover, since it is well known that the accuracy of WBC scintigraphy relies on the application of the correct acquisitions protocols, image display, and interpretation criteria, the secondary end point of this study was to evaluate, on a multicenter scale, the impact of recently published EANM guidelines [20] on the diagnosis of DFI.

2. Experimental Section

2.1. Materials and Methods

This retrospective multicenter study included five centers from The Netherlands, Italy, Israel, Greece, and Spain. Data from consecutive patients affected by diabetic foot complications between June 2008 and June 2014 were locally collected by each center, then merged in a single central database, and processed using SPSS statistic software. This study was approved by each local ethical committee and of the coordinating center (Groningen, the Netherlands).

2.1.1. Patients

Patients were retrospectively recruited by radiology and NM departments of each center where they were sent by the respective local diabetic foot units (DFUs), between 2008 and 2014, for the study of suspected DFI. The following inclusion and exclusion criteria were adopted in this study:

Inclusion criteria (the first four items were mandatory):

- Type 1 or type 2 diabetes treated with oral medications or insulin;
- Suspected DFI based on clinical presentation of foot wounds according to Perfusion, Extent, Depth, Infection, Sensation of Infectious Diseases Society of America (PEDIS/IDSA) classification [1];
- At least one out of the three imaging modalities performed for suspected DFI;
- Final diagnosis provided by gold standard;
- Bony abnormalities detected by plain radiographs;
- Palpable bone at "probe-to-bone test" (in presence of open wounds);
- Raised inflammatory markers.

Exclusion criteria:

- Lack of information on final diagnosis;
- Patients lost at clinical follow-up.

Demographic and laboratory data, including gender, age, type of diabetes, medical history, biochemistry, microbiology, histopathology, treatments, and final diagnosis, were collected by each center. In patients in whom more than one infection was investigated, each episode was considered as an individual event with corresponding imaging.

Patients were clinically or surgically managed by the DFUs of each center following their own protocols.

2.1.2. Imaging Modalities and Analysis

Information regarding the camera type, manufacturer, year of manufactory, the use of markers or contrast, details of the compounds, and sequences for MRI were recorded. For NM examinations, information on radiopharmaceutical, administered activity, type of gamma-camera, equipped or not with single-photon emission tomography/computed tomography (SPECT/CT), PET/CT camera systems, and exact protocols of acquisition were also specified by each center. All acquisition details and DICOM files had to be available in order to include the patients in the study. NM images were examined by two experienced NM physicians. Discordant cases were resolved by consensus. All MRI scans were evaluated by an experienced radiologist. All readers were blinded for clinical details. The following scoring method was used for each diagnostic tool in order to classify the outcome: 0 = negative/sterile inflammation; 1 = OM; 2 = STI; 3 = Charcot. If two or more conditions were concomitant in the same patient, the most clinically relevant was considered (e.g., OM + Charcot = OM; OM + STI = OM; STI + Charcot = STI).

For each scan, the location of disease (in forefoot or mid/hindfoot) was recorded.

2.1.3. Interpretation Criteria for WBC Scintigraphy

- Acquired according to EANM recommendations: Interpretation criteria were used as recommended by the guidelines [20] and obtained by both visual and, in equivocal cases, semi-quantitative analysis by drawing region of interests (ROIs) on target (T) and contralateral side as background (B) in order to calculate the T/B ratio. OM was defined when WBC focal accumulation at 20–24 h was higher in intensity than at 3–4 h. STI was defined when WBC focal or diffuse accumulation at 20–24 h was lower than at 3–4 h. Charcot was defined when diffuse WBC accumulation at 20–24 h was similar or decreased compared to the uptake at 3–4 h.
- Acquired not according to EANM recommendation: In the case scans were performed with only one time point acquisition, they were classified as follows: OM was defined when the WBC focal accumulation was higher than surrounding tissues. STI was defined when WBC accumulation (both focal or diffuse) was observed in the superficial regions of the foot. Charcot was defined when diffuse WBC accumulation at the mid/hindfoot was observed.

2.1.4. Interpretation Criteria for FDG PET/CT

FDG PET/CT assessment was performed using a visual analysis describing the target areas in terms of intensity (grade 0: no uptake; grade 1: uptake at foot location = contralateral side; grade 2: uptake at foot location > contralateral side), pattern of uptake (focal vs. diffuse), number of foci, and the exact localization of the increased uptake as provided by the CT. We also performed a semi-quantitative analysis using the maximum and mean standardized uptake values (SUVmax, SUVmean) of each area with increased uptake. The SUV_{max} ratio (SUV_{max} of target/SUV_{max} contralateral background) was also calculated. OM was defined when focal or diffuse FDG uptake higher than the contralateral side was visible on the bone structure with or without soft tissue involvement. STI was defined when focal or diffuse FDG uptake (grade 1 or 2) was visible only in the soft tissues without bony involvement. Charcot was defined when diffuse FDG uptake (grade 1 or 2) was visible involving tarsal and metatarsal joints and associated with bone destruction on CT.

2.1.5. Interpretation Criteria for MRI

MRI was evaluated for primary and secondary signs of OM, according to the literature [24–26]. Briefly, OM was defined in the presence of low medullary bone marrow signal in a geographic confluent pattern on T1-weighted imaging (T1w), concordant with abnormal (high) signal at fat-suppressed T2-weighted (T2w) and post-gadolinium (Gd) T1w imaging.

Secondary signs of OM were also evaluated [24]:

(a) Ulcer (skin interruption with raised margins and associated soft tissue defect);
(b) Sinus tract ("tram track" pattern post-Gd enhancement);
(c) Cellulitis (skin thickening and soft tissue edema with low T1 and T2 signal and post-Gd enhancement);
(d) Abscesses (signal intensity of fluid with post-Gd peripheral rim-like enhancement);
(e) Gangrene (post-Gd non-enhancing area of devitalized tissue that is sharply demarcated from surrounding viable tissue, without (dry gangrene) or with air bubbles in the soft tissue (wet gangrene));
(f) Tenosynovitis (area of post-Gd peri-tendinous enhancement coursing through an area of cellulitis and adjacent to an infected ulcer).

STI was considered present if at least one of the previously described findings was observed without any radiological signs of bone involvement. Charcot was defined as the presence of soft tissue edema, fluid collections, effusions, bone marrow abnormalities, post-Gd peri-articular soft-tissue, and bone marrow enhancement (typically in the tarsal-metatarsal and metatarsal-phalangeal joints), associated with deformities and osseous fragmentation.

2.1.6. Therapeutic Management

The different therapeutic strategies adopted by the DFUs of each local center were recorded when available, and were classified as follows:

- No treatment (including offloading);
- Conventional wound care and topic antibiotic treatment;
- Systemic antibiotic treatment;
- Surgery (debridement or amputation).

When possible, the results of the three imaging modalities were correlated with the treatment received by the patient.

2.1.7. Gold Standard

Bone biopsies were used as gold standard for the final diagnosis of OM and Charcot, independently by the availability of the isolated pathogen. Skin cultures were used for the diagnosis of STI. When bone biopsies or skin cultures were not available, a clinical follow-up of at least 12 months was used in order to confirm or rule out the diagnosis achieved with imaging modalities.

2.1.8. Statistical Analysis

All statistical analyses were performed using SAS version 9.4 and JMP version 14 (SAS Institute, Cary, NC, USA). Categorical variables are expressed as absolute frequencies and percentages. Continuous variables (SUV_{max} and SUV_{max} ratio) are presented in mean ± standard deviation (SD) mean differences across groups (OM, STI, and Charcot) and were compared by generalized linear models. The normality of the residuals was verified by Shapiro–Wilk test and homoscedasticity by the Levene and Brown–Forsythe test. Differences between the final diagnosis (no pathology, OM, and STI) vs. C-reactive protein (CRP) and erythrocytes sedimentation rate (ESR) were evaluated by the Kruskal–Wallis test and Steel–Dwass test using post hoc analysis. The sensitivity, specificity, and diagnostic accuracy of all the three imaging modalities in diagnosing OM, STI, and Charcot foot against the reference standard histology and/or clinical follow-up were performed by routine use of SAS. Comparisons of the sensitivity, specificity, and diagnostic accuracy between the three imaging modalities were performed using the Z test for the equality of two proportions. The Benjamini–Hochberg procedure was applied to check multiple comparisons. The results are reported in a percentage with 95% confidence intervals (CIs). A p-value <0.05 was considered statistically significant.

3. Results

A total of 251 patients were enrolled in the contributing five centers (Scheme 1). A descriptive analysis of our population is summarized in Table 1.

Post hoc analysis on median values of CRP and ESR showed that they were both significantly higher in patients with OM compared with patients without any infection ($p = 0.017$ and $p = 0.027$ respectively) as illustrated in Figure 1. No similar significant difference was observed between patients with STI and normal subjects and between patients with OM and STI.

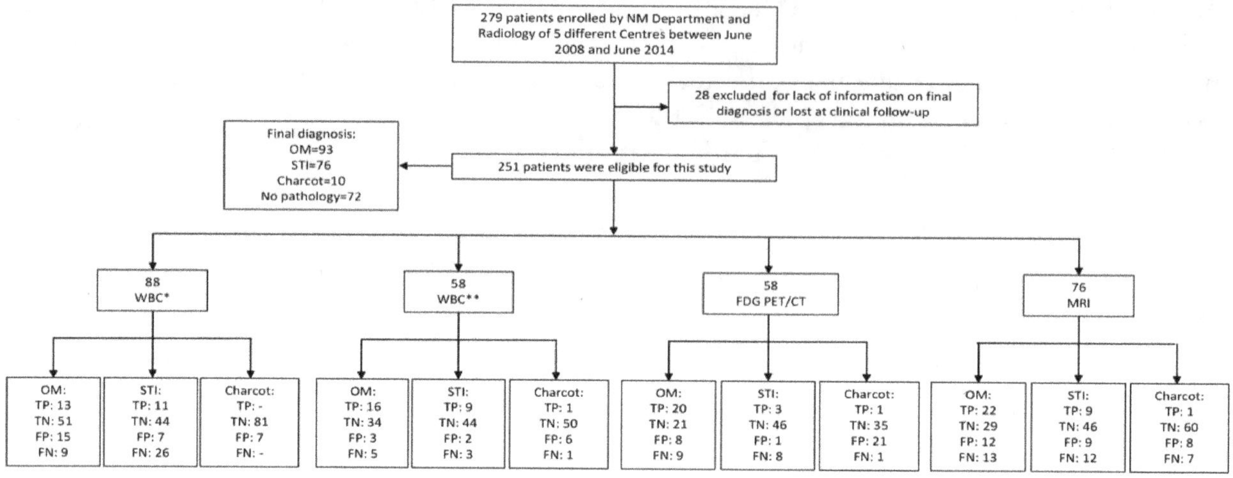

Scheme 1. Flow chart on patient selection and imaging modalities. NM: Nuclear Medicine; OM: osteomyelitis; STI: soft tissue infection; WBC: white blood cells scintigraphy; * WBC scans acquired without following European Association of Nuclear Medicine (EANM) guidelines; ** WBC scans acquired following EANM guidelines; ^{18}F-fluorodeoxyglucose positron emission tomography/computed tomography (FDG PET/CT); Magnetic Resonance Imaging (MRI); TP: true positives; TN: true negatives; FP: false positives; FN: false negatives; - no patients with a final diagnosis of Charcot foot were studied with * WBC scan.

Table 1. General characteristics of the study population.

	Age (Years) (Mean ± SD)	Gender (F/M) (%)	DM1/DM2 (%)	Glycaemia (mmol/L) (Mean ± SD)	Hb1Ac (%) (Mean ± SD)	ESR (mm/h) (Mean ± SD)	CRP (mg/L) (Mean ± SD)
All patients (251)	60.7 ± 10.8	34.3/65.7	17.1/82.9	9.1 ± 3.4	8.0 ± 1.9	47.3 ± 28.5	43.0 ± 73.1
WBC * (88)	64.2 ± 10.9	44.3/55.7	15.9/84.1	8.5 ± 2.8	7.7 ± 1.6	45.6 ± 28.0	14.3 ± 32.8
WBC ** (58)	57.2 ± 10.3	32.7/67.3	15.5/84.5	9.7 ± 4.2	9.2 ± 2.6	56.6 ± 35.9	73.4 ± 58.6
MRI (76)	59.2 ± 10.6	25.0/75.0	22.4/77.6	10.5 ± 4.0	8.2 ± 2. 2	48.2 ± 27.5	87.4 ± 100
FDG (58)	58.0 ± 9.0	29.3/70.7	10.3/89.7	7.8 ± 2.6	8.3 ± 1.9	n.r.	n.r.
OM (93)	59.6 ± 11.1	26.9/73.1	20.4/79.6	9.5 ± 3.3	8.4 ± 1.9	55.9 ± 32.1	68.3 ± 93.7
STI (76)	62.3 ± 10.01	38.1/61.9	19.7/80.3	9.0 ± 3.6	7.8 ± 1.7	46.7 ± 26.9	27.9 ± 53.4
Charcot (10)	56.5 ± 10.1	20.0/80.0	20.0/80.0	n.r.	7.4 ± 1.7	n.r.	42.8 ± 71.5
No pathology (72)	60.7 ± 10.9	43.0/57.0	9.7/90.3	8.5 ± 3.2	7.7 ± 1.9	37.6 ± 23.1	27.7 ± 53.7

In brackets: number of patients; SD: Standard Deviation; F: females; M: males; DM1: Type 1 Diabetes Mellitus; DM2: Type 2 Diabetes Mellitus; Hb1Ac: glycated hemoglobin; ESR: Erythrocytes Sedimentation Rate; CRP: C Reactive Protein; * WBC: scans acquired without following EANM guidelines; ** WBC: scans acquired following EANM guidelines; n.r: not reliable because data available in less than 10 patients. MRI, magnetic resonance imaging; FDG, fluorodeoxyglucose; OM: osteomyelitis; STI: soft tissue infection; WBC: white blood cells scintigraphy; EANM, European Society of Nuclear Medicine.

Causative pathogens were recorded in 67 patients that underwent skin cultures, and in 14 out of 50 patients who performed (pre- or intra-operative) biopsy; however, biopsy was used as a gold standard for final diagnosis in the other 36 patients in which we could not obtain information on the pathogen causing the infection. In the remaining 121 patients, final diagnosis was assessed with clinical follow-up (see Table 2). OM was found in 93 patients, STI in 76, and Charcot in 10 patients. The remaining 72 subjects had no pathology according the reference standard. Regarding the imaging modalities, 119 patients underwent a WBC scintigraphy, 46 FDG PET/CT, and 59 patients underwent MRI. In 10 patients, both WBC and FDG PET/CT were performed; in 15 patients, both WBC scintigraphy and MRI; and in 2 patients, all three imaging techniques were performed. The diagnostic performances of the three imaging modalities are summarized in Table 3.

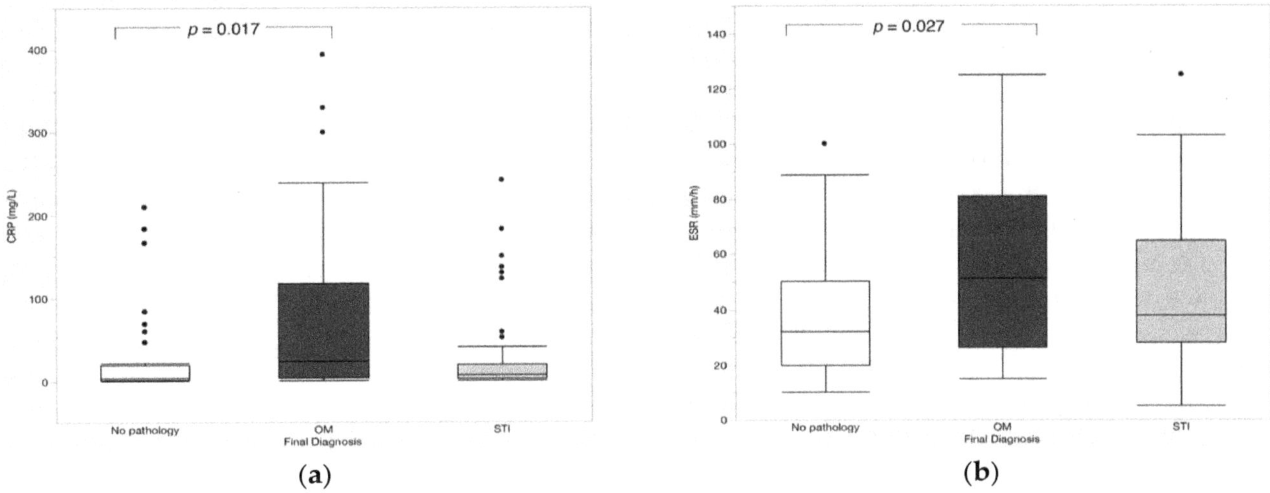

Figure 1. Box plots of C-reactive protein (CRP) (**a**) and erythrocyte sedimentation rate (ESR) (**b**) showing significantly higher values of CRP (median value 24.0 mg/L; min to max: 1–393.80) and ESR (median value 51.5 mm/h; min to max: 15.0–125) compared with non-infected patients (median values of CRP: 4.5 mg/L; min to max: 1–210); median values of ESR: 32.0; min to max: 10–100). OM: osteomyelitis; STI: soft tissue infection.

Table 2. Microbiology and histopathological findings.

Cultures from Aspirates (in 67 Patients)	Cultures from Bone Biopsies (in 14 Patients)
Negative: 13.4% *Staph. aureus*: 26.9% *Polymicrobial*: 23.8% *Strept. epidermidis*: 10.4% *P. aeruginosa*: 7.5% *Acinetobacter*: 4.5% *Staph. haemolyticus*: 4.5% *E. faecalis*: 3.0% *Proteus mirabilis*: 1.5% *E. coli*: 1.5% *Strept. agalactiae*: 1.5% *Citrobacter freundii*: 1.5%	Negative: 28.6% *Polymicrobial*: 28.6% *Staph. aureus*: 28.6% *Pseud. aeruginosa*: 14.2%

Table 3. Overview of the performance of diagnostic imaging tests in detecting OM, STI, and Charcot.

	Sensitivity (%) (95% CI)	Specificity (%) (95% CI)	Accuracy (%) (95% CI)
OM (WBC *)	59.1 (38.5–79.6)	77.3 (67.2–87.4)	72.7 (63.4–82.0)
STI (WBC *)	29.7 (15.0–44.5)	86.3 (76.8–95.7)	62.5 (52.4–72.6)
Charcot (WBC *)	n.c.	92.0 (86.4–97.7)	n.c.
OM (WBC-EANM **)	76.2 (58.0–94.4)	91.9 (83.1–100)	86.2 (77.3–95.1)
STI (WBC-EANM **)	75.0 (50.5–99.5)	95.7 (88.9–100)	91.4 (84.2–98.6)
Charcot (WBC-EANM **)	n.c.	89.3 (81.2–97.4)	87.9 (79.5–96.3)
OM (FDG PET/CT)	69.0 (52.1–85.8)	72.4 (56.1–88.7)	70.7 (59.0–82.4)
STI (FDG PET/CT)	27.3 (1.0–54.0)	97.9 (93.7–100)	84.5 (75.2–93.8)
Charcot (FDG PET/CT)	n.c.	62.5 (49.8–75.2)	62.1 (49.6–74.6)
OM (MRI)	62.9 (46.8–78.9)	70.7 (56.8–84.7)	67.1 (56.5–77.7)
STI (MRI)	42.9 (21.7–64.0)	83.6 (73.9–93.4)	72.4(62.3–82.4)
Charcot (MRI)	n.c.	88.2 (80.6–95.9)	80.3 (71.3–89.2)

* WBC scans acquired without following EANM guidelines; ** WBC scans acquired following EANM guidelines; n.c. = not calculated because of the low number of patients. FDG PET/CT, fluorodeoxyglucose positron emission tomography/computed tomography.

3.1. WBC Scintigraphy

The mean administered activity of ^{99m}Tc-radiolabelled leukocytes was 569.8 ± 116.5 MBq (15.4 ± 3.15 mCi).

Since a significant discrepancy was observed among the different centers regarding the acquisition procedure, we compared the results obtained by centers that applied EANM guidelines with those who did not follow these recommendations. Fifty-eight scans were acquired according to the EANM guidelines for WBC scintigraphy with acquisition times corrected for Tc-99m decay at two (4 and 24 h) or three times points (30′, 3 h, and 20 h) [20] (Figure 2). Eighty-eight scans did not follow these recommendations; in particular, 73 scans (83.0%) were acquired only 4 h post injection (p.i.) and 15 (17.0%) were acquired at 2 time points, 1 and 4 h p.i. Furthermore, given the low number of patients who performed combined SPECT/CT in these two groups that did not allow us to make a comparative analysis, we considered only planar images for the diagnosis, thus exploring the importance of multiple time-point acquisitions.

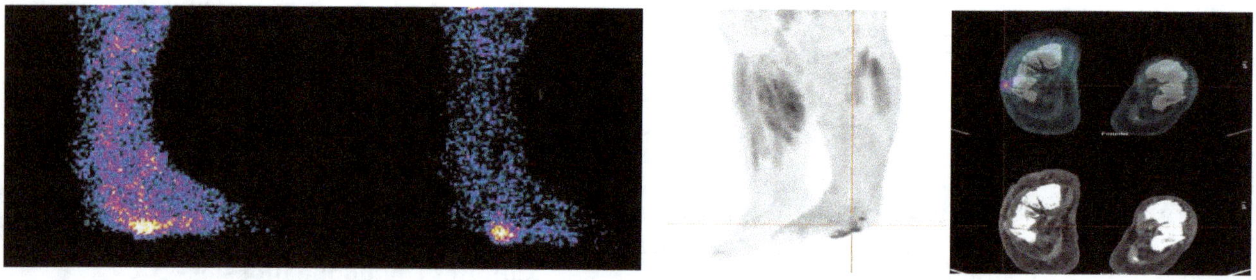

(a) (b)

Figure 2. (**a**) Planar images of the WBC scan acquired with correction for ^{99m}Technetium (^{99m}Tc) decay at 3 h (on the left) and 20 h (on the right). The focal uptake of labelled leukocytes detectable on the plantar surface of the left foot decreases between the 3 and 20 h images, being consistent with the diagnosis of STI; (**b**) Multi Intensity Projection (MIP) and transaxial views of FDG PET/CT, of the same patient, show the focal uptake in the plantar surface of the left foot in correspondence with a cutaneous/subcutaneous ulcer of the soft tissues. Bone and soft tissue biopsies confirmed the diagnosis of STI and the patient was treated with topic antibiotic therapy. WBC: white blood cells scintigraphy; FDG PET/CT, fluorodeoxyglucose positron emission tomography/computed tomography.

The sensitivity, specificity, and accuracy of the labelled WBC planar images of the two groups are reported in Table 3.

3.2. FDG PET/CT.

FDG PET/CT scans were generally acquired 60 min after the injection of approximately 3 MBq (0.08 mCi)/kg of FDG according to EANM guidelines [21]. Both qualitative assessment (intensity and pattern of uptake) and semiquantitative analysis of FDG uptake were performed (Table 4).

Table 4. Pattern of FDG PET/CT in the study population.

Final Diagnosis	Intensity		SUV_{max} (Mean ± SD [1])	SUV_{max} Ratio (Mean ± SD [1])
	Focal Uptake (%)	Diffuse Uptake (%)		
OM	62.1	37.9	5.3 ± 2.1	3.9 ± 2.4
STI	54.5	45.5	5.4 ± 1.8	4.2 ± 2.1
Charcot	0	100	4.9 ± 1.9	4.9 ± 1.6

[1] SD: Standard deviation.

In total, 96.5% of patients with a final diagnosis of OM (29 patients) showed "grade 2 uptake" that was focal in 62.1% (18 patients) of cases and diffuse in the remaining 37.9% (11 patients). The mean values of the SUV_{max} and SUV_{max} ratio were 5.3 ± 2.1 and 3.9 ± 2.4, respectively. All patients with STI (11) showed "grade 2 uptake" and it was focal in 54.5% of cases (6 patients) and diffuse in the remaining 45.5% of cases (5 patients). The mean values of the SUV_{max} and SUV_{max} ratio were respectively 5.4 ± 1.8 and 4.2 ± 2.1. Only two patients with Charcot were studied with FDG PET/CT and they all patients showed "grade 2" and diffuse uptake. The mean values of the SUV_{max} and SUV_{max} ratio were respectively 4.9 ± 1.9 and 4.9 ± 1.6. The semiquantitative analysis did not provide a significant difference in terms of both the SUV_{max} and SUV_{max} ratio between the three groups of patients ($p = 0.48$ and $p = 0.83$, respectively). The sensitivity, specificity, and accuracy for FDG PET/CT are reported in Table 3.

3.3. MRI

All centers used similar protocols of acquisitions that included at least T1w, fat-suppressed T2w, and post-Gd T1w sequences, with fat suppression or with subtraction of pre- and post-Gd T1w. Sequences were acquired in at least two perpendicular planes.

The sensitivity, specificity, and accuracy for MRI are reported in Table 3.

3.4. Comparison between WBC Scintigraphy, FDG PET/CT, and MRI in Suspected DFI

WBC scintigraphy, in particular if acquired according to EANM guidelines, showed significantly higher specificity and accuracy than MRI ($p < 0.0001$ and $p = 0.003$, respectively) in detecting OM. Moreover, the sensitivity, specificity, and accuracy of WBC scintigraphy were higher than FDG PET/CT, although not statistically significant. In STI, both FDG PET/CT and WBC scintigraphy achieved a significantly higher specificity than MRI ($p = 0.04$ and $p = 0.018$, respectively). The sensitivity of the three imaging modalities in detecting Charcot could not be calculated because of the low number of patients, but both MRI and WBC scintigraphy showed significantly higher specificity and accuracy than FDG PET/CT ($p = 0.0009$ and $p = 0.029$, respectively, for MRI and $p = 0.0009$ and $p = 0.003$, respectively, for the radiolabeled WBC scan). Moreover, WBC scintigraphy provided significantly higher specificity than MRI ($p < 0.0001$) in this condition. However, these results were based on only a small sample size.

3.5. Comparison between WBC Scintigraphy Performed according and not according to EANM Guidelines

In both OM and STI, using standardized protocols resulted in an overall increase of the sensitivity (from 59.1 to 76.2% and from 29.7% to 75%, respectively), specificity (from 77.3% to 91.9% and from 86.3% to 95.7%, respectively), and diagnostic accuracy (from 72.7% to 86.2% and from 62.5% to 91.4%, respectively) in comparison to those who did not use these protocols. Statistical significance was reached when comparing the sensitivity ($p = 0.006$) and diagnostic accuracy ($p < 0.0001$) in the evaluation of STI. In Charcot, due to the low number of the subjects (only two patients in the "EANM-approved protocols" group and none in the other), this comparison could not be done.

3.6. Comparison between WBC Scintigraphy, FDG PET/CT, and MRI according to the Location of Disease

We compared the performance of the three imaging modalities in the forefoot and mid/hindfoot disorders (Table 5).

Patients without any histopathology results (28.6%) according to the reference and patients with Charcot (only 3.9% of whole population) were excluded. FDG PET/CT was more specific than MRI in detecting STI in mid/hindfoot ($p = 0.03$). For the detection of OM, WBC scintigraphy showed significantly higher sensitivity in the forefoot rather than the mid/hindfoot ($p = 0.013$). Similarly, FDG showed significantly higher sensitivity and accuracy in detecting OM of the forefoot compared to the mid/hindfoot ($p = 0.026$ and $p = 0.015$, respectively).

Table 5. Comparison between the performance of WBC scintigraphy, FDG PET/CT, and MRI in detecting OM and STI according to the location.

	Sensitivity (%) (95% CI)		Specificity (%) (95% CI)		Accuracy (%) (95% CI)	
	Forefoot	Mid-Hindfoot	Forefoot	Mid-Hindfoot	Forefoot	Mid-Hindfoot
OM (WBC-EANM **)	78.6 (57.1–100)	71.4 (38.0–100)	88.9 (68.4–100)	85.7 (59.8–100)	82.6 (67.1–98.1)	78.6 (57.1–100)
STI (WBC-EANM **)	85.7 (59.8–100)	60.0 (17.1–100)	87.5 (71.3–100)	100 (100–100)	87.0 (73.2–100)	85.7 (67.4–100)
OM (FDG PET/CT)	91.7 (76.0–100)	52.9 (29.2–76.7)	60.0 (17.1–100)	72.7 (46.4–99.0)	82.4 (64.2–100)	60.7 (42.6–78.8)
STI (FDG PET/CT)	50.0 (1.0–99.0)	14.3 (0.0–40.2)	100 (100–100)	100 (100–100)	88.2 (75.9–100)	78.6 (63.4–93.8)
OM (MRI)	72.0 (54.0–89.6)	40.0 (9.6–70.4)	61.9 (41.1–82.7)	76.9 (54.0–99.8)	67.4 (53.8–80.9)	60.9 (40.9–80.8)
STI (MRI)	42.9 (16.9–68.8)	42.9 (6.2–79.5)	93.8 (85.4–100)	75.0 (53.8–96.2)	78.3 (66.3–90.2)	65.2 (45.7–84.7)

** WBC scans acquired following EANM guidelines.

3.7. *Correlation between the Findings of Diagnostic Tests and Therapeutic Management*

A descriptive analysis of the different therapeutic options conducted in the studied population, according to the final diagnosis, is summarized in Tables 6 and 7. Most patients with final diagnosis of OM (64.4%) underwent surgery and 32.8% were treated with antibiotics. WBC scintigraphy correctly identified 77% and 83% of these patients, FDG identified 83% and 50% of them, and MRI identified 65% and 73% of them.

Table 6. Different therapeutic strategies in patients with final imaging diagnosis of OM.

Therapeutic Strategy in OM	Imaging	Negative	OM	STI	Charcot
Conventional wound care and topic antibiotic treatment 2.8%	WBC	0%	100%	0%	0%
	FDG (no patients)				
	MRI	0%	0%	0%	100%
Systemic antibiotic treatment 32.8%	WBC	0%	83%	0%	17%
	FDG	0%	50%	0%	50%
	MRI	9%	73%	9%	9%
Surgery (debridement or amputation) 64.4%	WBC	3%	77%	10%	10%
	FDG	0%	83%	0%	17%
	MRI	20%	65%	5%	10%

Column heading over the diagnosis columns: Diagnosis according to Imaging Modalities (%)

Table 7. Different therapeutic strategies in patients with final imaging diagnosis of STI.

Therapeutic Strategy in STI	Diagnosis according to Imaging Modalities (%)				
		Negative	OM	STI	Charcot
No treatment 1.7%	WBC	0%	100%	0%	0%
	FDG (no patients)				
	MRI (no patients)				
Conventional wound care and topic antibiotic treatment 15%	WBC	78%	0%	22%	0%
	FDG (no patients)				
	MRI (no patients)				
Systemic antibiotic treatment 68.3%	WBC	19%	23%	39%	19%
	FDG (no patients)				
	MRI	15%	15%	47%	23%
Surgery (debridement or amputation) 15%	WBC	14%	0%	72%	14%
	FDG (no patients)				
	MRI	0%	33%	66%	0%

By contrast, most patients with a final diagnosis of STI (68.3%) were treated with antibiotics and only 15% underwent surgery. WBC scintigraphy correctly identified 39% and 72% of these patients while MRI identified 47% and 66% of them.

Since we did not observe any statistically significant difference between the three imaging modalities in therapy decision-making, we can conclude that they have similar accuracy in guiding clinicians for the correct management of patients affected by OM or STI.

4. Discussion

This retrospective multicenter study is, to the best of our knowledge, the first to compare the diagnostic value of WBC scintigraphy, FDG PET/CT, and MRI in a large population of patients with suspected DFI, with a particular emphasis on the ability of these imaging modalities to differentiate between OM, STI, and Charcot. At present, no similar studies are available in the literature, probably reflecting the heterogeneity in the diagnostic approaches used in patients from different countries. We believe that a consensus on the most appropriate imaging tool for the assessment of OM, STI, and Charcot is necessary in order to standardize the management of these patients in all centers.

Our analysis shows that the radiolabeled WBC scintigraphy, especially if acquired according to EANM guidelines, has an overall high diagnostic performance in OM, STI, and Charcot, in particular, in terms of the specificity and diagnostic accuracy.

It is well known that when adhering to standardized protocols for labelling, acquisition, image display, and interpretation, the accuracy of WBC scintigraphy in detecting different kinds of infection can be increased [20,27,28]. In our population, 58 patients were studied according to the EANM guidelines for WBC image acquisition and display, while 88 scans did not follow these recommendations.

In these 88 patients, clear superiority of the WBC scan over FDG PET/CT and MRI did not emerge neither in OM nor STI and Charcot. On the other hand, comparing the results of WBC scintigraphy acquired according to EANM guidelines with FDG PET/CT and MRI, we found that the WBC scan was more accurate and specific than MRI in OM, more specific than MRI in STI, and more specific and accurate than FDG in Charcot. These results emphasize the importance of using a standardized image acquisition protocol as suggested by EANM guidelines [20].

Furthermore, comparing the results of WBC scintigraphies acquired according to the EANM guidelines versus WBC acquired without following these recommendations, we found a statistically significant difference in the sensitivity ($p = 0.006$) and diagnostic accuracy ($p < 0.0001$) in the evaluation of STI. This is extremely important considering that STI in diabetics is a particular type of infection that cannot be managed as a common STI in other areas or in non-diabetic patients [29]. The presence of microangiopathy and neuropathy can impair tissue healing and treatment efficacy, with possible progression in OM. Therefore, the diagnosis of STI must be prompt and accurate. In OM, we also found a better specificity ($p = 0.06$) and accuracy ($p = 0.05$) in patients acquired with the EANM protocol than in patients acquired with non-EANM protocols, despite the statistical significance being low. ^{111}In-oxine could also be used as an alternative to ^{99m}Tc-HMPAO for the labelling of WBC and it is also able to provide a high accuracy in detecting an infection [19,20]; however, due to its physical characteristics and radiation burden, ^{99m}Tc remains the preferred agent.

FDG PET/CT has gained an important role in the diagnosis and follow-up of several infective and inflammatory diseases, but it is still unclear whether it could represent a valid alternative to WBC scintigraphy in DFI [15,21]. Moreover, the diagnostic performance of this modality mostly relies on the CT scan, which allows correct anatomical localization and evaluation of the extent of FDG uptake [30]. In our population, FDG PET/CT showed a higher specificity compared with MRI (respectively 95.7% vs. 83.6%) in detecting STI, especially in the mid/hindfoot. This may be explained by the use of CT, which improves the localization of the uptake to soft tissues, thus facilitating the achievement of a correct diagnosis and justifying the low number of false positive results with FDG PET/CT. Nevertheless, as explained above, in STI, the sensitivity is more important than the specificity and, to this regard, WBC showed better sensitivity than FDG. Moreover, we found a good sensitivity, specificity, and accuracy of FDG PET/CT in detecting pedal OM, especially in the forefoot. Although precise interpretative criteria exist for WBC scintigraphy, they are not applicable for FDG PET/CT. Several authors investigated the possible role of SUV measurements in the diagnosis of infectious processes, but the results are discordant among different studies [31–33]. For example, Basu et al. [31] found higher SUV_{max} values in patients with OM compared with patients with Charcot and uncomplicated DF (2.9–6.2 vs. 0.7–2.4 vs. 0.2–0.7), concluding that SUV could be a useful parameter for differentiating these conditions. Conversely, other authors did not find any significant correlation between SUV_{max} values and STI, OM, or Charcot, concluding that SUV alone is not sufficient for diagnosis [15,32,34]. In agreement with this view, in our population, SUV_{max} and SUV_{max} ratios did not significantly differ among patients with OM, STI, and Charcot. Qualitatively, we found a diffuse tracer uptake in all patients with Charcot and a focal uptake in the majority of patients affected by OM. In STI, we found more or less the same proportion of patients with focal and diffuse uptake, thus a precise pattern cannot be determined in this specific condition. Additionally, the evaluation of intensity was found to not be useful in discriminating between these three conditions since "grade 2 uptake" was present in almost all patients studied regardless of the final diagnosis.

In accordance with published meta-analysis and systematic reviews [23,34,35], we found that MRI was not superior to NM imaging modalities, showing high false positive and false negative rates. In the literature, the reported sensitivity of MRI in defining OM ranges between 77.0% and 100.0% [36–38], and, despite its the excellent spatial resolution and natural contrast between different structures, there are several conditions in which MRI is not accurate (e.g., in post-traumatic or post-operative phases or in the presence of lower limb ischemia). In this study, we did not exclude patients with peripheral ischemia, although this condition might have influenced the outcome of MRI [39] and, therefore, this aspect should be considered when comparing the diagnostic performance of the three different modalities. However, lower limb ischemia is a common diagnostic problem that also affects the correct interpretation of WBC scintigraphy, especially for the detection of STI, since a reduced vascular supply could impair leukocytes' recruitment into infected sites [29]. Moreover, in the diabetic foot, the possible presence of Charcot and mechanical stress can be responsible for changes in the bone marrow or soft tissue intensity that could be erroneously interpreted as an OM, thus impairing the specificity of MRI [40–42].

Although it was not a specific aim of our study, we also analyzed the relationship between inflammatory markers and the final diagnosis of infection and found significantly higher values of CRP and ESR in patients with OM compared to patients without any infection. However, we did not find a similar significant difference between patients with STI and normal subjects and between patients with OM and STI. Moreover, aiming to assess whether these values could be predictive of imaging outcomes, the analysis revealed that they are not reliable tools to predict a positive result of MRI, WBC scintigraphy, and FDG PET/CT. Indeed, the role of inflammatory markers is much debated and, although they are usually elevated in infections, they are not able to discriminate the kind of infection and to evaluate its severity, which could be accurately and non-invasively assessed only by advanced imaging.

Despite the large number of patients recruited, this study has several limitations. First, the retrospective nature resulted in a wide heterogeneity of patient selection and diagnostic and therapeutic approaches adopted among the different centers. Often, the choice of one imaging modality rather than another was based on local center availability or waiting lists for the scan, and this bias could of course reflect the comparability of different imaging modalities. Moreover, the different acquisition protocols adopted of both NM and radiological images could negatively affect the results, as shown in the group of patients who performed the WBC scan without following the EANM guideline. Another important limitation is the lack of completeness of the data. In several patients, we missed clinical or histopathological data. In addition, the lack of SPECT/CT in the majority of cases did not allow us to consider this imaging modality in the analysis, but only planar images. Finally, the low number of patients with Charcot does not allow final conclusions to be drawn regarding the best diagnostic approach in this condition. Moreover, it is well known that bone marrow scintigraphy has a central role in handling doubtful WBC scintigraphy, and this modality is particularly important in the evaluation of mid-hindfoot disorders in order to differentiate between an infection from a bone marrow expansion, which is typical of Charcot foot. Unfortunately, given the retrospective nature of this study, only a few patients performed bone marrow scintigraphy in addition to WBC scintigraphy, thus not allowing an evaluation of the added value of this combined approach on the diagnosis.

Nevertheless, retrospective multicenter studies are of clinical value because they consist of data from centers with different experiences, protocols, and equipment, thus representing the actual real situation in daily clinical practice for the diagnosis of DFI. In this context, our study underlines the need for the standardization of acquisition protocols and of interpretation criteria, aiming to correctly manage patients with suspected DFI. Professionals requesting these imaging tests should be specialists in the management of DF to reduce the diagnostic and therapeutic variability of IDFs.

The recent availability of PET/MRI may gain an important role in defining the different complications of the diabetic foot in the near future and it will hopefully solve these challenging clinical scenarios [43–45].

5. Conclusions

This retrospective study confirms the superiority of WBC scintigraphy over other imaging modalities in discriminating pedal OM, STI, and Charcot. In particular, when EANM guidelines are applied, this examination results in high sensitivity, specificity, and accuracy. Additional randomized powered prospective studies comparing these three imaging modalities, and possibly SPECT/CT and

PET/MRI in the same patient, are needed to provide a basis for a proper evidence-based multi-modality diagnostic algorithm.

Author Contributions: Conceptualization, A.W.J.M.G. and A.S.; methodology, A.W.J.M.G., R.H.J.A.S. and A.S.; formal analysis, C.L. and G.C.; investigation, C.L.; resources, A.W.J.M.G, Z.K. M.M.K., S.G., G.A. (Georgios Arsos) E.N.-Á. G.A. (Giuseppe Argento), T.C.K. R.H.J.A.S. and A.S.; data curation, C.L.; writing—original draft preparation, C.L.; writing—review and editing, C.L.; supervision, A.W.J.M.G, R.H.J.A.S. and A.S. All authors have read and agreed to the published version of the manuscript.

References

1. Lipsky, B.A.; Berendt, A.R.; Cornia, P.B.; Pile, J.C.; Peters, E.J.; Armstrong, D.G.; Deery, H.G.; Embil, J.M.; Joseph, W.S.; Karchmer, A.W.; et al. 2012 Infectious Diseases Society of America clinical practice guideline for the diagnosis and treatment of diabetic foot infections. *Clin. Infect. Dis.* **2012**, *54*, 132–173. [CrossRef]
2. Lipsky, B.A.; Aragón-Sánchez, J.; Diggle, M.; Embil, J.; Kono, S.; Lavery, L.; Senneville, É.; Urbančič-Rovan, V.; Van Asten, S. IWGDF guidance on the diagnosis and management of foot infections in persons with diabetes. *Diabetes Metab. Res. Rev.* **2016**, *32*, 45–74. [CrossRef]
3. Treglia, G.; Sadeghi, R.; Annunziata, S.; Zakavi, S.R.; Caldarella, C.; Muoio, B.; Bertagna, F.; Ceriani, L.; Giovannella, L. Diagnostic performance of Fluorine-18-Fluorodeoxyglucose positron emission tomography for the diagnosis of osteomyelitis related to diabetic foot: A systematic review and a meta-analysis. *Foot* **2013**, *23*, 140–148. [CrossRef]
4. Markakis, K.; Bowling, F.L.; Boulton, A.J. The diabetic foot in 2015: An overview. *Diabetes Metab. Res. Rev.* **2016**, *32*, 169–178. [CrossRef]
5. Zhang, P.; Lu, J.; Jing, Y.; Tang, S.; Zhu, D.; Bi, Y. Global epidemiology of diabetic foot ulceration: A systematic review and meta-analysis. *Ann. Med.* **2017**, *49*, 106–116. [CrossRef]
6. Brennan, M.B.; Hess, T.M.; Bartle, B.; Cooper, J.M.; Kang, J.; Huang, E.S.; Smith, M.; Sohn, M.W.; Crnich, C. Diabetic foot ulcer severity predicts mortality among veterans with type 2 diabetes. *J. Diabetes Complicat.* **2017**, *31*, 556–561. [CrossRef]
7. Capriotti, G.; Chianelli, M.; Signore, A. Nuclear medicine imaging of diabetic foot infection: Results of meta-analysis. *Nucl. Med. Commun.* **2006**, *27*, 757–764. [CrossRef]
8. Prompers, L.; Huijberts, M.; Apelqvist, J.; Jude, E.; Piaggesi, A.; Bakker, K.; Edmonds, M.; Holstein, P.; Jirkovska, A.; Mauricio, D.; et al. High prevalence of ischaemia, infection and serious comorbidity in patients with diabetic foot disease in Europe. Baseline results from the Eurodiale study. *Diabetologia* **2007**, *50*, 18–25. [CrossRef]
9. Lipsky, B.A. Osteomyelitis of the foot in diabetic patients. *Clin. Infect. Dis.* **1997**, *25*, 1318–1326. [CrossRef]
10. Lavery, L.A.; Armstrong, D.G.; Wunderlich, R.P.; Mohler, M.J.; Wendel, C.S.; Lipsky, B.A. Risk factors for foot infections in individuals with diabetes. *Diabetes Care* **2006**, *29*, 1288–1293. [CrossRef]
11. Gierbolini, R. Charcot's foot: Often overlooked complication of diabetes. *J. Am. Acad. Phys. Assist.* **1994**, *12*, 62–68.
12. Dinh, M.T.; Abad, C.L.; Safdar, N. Diagnostic accuracy of the physical examination and imaging tests for osteomyelitis underlying diabetic foot ulcers: Meta-analysis. *Clin. Infect. Dis.* **2008**, *47*, 519–527. [CrossRef]
13. Grayson, M.L.; Gibbons, G.W.; Balogh, K.; Levin, E.; Karchmer, A.W. Probing to bone in infected pedal ulcers: A clinical sign of underlying osteomyelitis in diabetic patients. *JAMA* **1995**, *273*, 721–723. [CrossRef]
14. Glaudemans, A.W.J.M.; Jutte, P.C.; Cataldo, M.A.; Cassar-Pullicino, V.; Gheysens, O.; Borens, O.; Trampuz, A.; Wörtler, K.; Petrosillo, N.; Winkler, H.; et al. Consensus document for the diagnosis of peripheral bone infection in adults: A joint paper by the EANM, EBJIS, and ESR (with ESCMID endorsement). *Eur. J. Nucl. Med. Mol. Imaging* **2019**, *46*, 957–970. [CrossRef]
15. Familiari, D.; Glaudemans, A.W.; Vitale, V.; Prosperi, D.; Bagni, O.; Lenza, A.; Cavallini, M.; Scopinaro, F.; Signore, A. Can sequential 18F-FDG PET/CT replace WBC imaging in the diabetic foot? *J. Nucl. Med.* **2011**, *52*, 1012–1019. [CrossRef]
16. Glaudemans, A.W.; Uçkay, I.; Lipsky, B.A. Challenges in diagnosing infection in the diabetic foot. *Diabet Med.* **2015**, *32*, 748–759. [CrossRef]

17. Tan, P.L.; The, J. MRI of the diabetic foot: Differentiation of infection from neuropathic change. *Br. J. Radiol.* **2007**, *80*, 939–948. [CrossRef]
18. De Vries, E.F.; Roca, M.; Jamar, F.; Israel, O.; Signore, A. Guidelines for the labelling of leucocytes with 99mTc-HMPAO. Inflammation/Infection Taskgroup of the European Association of Nuclear Medicine. *Eur J. Nucl. Med. Mol. Imaging* **2010**, *37*, 842–848. [CrossRef]
19. Roca, M.; de Vries, E.F.; Jamar, F.; Israel, O.; Signore, A. Guidelines for the labelling of leucocytes with 111In-oxine. Inflammation/Infection Taskgroup of the European Association of Nuclear Medicine. *Eur. J. Nucl. Med. Mol. Imaging* **2010**, *37*, 835–841. [CrossRef]
20. Signore, A.; Jamar, F.; Israel, O.; Buscombe, J.; Martin-Comin, J.; Lazzeri, E. Clinical indications, image acquisition and data interpretation for white blood cells and anti-granulocyte monoclonal antibody scintigraphy: An EANM procedural guideline. *Eur. J. Nucl. Med. Mol. Imaging* **2018**, *45*, 1816–1831. [CrossRef]
21. Jamar, F.; Buscombe, J.; Chiti, A.; Christian, P.E.; Delbeke, D.; Donohoe, K.J.; Israel, O.; Martin-Comin, J.; Signore, A. EANM/SNMMI guideline for 18F-FDG use in inflammation and infection. *J. Nucl. Med.* **2013**, *54*, 647–658. [CrossRef] [PubMed]
22. Signore, A.; Sconfienza, L.M.; Borens, O.; Glaudemans, A.W.J.M.; Cassar-Pullicino, V.; Trampuz, A.; Winkler, H.; Gheysens, O.; Vanhoenacker, F.M.H.M.; Petrosillo, N.; et al. Consensus document for the diagnosis of prosthetic joint infections: A joint paper by the EANM, EBJIS, and ESR (with ESCMID endorsement). *Eur. J. Nucl. Med. Mol. Imaging* **2019**, *46*, 971–988. [CrossRef] [PubMed]
23. Lauri, C.; Tamminga, M.; Glaudemans, A.W.J.M.; Juárez Orozco, L.E.; Erba, P.A.; Jutte, P.C.; Lipsky, B.A.; IJzerman, M.J.; Signore, A.; Slart, R.H.J.A. Detection of Osteomyelitis in the Diabetic Foot by Imaging Techniques: A Systematic Review and Meta-analysis Comparing MRI, White Blood Cell Scintigraphy, and FDG-PET. *Diabetes Care* **2017**, *40*, 1111–1120. [CrossRef] [PubMed]
24. Donovan, A.; Schweitzer, M.E. Use of MR imaging in diagnosing diabetes-related pedal osteomyelitis. *Radiographics* **2010**, *30*, 723–736. [CrossRef]
25. Ledermann, H.P.; Morrison, W.B.; Schweitzer, M.E. MR image analysis of pedal osteomyelitis: Distribution, patterns of spread, and frequency of associated ulceration and septic arthritis. *Radiology* **2002**, *223*, 747–755. [CrossRef]
26. Ahmadi, M.E.; Morrison, W.B.; Carrino, J.A.; Schweitzer, M.E.; Raikin, S.M.; Ledermann, H.P. Neuropathic arthropathy of the foot with and without superimposed osteomyelitis: MR imaging characteristics. *Radiology* **2006**, *238*, 622–631. [CrossRef]
27. Glaudemans, A.W.; de Vries, E.F.; Vermeulen, L.E.; Slart, R.H.; Dierckx, R.A.; Signore, A. A large retrospective single-centre study to define the best image acquisition protocols and interpretation criteria for white blood cell scintigraphy with (99)mTc-HMPAO-labelled leucocytes in musculoskeletal infections. *Eur. J. Nucl. Med. Mol. Imaging* **2013**, *40*, 1760–1769. [CrossRef]
28. Erba, P.A.; Glaudemans, A.W.; Veltman, N.C.; Sollini, M.; Pacilio, M.; Galli, F.; Dierckx, R.A.; Signore, A. Image acquisition and interpretation criteria for 99mTc-HMPAO-labelled white blood cell scintigraphy: Results of a multicenter study. *Eur. J. Nucl Med. Mol. Imaging* **2014**, *41*, 615–623. [CrossRef]
29. Lauri, C.; Glaudemans, A.W.J.M.; Signore, A. Leukocyte Imaging of the Diabetic Foot. *Curr. Pharm. Des.* **2018**, *24*, 1270–1276. [CrossRef]
30. Keidar, Z.; Militianu, D.; Melamed, E.; Bar-Shalom, R.; Israel, O. The diabetic foot: Initial experience with 18F-FDG PET/CT. *J. Nucl. Med.* **2005**, *46*, 444–449.
31. Basu, S.; Chryssikos, T.; Houseni, M.; Scot Malay, D.; Shah, J.; Zhuang, H.; Alavi, A. Potential role of FDG PET in the setting of diabetic neuro-osteoarthropathy: Can it differentiate uncomplicated Charcot's neuroarthropathy from osteomyelitis and soft-tissue infection? *Nucl. Med. Commun.* **2007**, *28*, 465–472. [CrossRef] [PubMed]
32. Kagna, O.; Srour, S.; Melamed, E.; Militianu, D.; Keidar, Z. FDG PET/CT imaging in the diagnosis of osteomyelitis in the diabetic foot. *Eur. J. Nucl. Med. Mol Imaging* **2012**, *39*, 1545–1550. [CrossRef] [PubMed]
33. Shagos, G.S.; Shanmugasundaram, P.; Varma, A.K.; Padma, S.; Sarma, M. 18-F flourodeoxy glucose positron emission tomography-computed tomography imaging: A viable alternative to three phase bone scan in evaluating diabetic foot complications? *Indian J. Nucl. Med.* **2015**, *30*, 97–103. [CrossRef] [PubMed]
34. Nawaz, A.; Torigian, D.A.; Siegelman, E.S.; Basu, S.; Chryssikos, T.; Alavi, A. Diagnostic performance of FDG-PET, MRI, and plain film radiography (PFR) for the diagnosis of osteomyelitis in the diabetic foot. *Mol. Imaging Biol.* **2010**, *12*, 335–342. [CrossRef]

35. Newman, L.G.; Waller, J.; Palestro, C.J.; Hermann, G.; Klein, M.J.; Schwartz, M.; Harrington, E.; Harrington, M.; Roman, S.H.; Stagnaro-Green, A. Leukocyte scanning with ^{111}In is superior to magnetic resonance imaging in diagnosis of clinically unsuspected osteomyelitis in diabetic foot ulcers. *Diabetes Care.* **1992**, *15*, 1527–1530. [CrossRef]
36. Craig, J.G.; Amin, M.B.; Wu, K.; Eyler, W.R.; van Holsbeeck, M.T.; Bouffard, J.A.; Shirazi, K. Osteomyelitis of the diabetic foot: MR imaging-pathologic correlation. *Radiology* **1997**, *203*, 849–855. [CrossRef]
37. Erdman, W.A.; Tamburro, F.; Jayson, H.T.; Weatherall, P.T.; Ferry, K.B.; Peshock, R.M. Osteomyelitis: Characteristics and pitfalls of diagnosis with MR imaging. *Radiology* **1991**, *180*, 533–539. [CrossRef]
38. Lipman, B.T.; Collier, B.D.; Carrera, G.F.; Timins, M.E.; Erickson, S.J.; Johnson, J.E.; Mitchell, J.R.; Hoffmann, R.G.; Finger, W.A.; Krasnow, A.Z.; et al. Detection of osteomyelitis in the neuropathic foot: Nuclear medicine, MRI and conventional radiography. *Clin. Nucl. Med.* **1998**, *23*, 77–82. [CrossRef]
39. Fujii, M.; Armstrong, D.G.; Terashi, H. Efficacy of magnetic resonance imaging in diagnosing diabetic foot osteomyelitis in the presence of ischemia. *J. Foot Ankle Surg.* **2013**, *52*, 717–723. [CrossRef]
40. Morrison, W.B.; Schweitzer, M.E.; Wapner, K.L.; Hecht, P.J.; Gannon, F.H.; Behm, W.R. Osteomyelitis in feet of diabetics: Clinical accuracy, surgical utility, and cost-effectiveness of MR imaging. *Radiology* **1995**, *196*, 557–564. [CrossRef]
41. Ledermann, H.P.; Schweitzer, M.E.; Morrison, W.B. Non-enhancing tissue on MR imaging of pedal infection: Characterization of necrotic tissue and associated limitations for diagnosis of osteomyelitis and abscess. *Am. J. Roentgenol.* **2002**, *178*, 215–222. [CrossRef] [PubMed]
42. Leone, A.; Cassar-Pullicino, V.N.; Semprini, A.; Tonetti, L.; Magarelli, N.; Colosimo, C. Neuropathic osteoarthropathy with and without superimposed osteomyelitis in patients with a diabetic foot. *Skeletal Radiol.* **2016**, *45*, 735–754. [CrossRef] [PubMed]
43. Glaudemans, A.W.; Prandini, N.; Di Girolamo, M.; Argento, G.; Lauri, C.; Lazzeri, E.; Muto, M.; Sconfienza, L.M.; Signore, A. Hybrid imaging of musculoskeletal infections. *Q. J. Nucl. Med. Mol. Imaging* **2018**, *62*, 3–13. [CrossRef] [PubMed]
44. Catalano, O.; Maccioni, F.; Lauri, C.; Auletta, S.; Dierckx, R.; Signore, A. Hybrid imaging in Crohn's disease: From SPECT/CT to PET/MR and new image interpretation criteria. *Q. J. Nucl. Med. Mol. Imaging* **2018**, *62*, 40–55. [CrossRef]
45. Heiba, S.; Knešaurek, K. Evaluation of diabetic foot infection in nuclear medicine. *Q. J. Nucl. Med. Mol. Imaging* **2017**, *61*, 283–291. [CrossRef]

11

Imaging Bacteria with Radiolabelled Probes: Is it Feasible?

Alberto Signore [1,*], Vera Artiko [2], Martina Conserva [1], Guillermina Ferro-Flores [3], Mick M. Welling [4], Sanjay K. Jain [5], Søren Hess [6] and Mike Sathekge [7]

1 Nuclear Medicine Unit, Department of Medical-Surgical Sciences and of Translational Medicine, Faculty of Medicine and Psychology, Sapienza University of Rome, 00189 Rome, Italy; martina.conserva977@gmail.com
2 Center for Nuclear Medicine, Clinical Center of Serbia, Faculty of Medicine, University of Belgrade, 101801 Beograd, Serbia; vera.artiko@gmail.com
3 Department of Radioactive Materials, Instituto Nacional de Investigaciones Nucleares, Carretera Mexico-Toluca S/N, La Marquesa, Ocoyoacac 52750, Estado de Mexico, Mexico; guillermina.ferro@inin.gob.mx
4 Interventional Molecular Imaging Laboratory, Department of Radiology, Leiden University Medical Center, 2333 ZA Leiden, The Netherlands; m.m.welling@lumc.nl
5 Center for Infection and Inflammation Imaging Research, Johns Hopkins University School of Medicine, Baltimore, MD 21205, USA; sjain5@jhmi.edu
6 Department of Radiology and Nuclear Medicine, Hospital South West Jutland, University Hospital of Southern Denmark, 6700 Esbjerg, Denmark; soren.hess@rsyd.dk
7 Nuclear Medicine Department, University of Pretoria, Pretoria 0001, South Africa; Mike.Sathekge@up.ac.za
* Correspondence: alberto.signore@uniroma1.it

Abstract: Bacterial infections are the main cause of patient morbidity and mortality worldwide. Diagnosis can be difficult and delayed as well as the identification of the etiological pathogen, necessary for a tailored antibiotic therapy. Several non-invasive diagnostic procedures are available, all with pros and cons. Molecular nuclear medicine has highly contributed in this field by proposing several different radiopharmaceuticals (antimicrobial peptides, leukocytes, cytokines, antibiotics, sugars, etc.) but none proved to be highly specific for bacteria, although many agents in development look promising. Indeed, factors including the number and strain of bacteria, the infection site, and the host condition, may affect the specificity of the tested radiopharmaceuticals. At the Third European Congress on Infection/Inflammation Imaging, a round table discussion was dedicated to debate the pros and cons of different radiopharmaceuticals for imaging bacteria with the final goal to find a consensus on the most relevant research steps that should be fulfilled when testing a new probe, based on experience and cumulative published evidence.

Keywords: infection; bacteria; radiopharmaceutical; molecular imaging; nuclear medicine

---

1. Introduction

The diagnosis of bacterial infections remains a serious medical challenge, as they are among the main causes of mortality and morbidity worldwide. Nuclear medicine lacks specific radiopharmaceuticals to discriminate infection from sterile inflammation, and radiology often has poor sensitivity in detecting infective foci, especially in the early phases or in deeply seated infections. The diagnosis of infection often relies on serological markers and clinical symptoms, the gold standard being the isolation of the pathogen [1,2].

Indeed, radiological imaging modalities, such as X-rays, ultrasound (US), computed tomography (CT) and magnetic resonance imaging (MRI) provide an indication of the anatomical area of lesion only after the formation of a morphological alteration.

For Nuclear medicine imaging, many radiopharmaceuticals have been synthetized to detect physiological and biochemical changes at the early stages of infection, but to date, none have been made commercially available. Appropriate radiopharmaceuticals should enable early diagnostic imaging, identifying the pathogen and its biological characteristics, thus monitoring the therapy response as well as identifying drug-resistant strains, and the prognosis. The ideal one should have fast accumulation, high retention at the site of infection with fast clearance from non-infected tissues, with low absorbed radiation dose. In addition, it must be readily available, with simple labelling, inexpensive, repeatable and safe [3].

Nowadays, according to these criteria, the detection of infection by non-specific radiopharmaceuticals could be performed with metabolism-based particles (nucleoside analogues, sugars, cell wall components, components based in iron metabolism), antimicrobial peptides, antibiotics (fluoroquinolones, cephalosporins, antifolates), immunoglobulins and cytokines labelled with gamma- or positron-emitting isotopes (^{18}F, ^{64}Cu, ^{68}Ga, ^{99m}Tc, ^{111}In, ^{67}Ga etc.), aptamers/oligomers, bacteriophages, and vitamins (Figure 1), [4–7]. However, each approach has its limitations and investigations lack standardization.

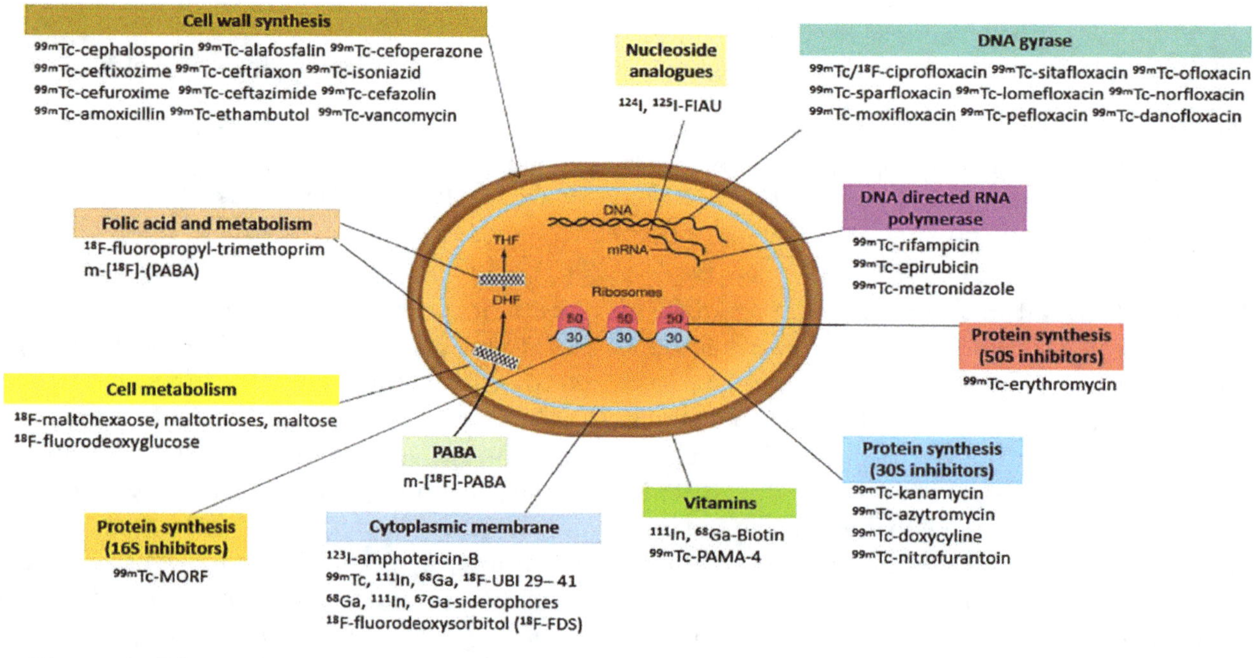

Figure 1. Schematic representation of most radiopharmaceuticals proposed for targeting bacteria, according to their mechanism of action. However, none are able, in humans, to differentiate between infection and inflammation with high diagnostic accuracy (>95%).

It is now well known that [^{18}F]-fluorodeoxyglucose ([^{18}F]FDG) is taken up by the cells involved in the inflammatory response (e.g., neutrophils, macrophages and activated leukocytes) because they express high levels of glucose transporters like malignant cells (albeit not to the same extent), and in addition, circulating cytokines seem to increase the affinity of these glucose transporters for [^{18}F]FDG [8] and it has recently been shown that some bacterial strain can also bind [^{18}F]FDG [9].

Nonetheless, the non-specific nature of [^{18}F]FDG may also be a hindrance in other settings, as the distinction between aseptic inflammation and infectious foci is difficult. Much work has been invested in optimizing the use of [^{18}F]FDG.

On the other hand, in recent years, some more specific radiopharmaceuticals were developed in different nuclear medicine fields, such as the oncological one (e.g., prostate-specific membrane antigen (PSMA)-imaging for prostate cancer and various radiopharmaceuticals for neuroendocrine tumours). Just as tumour imaging, more specific radiopharmaceuticals are also being investigated for infection, even if ^{99m}Tc and ^{111}In-labelled white-blood-cells (WBC) remain the gold standard technique for the nuclear medicine imaging of infections [10].

Possible reasons for not having a commercially available radiopharmaceutical yet for imaging bacteria, could be the high costwith respect to the available market, but more likely, the lack of reproducibility of the published data. This is because different animal models are often used, different bacteria, different methods of image acquisition and interpretation, different quality controls on radiopharmaceuticals, etc.

Based on the active discussion during the round table session on "Bacteria imaging" at the Third European Congress on Infection/Inflammation Imaging, we aimed with this paper to generate a consensus document on the minimum requirements needed for more infection-specific radiopharmaceuticals for bacteria imaging (i.e., radiopharmaceuticals aimed directly at the microorganism and not only at the secondary inflammatory response), looking also at the upcoming technologies that could improve diagnosis and patient comfort, especially in areas not readily accessible for sampling or biopsies.

The Role of Pathogenic Bacteria in Infections and Bacteria-Specific Features for Targeting

Planktonic bacteria are free-living bacteria, which are generally treatable with antibiotics, but when they adhere to a surface, develop a biofilm.

Bacterial biofilms are groups of bacteria that are embedded in a self-produced matrix of extracellular polymeric substances (EPS), adhering to each other and usually to a surface, thus, allowing intense interactions to occur, including cell–cell communication, altered phenotypes with respect to growth rate and gene transcription [11]. Biofilm-embedded bacteria represent a serious clinical problem in medicine, because their infections are notoriously difficult to treat due to extreme resistance to antibiotics.

Antibiotics are drugs of natural or synthetic origin that can kill (bactericidal drugs) or inhibit (bacteriostatic drugs) cell growth. Most bactericidal antimicrobials are: cephalosporins, carbapenems, glycopeptides, fluoroquinolones, polymyxins that inhibit DNA synthesis, RNA synthesis, cell wall synthesis, or bacterial protein synthesis.

Fluoroquinolones (FQs) are bactericidal antibiotics effective for both Gram-negative and Gram-positive bacteria, and ciprofloxacin is the most widely used antimicrobial agent among FQs. The action of ciprofloxacin results from the inhibition of the enzymes topoisomerase II (DNA gyrase, gyrA and B) and topoisomerase IV (grlA and B), which are required for bacterial DNA replication, transcription, repair, strand super coiling repair, and recombination. Resistance to FQs in bacteria is mainly mediated by alterations in DNA gyrase and topoisomerase IV with specific amino acid substitutions in the "quinolone-resistance determining region" (QRDR) in gyrA and B subunits of DNA gyrase and parC and parE subunits of topoisomerase IV. Other common mechanisms are the reduced permeability/increased efflux of ciprofloxacin across bacterial membranes, and plasmids that protect cells from the lethal effects of FQs [12,13].

Toxic effects of FQs on humans have been attributed to their interactions with different receptor complexes, such as the blockade of the GABAa receptor complex within the central nervous system, leading to excitotoxic type effects and oxidative stress [14]. These toxic effects, however, are unlikely to be noted at a tracer dose that is used for PET/SPECT imaging because of the relatively high IC50 of FQs with respect to the micromolar quantities injected as radiopharmaceuticals.

Cephalosporins are one of the largest families of β-lactam antibiotics. They are bactericidal agents and have the same mode of action as other beta-lactam antibiotics (such as penicillin). Cephalosporins disrupt the synthesis of the peptidoglycan layer of bacterial cell walls by binding to penicillin-binding proteins (PBPs), causing the walls to break down and eventually the bacteria die. The three fundamental mechanisms of antimicrobial resistance are: the enzymatic degradation of antibacterial drugs, changes in PBPs, and changes in membrane permeability to antibiotics. The most important mechanism of resistance to cephalosporins is the destruction of beta-lactam rings by β-lactamase enzymes. Mutational changes in original PBPs or the acquisition of different PBPs will lead to the inability of the antibiotic to bind to the PBPs and inhibit cell wall synthesis. A change in the number or function of the general diffusion porin channels can reduce the permeability.

Since antimicrobial compounds act on processes that are unique to bacteria, it has been proposed that radiolabelled antibiotics should be able to distinguish microbial from non-microbial inflammation, because of their specific binding to the causative agents.

Another important problem of antibiotics is the risk of a resistance mechanism in bacteria that are increasingly common and could prevent the specific binding of the antibiotic ligand, leading to poor uptake. Furthermore, since antibiotics are designed to kill or disable the bacteria with high potency, many radiolabelled antibiotics do not accumulate in the bacteria, and thus may not provide a high enough contrast from the surrounding mammalian cells [2]. For these reasons the gold standard for bacterial infection imaging has not yet been found. Further in understanding the pathogenesis of infectious diseases goes beyond identifying the site of infection and disease-causing pathogen. Infectious lesions are characterized by a heterogeneous microenvironment which may include spatial physical and chemical differences as well as varied immune responses. These non-specific radiotracers targeted at these microenvironment biomarkers may provide valuable information regarding the heterogeneity of infection sites and have the potential to inform on the efficacy of antimicrobial treatments [14,15] as well as host-directed therapies [13,16,17]. Hopefully in the future we will have many radiopharmaceuticals available, tailored for specific pathogens, and clinical conditions, thus having the maximum specificity (see Table 1).

Table 1. Aspects to be considered for the improvement of bacteria imaging.

Pathogen-Specific Radiopharmaceuticals	
✓	Sensitivity for a broader range of microbes rather than species-specific probes
✓	Screen potential radiopharmaceuticals in whole bacterial cell
✓	Always use referenced bacterial strains and specify Colony Forming Units (CFUs)
Antimicrobial Radiopharmaceuticals	
✓	Library of antibiotics—very high affinity to targets (accumulation and slow clearance)
✓	Radiochemistry to balance T1/2 of the radioisotope and the parent drug
Vitamins and Sugars	
✓	Define the metabolic role and pathway of new radiopharmaceuticals derived from vitamin's or sugar's analogues
✓	Test specificity in different bacteria strain and binding to eukaryotic cells
Optimize Labelling Protocols and Quality Controls	
✓	Consensus guidelines on minimal required in vitro quality controls to better characterize the new radiopharmaceuticals (labelling efficiency, specific activity, mass spectroscopy, chromatography data, radiopharmaceutical stability in saline and plasma, etc.)
✓	Determine the Kd for tracer target specificity
✓	Test on living bacteria in vitro (binding at 37 °C and 4 °C, binding to living and killed bacteria, competitive binding assay, etc.)

Table 1. *Cont.*

	Optimize Animal Models (Figure 2)
✓	Standardized protocols and consensus guidelines regarding animal models of infection are needed
✓	Trials with new probes compared with commonly used radiopharmaceuticals in clinical settings and other modalities (e.g., fluorescence imaging)
✓	Include positive and negative control tracers like D,L analogues or scrambled peptides, etc.
✓	Consider competition studies
✓	Always provide information about the model (injected CFUs, time of imaging and sacrifice, CFU recruited from infected site at different time points, etc.)
✓	Provide information on the animal used (strain, culture, food, drinking water, age, sex, body weight, etc.)

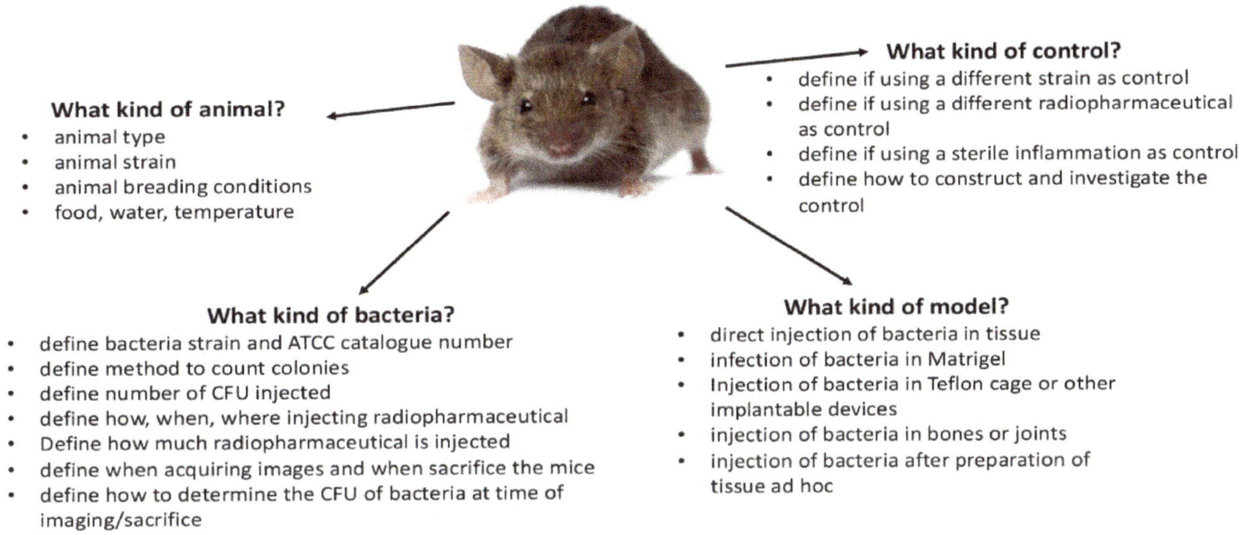

Figure 2. Schematic representation of the most relevant aspects to be taken in consideration when planning new experiments in animal models for targeting bacteria.

2. Imaging Bacteria in Animal Models

Nuclear medicine imaging improved the diagnosis of infections through the development of several radiopharmaceuticals that are constituted by different molecules such as "antibodies or fragments, antibiotics, antimicrobial peptides, bacteriophages", but none of these are really "infection specific". The main limits include a low specificity, low bacterial mass, unclear mechanisms of action, the presence of biofilm that limits their penetration and the host immune response. Moreover, the location of the bacterial target influences the choice of radiopharmaceuticals and its development [18–21].

For this purpose, for imaging infections, several steps should be followed to develop an efficient radiopharmaceutical to target bacteria. Firstly, test the specificity through in vitro binding assays and, secondly, evaluate the specificity in vivo choosing the best animal model. Then, translate the preclinical results to humans.

The Teflon cage model is an example of a standardized reproducible model to study bacterial infections in animals. In this model, a Teflon cage is implanted into the back of the mouse under the skin, by easy surgical procedure with a small incision of 5 mm. Despite that this model requires surgical intervention, it provides several advantages such as: the possibility to locally inject a known number of bacteria; the possibility to accurately evaluate the bacterial mass; the possibility to withdraw samples of fluids or cage to measure the bacteria and radiopharmaceutical concentration over time; the possibility to study biofilm formation [22].

The following radiopharmaceuticals might be considered the progenitors for bacterial infections by SPECT imaging because there are more data both in animals and in humans: 99mTc/18F-UBI 29-41, 111In-biotin [23,24]. Ubiquicidin (UBI) is a cationic human antimicrobial peptide fragment.

However, radiolabelled UBI 29-41 is not widely used as a clinical agent due to the lack of a commercial kit approved worldwide for human studies (only available in Mexico), however, there are over 30 clinical studies performed underlying its usefulness in imaging infections [25,26]. Radiolabelled ciprofloxacin, after promising results in animals, when tested in humans, showed very discordant results in terms of specificity and sensibility [24]. In the majority of papers on Gram-negative bacteria, promising results were reported by using radiolabelled sugars (glucose, sorbitol, maltose, maltohexaose and ^{18}F-fluoromaltotriose and ^{18}F-fluoroacetamido-D-glucopyranose (FAG)) [27]. Indeed, several groups showed a high specificity of [^{18}F]FDS binding to *E. coli* or *K. pneumoniae* [28] in animals. Several other studies have demonstrated similar results, but always in animal models [29,30]. In addition, other sugars such as ^{18}F-fluoromaltohexaose (FMH) [31], 6′′-^{18}F-fluoromaltotriose and ^{18}F-fluoroacetamido-D-glucopyranose (FAG), [32] were revealed to be sensitive and specific radiopharmaceuticals for the detection of *E. coli* [33]. In addition, a new Gram-negative bacterial infection-specific radiopharmaceutical has been developed: ^{99m}Tc-polymyxin B. The polymyxin B is an antibiotic, usually used for multidrug-resistant Gram-negative bacteria, that acts like an amphipathic antimicrobial peptide. Similarly, D-amino acids, molecules targeting the folate pathway in bacteria and siderophores have also been studied as bacterial specific imaging agents [34–39].

In conclusion, the results highlighted the availability of many promising PET radiopharmaceuticals for bacterial imaging, even if imaging bacteria is still a difficult and challenging task. Animal models should be carefully selected and standardized, as well as bacteria strains. Experimental design should include in vitro and in vivo studies with appropriate controls and details of *S. aureus*, injected dose and bacterial number. A consensus document about how to test (in vitro and in animals) new bacterial imaging agents may allow a standardization of procedures and a better comparison between different agents.

There is a lack of knowledge whether it is possible to develop an all-purpose radiopharmaceutical to image all bacterial strains. Nowadays, this remains an open goal, difficult to achieve, however, at the same time, crucial for the management, treatment and follow-up of patients with suspected bacterial infections.

3. Imaging Bacteria in Humans

Despite excellent pre-clinical studies, radiopharmaceuticals for imaging bacteria in humans are still under development [40]. An unmet need, therefore, remains in the clinical differentiation of inflammation from infection. Bacterial-specific imaging is a viable attempt to cater for this need, and efforts in this regard must be encouraged, especially given the significant morbidity and mortality burden that infections continue to cause.

In humans, following the target-based classification, the best radiopharmaceuticals for bacteria imaging are: pathogen-specific tracers, antimicrobial tracers and microenvironment tracers.

In particular, tracers with the highest translational potential are antimicrobial peptides such as UBI 29-41, bacterial carbohydrates, nucleoside/thymidine analogue, folic acid, siderophores and antibiotics such as Trimethoprim and Vancomycin.

Antimicrobial peptides have been successfully radiolabelled and tested for infection imaging in animal models and humans. The first radiolabelled antimicrobial agent evaluated for human use was ^{99m}Tc-ciprofloxacin [41]. Disappointing results from its application in humans led to its withdrawal from the market. In particular, its specificity and sensitivity for infections were questioned in several studies, probably due to the formation of several radiolabelled chemical species with different biodistribution profiles [42–44]. Imaging time-points were also questioned, up to 4 h in one study and up to 24 h in another. Many other antibiotics, including fluoroquinolones, cephalosporins, and anti-tuberculosis drugs, have since been successfully labelled with a suitable radionuclide and tested in preclinical studies [45].

A radiolabelled antimicrobial peptide that has gained popularity in the clinic is radiolabelled ubiquicidin, a human antimicrobial peptide present in the respiratory epithelium. Its fragments have been successfully labelled with ^{68}Ga for PET imaging and ^{99m}Tc for SPECT imaging [46]. The basis for the use of the fragment UBI 29-41 is its ability to be attracted to the negatively charged bacterial cell wall, itself being positively charged. ^{99m}Tc-UBI 29-41 scintigraphy has an excellent diagnostic performance in the evaluation of musculoskeletal infection. The addition of CT morphologic imaging to planar and SPECT-only imaging led to an increase in diagnostic performance and an improvement in diagnostic confidence in differentiating soft tissue from bone infection, as well as a higher inter-observer agreement [26].

Moreover, gallium-68-based infection-imaging agents are in demand to detect infection foci with high spatial resolution and sensitivity. ^{68}Ga-NOTA-UBI 29-41 is an efficient and sensitive radiopharmaceutical of the in vivo imaging of infection and has exhibited significant uptake ratios between muscular infection and inflammation [47]. Further clinical evaluation of this novel metabolic tracer is warranted to investigate its potential use as a first-line PET/CT infection-imaging agent. ^{68}Ga-UBI prepared using the NOTA-UBI kit is a potential agent in targeting infections associated with disease conditions including diabetic foot, cellulitis and fracture. Indeed, biodistribution studies with ^{68}Ga-NOTA-UBI 31-38 revealed a specific uptake of the complex in infected muscle, compared to inflamed muscle. This was the first report on ^{68}Ga labelled NOTA-UBI 31-38 fragment for prospective infection imaging [48].

Furthermore, ^{18}F-fluorodeoxysorbitol has been successfully synthesized from ^{18}F-FDG, and it showed specific uptake in the cultures of *E. coli* and *K. pneumoniae*. No uptake of ^{18}F-fluorodeoxysorbitol was seen in Gram-positive organisms, normal human cells, or cancer cells. The probe was able to differentiate the infection due to Enterobacteriaceae from sterile inflammation, and the PET signal disappeared after successful treatment [28].

Antibiotics such as ^{99m}Tc-vancomycin and ^{18}F-fluoropropyl-trimethoprim target peptidoglycan precursors on bacterial (Gram-positive bacteria) membrane and inhibit the bacterial cell wall synthesis [49]. Although they are bacteria-specific and -targeting drug-resistant Gram-positive bacteria, biodistribution studies revealed a high liver uptake, high background activity and low sensitivity. Therefore, they are not used for routine clinical application yet.

Fialuridine is a nucleoside analogue that is a substrate for the bacterial thymidine kinase enzyme but is not acted on by the human form of the enzyme. This is its basis for use as a potential molecular probe for infection imaging. However, ^{124}I-FIAU lacks specificity in patients with prosthetic joint infections, and it has a high background signal in uninfected muscle, presumably due to host mitochondrial metabolism [50].

4. Conclusions

To conclude, the metabolic imaging of infection holds great promise. The focus of its application is shifting from mere diagnosis of infection to prognostication, to predict the response to treatment, to identify resistant strains and to identify and target at-risk patients for prevention.

New possibilities emerge also by the application of dual-isotope imaging after the simultaneous administration of two radiopharmaceuticals or one radiolabelled and one fluorescent or one paramagnetic.

It is hoped that when PET/MRI and SPECT/MRI achieve greater clinical utility, these hybrid systems may have even more applications in infection imaging due to the high sensitivity of MRI for soft tissues and oedema. It is also hoped that hybrid molecular probes for multimodality imaging soon may gain clinical relevance for infection imaging. Focused research is pointing toward a time when molecular probes will be able not only to detect infection but also to identify the offending organism and its biologic characteristics [47].

Overall, this article highlights that standardized protocols and consensus guidelines regarding animal models of infection are needed, preferably written by a joint technical committee. The optimization of preclinical research should be directed in improving the sensitivity for a broader range of microbes rather than species-specific probes. This broader range approach, in combination with the growing opportunities for imaging the microenvironment at infection sites, may help to resolve the challenges in the development of the radiopharmaceuticals that can differentiate sterile inflammation from infection, and thus, making the imaging of bacteria a viable option for future clinical studies.

Author Contributions: Conceptualization of this paper was made by A.S. and M.S.; data were obtained and analyzed by G.F.-F., M.M.W. and S.K.J. and S.H.; draft preparation by M.C. and A.S.; review and editing by A.S., V.A., M.C., G.F.-F., M.M.W., S.K.J., S.H. and M.S. All authors have read and agreed to the published version of the manuscript.

References

1. Drago, L.; Clerici, P.; Morelli, I.; Ashok, J.; Benzakour, T.; Bozhkova, S.; Alizadeh, C.; Del Sel, H.; Sharma, H.K.; Peel, T.; et al. The World Association against Infection in Orthopaedics and Trauma (WAIOT) procedures for Microbiological Sampling and Processing for Periprosthetic Joint Infections (PJIs) and other Implant-Related Infections. *J. Clin. Med.* **2019**, *8*, 933. [CrossRef] [PubMed]
2. Ordonez, A.A.; Sellmyer, M.A.; Gowrishankar, G.; Ruiz-Bedoya, C.A.; Tucker, E.W.; Palestro, C.J.; Hammoud, D.A.; Jain, S.K. Molecular imaging of bacterial infections: Overcoming the barriers to clinical translation. *Sci. Transl. Med.* **2019**, *11*. [CrossRef] [PubMed]
3. Jain, S.K. The Promise of Molecular Imaging in the Study and Treatment of Infectious Diseases. *Mol. Imaging Biol.* **2017**, *19*, 341–347. [CrossRef] [PubMed]
4. Lambrecht, F.Y. Evaluation of 99mTc-labeled antibiotics for infection detection. *Ann. Nucl. Med.* **2011**, *25*, 1–6. [CrossRef] [PubMed]
5. Oyen, W.J.G.; Corstens, F.H.M.; Boerman, O.C. Discriminating infection from sterile inflammation: Can radiolabelled antibiotics solve the problem? *Eur. J. Nucl. Med. Mol. Imaging* **2005**, *32*, 151–152. [CrossRef]
6. Palestro, C.J.; Glaudemans, A.W.J.M.; Dierckx, R.A.J.O. Multiagent imaging of inflammation and infection with radionuclides. *Clin. Transl. Imaging* **2013**, *1*, 385–396. [CrossRef]
7. Shah, M.; Garg, G.; Dadachova, E. Preclinical testing of radiopharmaceuticals for novel applications in HIV, bacterial and fungal infectious diseases. *Q. J. Nucl. Med. Mol. Imaging* **2015**, *59*, 317–326.
8. Zhuang, H.; Alavi, A. 18-Fluorodeoxyglucose positron emission tomographic imaging in the detection and monitoring of infection and inflammation. *Semin. Nucl. Med.* **2002**, *32*, 47–59. [CrossRef]
9. Heuker, M.; Sijbesma, J.W.A.; Aguilar Suárez, R.; de Jong, J.R.; Boersma, H.H.; Luurtsema, G.; Elsinga, P.H.; Glaudemans, A.W.J.M.; van Dam, G.M.; van Dijl, J.M.; et al. In vitro imaging of bacteria using 18F-fluorodeoxyglucose micro positron emission tomography. *Sci. Rep.* **2017**, *7*, 4973. [CrossRef]
10. Signore, A.; Jamar, F.; Israel, O.; Buscombe, J.; Martin-Comin, J.; Lazzeri, E. Clinical indications, image acquisition and data interpretation for white blood cells and anti-granulocyte monoclonal antibody scintigraphy: An EANM procedural guideline. *Eur. J. Nucl. Med. Mol. Imaging* **2018**, *45*, 1816–1831. [CrossRef]
11. Flemming, H.C.; Wingender, J.; Szewzyk, U.; Steinberg, P.; Rice, S.A.; Kjelleberg, S. Biofilms: An emergent form of bacterial life. *Nat. Rev. Microbiol.* **2016**, *14*, 563–575. [CrossRef] [PubMed]
12. Jacoby, G.A. Mechanisms of Resistance to Quinolones. *Clin. Infect. Dis.* **2005**, *41*, S120–S126. [CrossRef]
13. Hooper, D.C. Mechanisms of quinolone resistance. In *Quinolone Antimicrobial Agents*, 3rd ed.; American Society for Microbiology Press: Washington, DC, USA, 2003; pp. 41–67.
14. Ordonez, A.A.; Wang, H.; Magombedze, G.; Ruiz-Bedoya, C.A.; Srivastava, S.; Chen, A.; Tucker, E.W.; Urbanowski, M.E.; Pieterse, L.; Fabian Cardozo, E.; et al. Dynamic imaging in patients with tuberculosis reveals heterogeneous drug exposures in pulmonary lesions. *Nat. Med.* **2020**, *26*, 529–534. [CrossRef] [PubMed]
15. DeMarco, V.P.; Ordonez, A.A.; Klunk, M.; Prideaux, B.; Wang, H.; Zhuo, Z.; Tonge, P.J.; Dannals, R.F.; Holt, D.P.; Lee, C.K.K.; et al. Determination of [^{11}C]Rifampin Pharmacokinetics within Mycobacterium tuberculosis-Infected Mice by Using Dynamic Positron Emission Tomography Bioimaging. *Antimicrob. Agents Chemother.* **2015**, *59*, 5768–5774. [CrossRef] [PubMed]

16. Ordonez, A.A.; Abhishek, S.; Singh, A.K.; Klunk, M.H.; Azad, B.B.; Aboagye, E.O.; Carroll, L.; Jain, S.K. Caspase-Based PET for Evaluating Pro-Apoptotic Treatments in a Tuberculosis Mouse Model. *Mol. Imaging Biol.* **2020**. [CrossRef] [PubMed]
17. Mota, F.; Ordonez, A.A.; Firth, G.; Ruiz-Bedoya, C.A.; Ma, M.T.; Jain, S.K. Radiotracer Development for Bacterial Imaging. *J. Med. Chem.* **2020**, *63*, 1964–1977. [CrossRef]
18. Monsel, A.; Zhu, Y.; Gennai, S.; Hao, Q.; Liu, J.; Lee, J.W. Cell-based Therapy for Acute Organ Injury: Preclinical Evidence and Ongoing Clinical Trials Using Mesenchymal Stem Cells. *Anesthesiology* **2014**, *121*, 1099–1121. [CrossRef]
19. Signore, A. About inflammation and infection. *EJNMMI Res.* **2013**, *3*, 8. [CrossRef]
20. Northrup, J.D.; Mach, R.H.; Sellmyer, M.A. Radiochemical Approaches to Imaging Bacterial Infections: Intracellular versus Extracellular Targets. *IJMS* **2019**, *20*, 5808. [CrossRef]
21. Ordonez, A.A.; Weinstein, E.A.; Bambarger, L.E.; Saini, V.; Chang, Y.S.; DeMarco, V.P.; Klunk, M.H.; Urbanowski, M.E.; Moulton, K.L.; Murawski, A.M.; et al. A Systematic Approach for Developing Bacteria-Specific Imaging Tracers. *J. Nucl. Med.* **2017**, *58*, 144–150. [CrossRef]
22. Baldoni, D.; Waibel, R.; Bläuenstein, P.; Galli, F.; Iodice, V.; Signore, A.; Schibli, R.; Trampuz, A. Evaluation of a Novel Tc-99m Labelled Vitamin B12 Derivative for Targeting Escherichia coli and Staphylococcus aureus In Vitro and in an Experimental Foreign-Body Infection Model. *Mol. Imaging Biol.* **2015**, *17*, 829–837. [CrossRef] [PubMed]
23. Auletta, S.; Baldoni, D.; Varani, M.; Galli, F.; Hajar, I.A.; Duatti, A.; Ferro-Flores, G.; Trampuz, A.; Signore, A. Comparison of 99mTc-UBI 29-41, 99mTc-ciprofloxacin, 99mTc-ciprofloxacin dithiocarbamate and 111In-biotin for targeting experimental Staphylococcus aureus and Escherichia coli foreign-body infections: An ex-vivo study. *Q. J. Nucl. Med. Mol. Imaging* **2019**, *63*, 37–47. [CrossRef] [PubMed]
24. Signore, A.; Glaudemans, A.W.J.M. The molecular imaging approach to image infections and inflammation by nuclear medicine techniques. *Ann. Nucl. Med.* **2011**, *25*, 681–700. [CrossRef] [PubMed]
25. Ferro-Flores, G.; Arteaga de Murphy, C.; Pedraza-López, M.; Meléndez-Alafort, L.; Zhang, Y.M.; Rusckowski, M.; Hnatowich, D.J. In vitro and in vivo assessment of 99mTc-UBI specificity for bacteria. *Nucl. Med. Biol.* **2003**, *30*, 597–603. [CrossRef]
26. Sathekge, M.; Garcia-Perez, O.; Paez, D.; El-Haj, N.; Kain-Godoy, T.; Lawal, I.; Estrada-Lobato, E. Molecular imaging in musculoskeletal infections with 99mTc-UBI 29-41 SPECT/CT. *Ann. Nucl. Med.* **2018**, *32*, 54–59. [CrossRef] [PubMed]
27. Ning, X.; Seo, W.; Lee, S.; Takemiya, K.; Rafi, M.; Feng, X.; Weiss, D.; Wang, X.; Williams, L.; Camp, V.M.; et al. PET Imaging of Bacterial Infections with Fluorine-18-Labeled Maltohexaose. *Angew. Chem. Int. Ed.* **2014**, *53*, 14096–14101. [CrossRef]
28. Weinstein, E.A.; Ordonez, A.A.; DeMarco, V.P.; Murawski, A.M.; Pokkali, S.; MacDonald, E.M.; Klunk, M.; Mease, R.C.; Pomper, M.G.; Jain, S.K. Imaging Enterobacteriaceae infection in vivo with 18F-fluorodeoxysorbitol positron emission tomography. *Sci. Transl. Med.* **2014**, *6*. [CrossRef]
29. Kang, S.R.; Jo, E.J.; Nguyen, V.H.; Zhang, Y.; Yoon, H.S.; Pyo, A.; Kim, D.Y.; Hong, Y.; Bom, H.S.; Min, J.J. Imaging of tumor colonization by *Escherichia coli* using ^{18} F-FDS PET. *Theranostics* **2020**, *10*, 4958–4966. [CrossRef]
30. Li, J.; Zheng, H.; Fodah, R.; Warawa, J.M.; Ng, C.K. Validation of 2- ^{18} F-Fluorodeoxysorbitol as a Potential Radiopharmaceutical for Imaging Bacterial Infection in the Lung. *J. Nucl. Med.* **2018**, *59*, 134–139. [CrossRef]
31. Takemiya, K.; Ning, X.; Seo, W.; Wang, X.; Mohammad, R.; Joseph, G.; Titterington, J.S.; Kraft, C.S.; Nye, J.A.; Murthy, N.; et al. Novel PET and near infrared imaging probes for the specific detection of bacterial infections associated with cardiac devices. *JACC Cardiovasc. Imaging* **2018**. [CrossRef]
32. Martìnez, M.E.; Kiyono, Y.; Noriki, S.; Inai, K.; Mandap, K.S.; Kobayashi, M.; Mori, T.; Tokunaga, Y.; Tiwari, V.N.; Okazawa, H.; et al. New radiosynthesis of 2-deoxy-2-[18F]fluoroacetamido-D-glucopyranose and its evaluation as a bacterial infections imaging agent. *Nucl. Med. Biol.* **2011**, *38*, 807–817. [CrossRef] [PubMed]
33. Gowrishankar, G.; Hardy, J.; Wardak, M.; Namavari, M.; Reeves, R.E.; Neofytou, E.; Srinivasan, A.; Wu, J.C.; Contag, C.H.; Gambhir, S.S. Specific Imaging of Bacterial Infection Using 6″- ^{18} F-Fluoromaltotriose: A Second-Generation PET Tracer Targeting the Maltodextrin Transporter in Bacteria. *J. Nucl. Med.* **2017**, *58*, 1679–1684. [CrossRef] [PubMed]

34. Neumann, K.D.; Villanueva-Meyer, J.E.; Mutch, C.A.; Flavell, R.R.; Blecha, J.E.; Kwak, T.; Sriram, R.; VanBrocklin, H.F.; Rosenberg, O.S.; Ohliger, M.A.; et al. Imaging Active Infection in vivo Using D-Amino Acid Derived PET Radiotracers. *Sci. Rep.* **2017**, *7*, 7903. [CrossRef] [PubMed]
35. Parker, M.F.L.; Luu, J.M.; Schulte, B.; Huynh, T.L.; Stewart, M.N.; Sriram, R.; Yu, M.A.; Jivan, S.; Turnbaugh, P.J.; Flavell, R.R.; et al. Sensing Living Bacteria in Vivo Using D -Alanine-Derived ^{11} C Radiotracers. *ACS Cent. Sci.* **2020**, *6*, 155–165. [CrossRef]
36. Petrik, M.; Umlaufova, E.; Raclavsky, V.; Palyzova, A.; Havlicek, V.; Haas, H.; Novy, Z.; Dolezal, D.; Hajduch, M.; Decristoforo, C. Imaging of Pseudomonas aeruginosa infection with Ga-68 labelled pyoverdine for positron emission tomography. *Sci. Rep.* **2018**, *8*, 15698. [CrossRef]
37. Mutch, C.A.; Ordonez, A.A.; Qin, H.; Parker, M.; Bambarger, L.E.; Villanueva-Meyer, J.E.; Blecha, J.; Carroll, V.; Taglang, C.; Flavell, R.; et al. [^{11} C]Para-Aminobenzoic Acid: A Positron Emission Tomography Tracer Targeting Bacteria-Specific Metabolism. *ACS Infect. Dis.* **2018**, *4*, 1067–1072. [CrossRef]
38. Sellmyer, M.A.; Lee, I.; Hou, C.; Weng, C.C.; Li, S.; Lieberman, B.P.; Zeng, C.; Mankoff, D.A.; Mach, R.H. Bacterial infection imaging with [^{18} F]fluoropropyl-trimethoprim. *Proc. Natl. Acad. Sci. USA* **2017**, *114*, 8372–8377. [CrossRef]
39. Zhang, Z.; Ordonez, A.A.; Wang, H.; Li, Y.; Gogarty, K.R.; Weinstein, E.A.; Daryaee, F.; Merino, J.; Yoon, G.E.; Kalinda, A.S.; et al. Positron Emission Tomography Imaging with 2-[^{18} F]F- *p* -Aminobenzoic Acid Detects *Staphylococcus aureus* Infections and Monitors Drug Response. *ACS Infect. Dis.* **2018**, *4*, 1635–1644. [CrossRef]
40. Foss, C.A.; Harper, J.S.; Wang, H.; Pomper, M.G.; Jain, S.K. Noninvasive Molecular Imaging of Tuberculosis-Associated Inflammation with Radioiodinated DPA-713. *J. Infect. Dis.* **2013**, *208*, 2067–2074. [CrossRef]
41. Britton, K.E. Imaging bacterial infection with 99mTc-ciprofloxacin (Infecton). *J. Clin. Pathol.* **2002**, *55*, 817–823. [CrossRef]
42. Dumarey, N.; Blocklet, D.; Appelboom, T.; Tant, L.; Schoutens, A. Infecton is not specific for bacterial osteo-articular infective pathology. *Eur. J. Nucl. Med. Mol. Imaging* **2002**, *29*, 530–535. [CrossRef] [PubMed]
43. Sarda, L.; Cremieux, A.C.; Lebellec, Y.; Meulemans, A.; Lebtahi, R.; Hayem, G.; Genin, R.; Delahaye, N.; Huten, D.; Le Guludec, D. Inability of Tc-99m-ciprofloxacin scintigraphy to discriminate between septic and sterile osteoarticular diseases. *J. Nucl. Med.* **2003**, *44*, 920–926. [PubMed]
44. Palestro, C.J.; Love, C.; Caprioli, R.; Marwin, S.E.; Richardson, H.; Haight, J.; Tronco, G.G.; Pugliese, P.V.; Bhargava, K.K. Phase II study of 99mTc-ciprofloxacin uptake in patients with high suspicion of osteomyelitis [abstract]. *J. Nucl. Med.* **2007**, *47*, 152.
45. Ankrah, A.O.; van der Werf, T.S.; de Vries, E.F.J.; Dierckx, R.A.J.O.; Sathekge, M.M.; Glaudemans, A.W.J.M. PET/CT imaging of Mycobacterium tuberculosis infection. *Clin. Transl. Imaging* **2016**, *4*, 131–144. [CrossRef]
46. Ebenhan, T.; Zeevaart, J.R.; Venter, J.D.; Govender, T.; Kruger, G.H.; Jarvis, N.V.; Sathekge, M.M. Preclinical Evaluation of 68Ga-Labeled 1,4,7-Triazacyclononane-1,4,7-Triacetic Acid-Ubiquicidin as a Radioligand for PET Infection Imaging. *J. Nucl. Med.* **2014**, *55*, 308–314. [CrossRef]
47. Lawal, I.; Zeevaart, J.; Ebenhan, T.; Ankrah, A.; Vorster, M.; Kruger, H.G.; Govender, T.; Sathekge, M. Metabolic Imaging of Infection. *J. Nucl. Med.* **2017**, *58*, 1727–1732. [CrossRef]
48. Bhatt, J.; Mukherjee, A.; Shinto, A.; Koramadai Karuppusamy, K.; Korde, A.; Kumar, M.; Sarma, H.D.; Repaka, K.; Dash, A. Gallium-68 labeled Ubiquicidin derived octapeptide as a potential infection imaging agent. *Nucl. Med. Biol.* **2018**, *62*, 47–53. [CrossRef]
49. Van Oosten, M.; Schäfer, T.; Gazendam, J.A.C.; Ohlsen, K.; Tsompanidou, E.; de Goffau, M.C.; Harmsen, H.J.M.; Crane, L.M.A.; Lim, E.; Francis, K.P.; et al. Real-time in vivo imaging of invasive- and biomaterial-associated bacterial infections using fluorescently labelled vancomycin. *Nat. Commun.* **2013**, *4*, 2584. [CrossRef]
50. Zhang, X.M.; Zhang, H.H.; McLeroth, P.; Berkowitz, R.D.; Mont, M.A.; Stabin, M.G.; Siegel, B.A.; Alavi, A.; Barnett, T.M.; Gelb, J.; et al. [^{124}I]FIAU: Human dosimetry and infection imaging in patients with suspected prosthetic joint infection. *Nucl. Med. Biol.* **2016**, *43*, 273–279. [CrossRef]

12

The Role of Imaging Techniques to Define a Peri-Prosthetic Hip and Knee Joint Infection: Multidisciplinary Consensus Statements

Carlo Luca Romanò [1], Nicola Petrosillo [2], Giuseppe Argento [3], Luca Maria Sconfienza [4,5], Giorgio Treglia [6,7], Abass Alavi [8], Andor W.J.M. Glaudemans [9], Olivier Gheysens [10], Alex Maes [11], Chiara Lauri [12], Christopher J. Palestro [13] and Alberto Signore [12,*]

1 Gruppo di Studio SIOT Infezioni-Clinica San Gaudenzio-Novara-Gruppo Policlinico di Monza, University of Milan, 20100 Milan, Italy; carlo.romano@unimi.it
2 Clinical and Research Department for Infectious Diseases, National Institute for Infective Diseases "L. Spallanzani", 00144 Rome, Italy; nicola.petrosillo@inmi.it
3 Radiology Unit, AOU Sant'Andrea, 00189 Rome, Italy; giuseppe.argento@uniroma1.it
4 IRCCS Istituto Ortopedico Galeazzi, 20161 Milan, Italy; io@lucasconfienza.it
5 Department of Biomedical Sciences for Health, University of Milan, 20123 Milan, Italy
6 Nuclear Medicine and PET/CT Center, Imaging Institute of Southern Switzerland, Ente Ospedaliero Cantonale Via Lugano 4F, CH-6500 Bellinzona, Switzerland; giorgiomednuc@libero.it
7 Department of Nuclear Medicine and Molecular Imaging, Lausanne University Hospital and University of Lausanne, 1011 Lausanne, Switzerland
8 Division of Nuclear Medicine, Department of Radiology, Hospital of the University of Pennsylvania, Philadelphia, PA 1904, USA; abass.alavi@pennmedicine.upenn.edu
9 Department of Nuclear Medicine and Molecular Imaging, University of Groningen, University Medical Center Groningen, 9713 GZ Groningen, The Netherlands; a.w.j.m.glaudemans@umcg.nl
10 Department of Nuclear Medicine, Cliniques Universitaires Saint-Luc, 1200 Brussels, Belgium; olivier.gheysens@uclouvain.be
11 Department of Nuclear Medicine, AZ Groeninge, Kortrijk Belgium and Department of Imaging and Pathology @ KULAK, KU Leuven campus Kulak, 8500 Kortrijk, Belgium; alex.maes@azgroeninge.be
12 Nuclear Medicine Unit Department of Medical-Surgical Sciences and of Translational Medicine, Faculty of Medicine and Psychology, "Sapienza" University of Rome, 00161 Rome, Italy; chialau84@hotmail.it
13 Department of Radiology Donald and Barbara Zucker School of Medicine at Hofstra/Northwell, Hempstead, NY 11549, USA; palestro@northwell.edu
* Correspondence: alberto.signore@uniroma1.it

Abstract: Diagnosing a peri-prosthetic joint infection (PJI) remains challenging despite the availability of a variety of clinical signs, serum and synovial markers, imaging techniques, microbiological and histological findings. Moreover, the one and only true definition of PJI does not exist, which is reflected by the existence of at least six different definitions by independent societies. These definitions are composed of major and minor criteria for defining a PJI, but most of them do not include imaging techniques. This paper highlights the pros and cons of available imaging techniques—X-ray, ultrasound, computed tomography (CT), Magnetic Resonance Imaging (MRI), bone scintigraphy, white blood cell scintigraphy (WBC), anti-granulocyte scintigraphy, and fluorodeoxyglucose positron emission tomography/computed tomography (FDG-PET/CT), discusses the added value of hybrid camera systems—single photon emission tomography/computed tomography (SPECT/CT), PET/CT and PET/MRI and reports consensus answers on important clinical questions that were discussed during the Third European Congress on Inflammation/Infection Imaging in Rome, December 2019.

Keywords: prosthetic joint infection; nuclear imaging; SPECT/CT; PET/CT; radiology

1. Introduction

The definition and the diagnosis of peri-prosthetic joint infection (PJI) and, more generally, of implant-related infections, remains a challenge of modern orthopaedics.

In fact, while it seems relatively straightforward to diagnose an infection in the presence of a draining sinus, an exposed implant, or classical signs and symptoms of an acute inflammatory process, the differential diagnosis between septic and aseptic implant failure becomes much more challenging when unspecific clinical symptoms—most often a variable degree of pain and reduced function—are reported, and laboratory tests yield nonspecific or conflicting results.

Clinical presentations of peri-prosthetic infection are extremely varied, ranging from the acute, high-grade inflammatory cases to the subclinical low-grade ones [1–3]. The lack of a single accepted reference test or benchmark makes the evaluation and comparison of the diagnostic accuracy of both old and new markers, as well as other diagnostic tools, particularly difficult [4–6].

The diagnostic challenge is mirrored by the absence of a universally accepted definition of PJI. In the last decade, at least six different definitions of PJI have been released by well-respected scientific societies, including the Musculo-Skeletal Infection Society (MSIS) [7], the Infectious Disease Society of America (IDSA) [8], two International Consensus Meetings [9–11], the European Bone and Joint Infection Society (EBJIS) [1], (Table 1) and, more recently, the World Association against Infection in Orthopaedics and Trauma (WAIOT) (Table 2) [12].

Table 1. Comparison of the diagnostic criteria adopted by five peri-prosthetic joint infection (PJI) definitions, published from 2011 to 2018 (modified from [13]). MSIS: Musculo-Skeletal Infection Society; IDSA: Infectious Disease Society of America; ICM: International Consensus Meeting; EBJIS: European Bone and Joint Infection Society.

Definition Source	MSIS 2011	IDSA 2013	ICM 2013	ICM 2018	Proposed EBJIS 2018
Scoring System	1 of the 2 major criteria OR ≥4 of 6 minor criteria [1]	≥1 positive criteria [2]	1 of the 2 major criteria OR ≥3 of 5 minor criteria [3]	1 of the 2 major criteria OR minor criteria scoring ≥6 infected 3–5 possibly infected ("consider further molecular diagnostics such as next-generation sequencing") <3 not infected [4]	≥1 positive criteria
Criteria	Major: 1. sinus tract communicating with the prosthesis; 2. A pathogen is isolated by culture from at least two separate tissue or fluid samples obtained from the affected prosthetic joint Minor: (a) Elevated ESR (>30 mm/hr) and CRP (>10 mg/L) concentration (b) Elevated synovial leukocyte count (c) Elevated PMN% (d) Purulence in the affected joint (e) Isolation of a microorganism in one culture of periprosthetic tissue or fluid (f) Greater than five neutrophils per high-power field in five high-power fields observed from histologic analysis of periprosthetic tissue at 400× magnification	1. Sinus tract communicating with the prosthesis 2. Purulence without other aetiology surrounding the prosthesis 3. Acute inflammation seen on histopathological examination of the periprosthetic tissue 4. ≥2 intraoperative cultures or combination of preoperative aspiration and intraoperative cultures yielding an indistinguishable organism (the growth of a virulent microorganism (e.g., *Staphylococcus aureus*) in a single specimen of a tissue biopsy or synovial fluid is also considered as indicative of a PJI)	Major: 1. A sinus tract communicating with the joint 2. Two positive periprosthetic cultures with phenotypically identical organisms, Minor: (a) Elevated ESR (>30 mm/hr) and CRP (>100 mg/L for acute infections; >10 mg/L for chronic infections) (b) Elevated synovial fluid WBC count (>10,000 cells/mL for acute infections; >3000 cells/mL for chronic infections) or ++ change on leukocyte esterase test strip (c) Elevated PMN% (>90% for acute infections; >80% for chronic infections) (d) Positive histological analysis of periprosthetic tissue (>5 neutrophils per high-power field in five high-power fields observed on periprosthetic tissue at 400× magnification) (e) A single positive culture	Major: 1. Sinus tract with evidence of communication to the joint or visualization of the prosthesis 2. Two positive growths of the same organism using standard culture methods Minor: (a) Elevated CRP (>100 mg/L for acute infections; >10 mg/L for chronic infections) or D-dimer (unknown threshold for acute infection; >860 ug/L for chronic infection) (score 2) (b) Elevated ESR (no role for acute infections; >30 mm/hr for chronic infections) (score 1) (c) Elevated synovial WBC count (>10,000 cells/mL for acute infections; >3000 cells/mL for chronic infections) OR leukocyte esterase (++ for acute and chronic infections) OR positive alpha-defensin (score 3) (d) Elevated synovial PMN% (>90% for acute infections; >70% for chronic infections) (score 2) (e) Single positive culture (score 2) (f) Positive histology (score 3) (g) Positive intraoperative purulence (score 3)	1. Purulence around the prosthesis or sinus tract 2. Increased synovial fluid leukocyte count (>2000 cells/mL or >70% granulocytes) 3. Positive histopathology 4. Confirmatory microbial growth in synovial fluid, periprosthetic tissue, or sonication culture ("confirmatory microbial growth in periprosthetic tissue: if positive in ≥1 specimen in highly virulent organisms or ≥2 in low virulent pathogens; sonication culture considered positive if >50 colony-forming units/mL of sonication fluid.")

Abbreviations: ESR: erythrocyte sedimentation rate; CRP: C-reactive protein; PMN: polymorphonuclear leukocytes; WBC: white blood cells; ++: positive. [1] PJI may be present if fewer than four of these criteria are met. [2] The presence of PJI is possible even if the above criteria are not met. [3] PJI may be present without meeting these criteria. [4] Proceed with caution in adverse local tissue reaction, crystal deposition disease, slow growing organisms.

Table 2. World Association against Infection in Orthopaedics and Trauma (WAIOT) proposed definition of peri-prosthetic joint infection (PJI). Pre- and intra-operative tests, classified according to their sensitivity and specificity and hence their ability to exclude ("rule OUT") or to confirm ("rule IN") a PJI. In parenthesis, the reference cut-off value considered here (modified from [13]).

	No Infection	Contamination	BIM	LG-PJI	HG-PJI
Clinical presentation	One or more condition(s), other than infection, can cause the symptoms or the reason for reoperation (e.g., wear debris, metallosis, recurrent dislocation or joint instability, fracture, malposition, neuropathic pain)		One or more of the following: otherwise "unexplained" pain, swelling, stiffness		Two or more of the following: pain, swelling, redness, warmth, functio laesa
(Number of positive rule IN tests)-(number of negative rule OUT tests)	<0	<0	<0	≥0	≥1
Post-operatively confirmed if	Negative cultural examination	One pre- or intra-operative positive culture, with negative histology	Positive cultural examination (preferably with antibiofilm techniques) and/or positive histology		
Rule OUT Tests (Sensitivity > 90%) EACH NEGATIVE TEST Scores − 1 (Positive Rule OUT Test Score 0)					
Serum	ESR (>30 mm/h) CRP (>10 mg/L)				
Synovial fluid	WBC (>1500/μL) LE (++) Alpha-defensin immunoassay (>5.2 mg/L)				
Imaging	^{99m}Tc bone scan				
Rule IN Tests (Specificity > 90%) EACH POSITIVE TEST Scores + 1 (Negative Rule IN Test Score 0)					
Clinical examination	Purulence or draining sinus or exposed joint prosthesis				
Serum	IL-6 (>10 pg/mL) PC (>0.5 ng/mL) D-Dimer (>850 ng/mL)				
Synovial fluid	Cultural examination WBC (>3000/mL) LE (++) Alpha-defensin immunoassay (>5.2 mg/L) or lateral flow test				
Imaging	Radio-labelled leukocyte scintigraphy (if necessary, with combined bone marrow scintigraphy)				
Histology	Frozen section (5 neutrophils in at least 3 HPFs)				

Abbreviations: BIM: biofilm-related implant malfunction; LG-PJI: low-grade peri-prosthetic joint infection; HG-PJI: high-grade peri-prosthetic joint infection. ESR: erythrocyte sedimentation rate; CRP: C-reactive protein; IL-6: interleukin-6; WBC: white blood cell count; PC: procalcitonin; LE: leukocyte esterase strip (++); HPFs: high power fields (400×); ^{99m}Tc: 99 metastable Technetium.

These six definitions differ greatly in their diagnostic criteria, scoring systems and reference values (Tables 1 and 2), while even the most complex scores may result as "inconclusive" in a given patient [10]. Of note, with the exception of the WAIOT's definition, all other proposed definitions of PJI include only a selection of diagnostic tests while systematically excluding any role of imaging, in spite of their reported diagnostic value (Table 2) [14]. In doing so, none of them provide a clear scientific explanation for this exclusion, while on the other hand, it is a common observation that most clinicians do prescribe some imaging investigations when dealing with a (suspected case of) PJI. In this complex panorama, to further understand the role of imaging techniques in the diagnostic protocol of peri-prosthetic joint infections, a multidisciplinary group met from December 9 to 12, 2019 in Rome, during the Third European Congress on Inflammation/Infection Imaging.

The results of the discussions, held during those days and thereafter through online consultations, are reported here in the form of clinical questions with consensus answers. These are also based on the previously published Italian Guidelines to Diagnose Peri-Prosthetic Joint Infections [15] and joint European guidelines on PJI published by European Association of Nuclear Medicine (EANM), European Bone and Joint Infection Society (EBJIS) and European Society of Radiology (ESR), with the endorsement of European Society of Clinical Microbiology and Infectious Disease (ESCMID) [14,16], to which we refer that contain details about all imaging modalities.

2. Assessment Parameters of Peri-Prosthetic Joint According to PJI Definitions

Current PJI definitions rely on four diagnostic classes of investigations: (1) clinical presentation, (2) serum and synovial markers, (3) imaging techniques and (4) microbiological and histological findings (Tables 1 and 2).

Concerning clinical presentation, the presence of a draining sinus or of an exposed implant is considered as pathognomonic or highly specific by all the available definitions [7–12]. However, this sign may be totally absent in more than 70% of peri-prosthetic joint infections, thus featuring a quite low sensitivity [17].

Serum and synovial fluid markers are variably included in all the available PJI definitions, apart from the one released by IDSA, while the proposed EBJIS definition only considers synovial leukocyte cell count. No single biomarker has been shown to be 100% accurate in diagnosing PJI, and therefore all definitions introduced a scoring system based on combining the results of different tests. These scoring systems not only vary greatly among the definitions, but also differ in cut-off values that are chosen for the various definitions, which limits their comparability. Furthermore, most of the definition systems acknowledge the fact that serum and synovial biomarkers results should be interpreted with caution within the first three months after surgery and in patients under antibiotic treatment or patients with concomitant systemic inflammatory diseases.

Concerning imaging, no available PJI definition includes any of these investigations, except for the recently released WAIOT definition (Table 2).

The WAIOT definition, validated in a large clinical, multi-institutional and international trial [13], includes only two imaging techniques, 99metastable Technetium (^{99m}Tc)-bone scan and ^{99m}Tc-leukocyte scan, chosen according to the available literature, respectively as a 'rule out' and 'rule in' test to define PJI. In this regard, it should be noted that the WAIOT definition provides a set of rule out and rule in tests, among which the clinician is left free to choose. The final definition is based on the relative balance of positive rule in tests and negative rule out tests. Microbiological and histological findings are considered relevant investigations by all the available definitions to confirm PJI. More specifically, positive cultures, even if criteria and recommendations vary across definitions, are considered pathognomonic by all of the classification systems examined in Tables 1 and 2. However, limitations do apply with regard to the interpretation of a single positive culture and for suboptimal procedural investigations. In fact, falsely negative cultures are reported in approximately 20% of PJIs, according to a recent review [18]. Therefore, microbiological sampling, transport and processing should be performed according to the best available microbiological standards, which includes the preparation of four to six peri-prosthetic tissue cultures and the analysis of the removed implant, transported in closed systems processing with antibiofilm techniques (sonication or dithiothreitol) and with prolonged cultures. In selected cases, genomic pathogen identification may also be advisable [19].

Similarly, histology is ranked among the most specific examinations to differentiate a PJI from other causes and is highly scored or plays a confirmatory role in five out of six of the examined PJI definitions, even if its sensitivity may by be as low as 57% and it may be prone to interpretation bias, according to the experience of the pathologist [20].

3. Conventional Techniques for Diagnosis of PJI

The first diagnostic imaging modality is generally conventional radiography.

X-ray examinations are the standard examination to perform after arthroplasty and for follow-up to assess the presence of displacement, mobilization of the implant components, periprosthetic bone resorption and other causes of pain.

However, diagnostic performance of conventional radiography in detecting PJI is very low. Furthermore, conventional radiography may show demineralization only when more than 30–50% of bone mass has been lost, and abnormalities of bone around the implant are usually non-specific for infection. In addition, up to 50% of conventional *X*-ray exams give negative results.

Regarding ultrasound (US), disputable results have been reported for the detection of PJI. US may be used to guide aspiration procedures of infectious materials in PJI and can be effectively used to evaluate peri-prosthetic fluid collections, attempting to differentiate abscesses from aseptic collections [21], and to track the presence of sinus tracts within soft tissues. The main advantages of US are its wide availability, low cost, the possibility to perform it bedside and repeated imaging without radiation burden [21].

Computed tomography (CT) has been reported to have a good diagnostic performance in the detection of PJI, with accuracy of up to 84% (Figure 1). CT is also the imaging modality of choice perform image-guided bone biopsies [22].

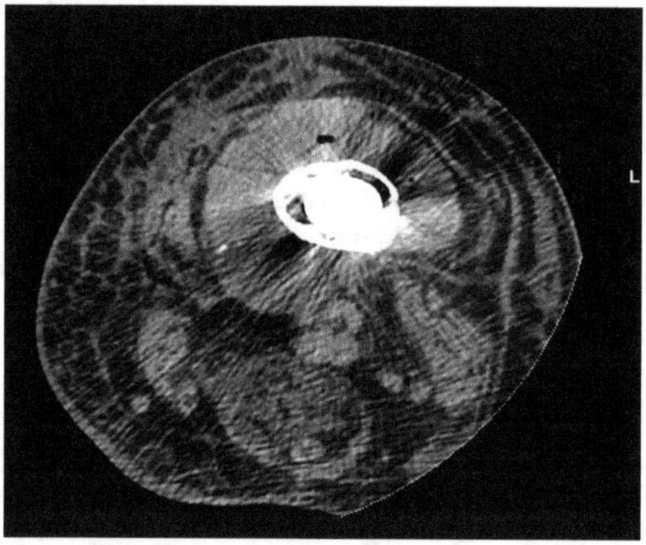

Figure 1. Computed tomography (CT) features: axial scan showing a fluid collection with increasd density surrounding infected bone with a prosthetic implant. Note the swelling and hyperdensity of soft tissues due to edema.

Most papers dealing with magnetic resonance imaging (MRI) in the field of PJI have been focused on technical feasibility and metallic artefact reduction.

For knee arthroplasty, MRI has been shown to be highly sensitive (92%) and specific (99%) for diagnosing PJI. Only one paper has been published in patients with hip arthroplasty showing that the presence of periosteal reaction, capsule edema, and intramuscular edema has a high accuracy for evaluating PJI [23], (Figure 2). Similar to US, MRI has the advantage of not using ionizing radiation or contrast agents [24–26].

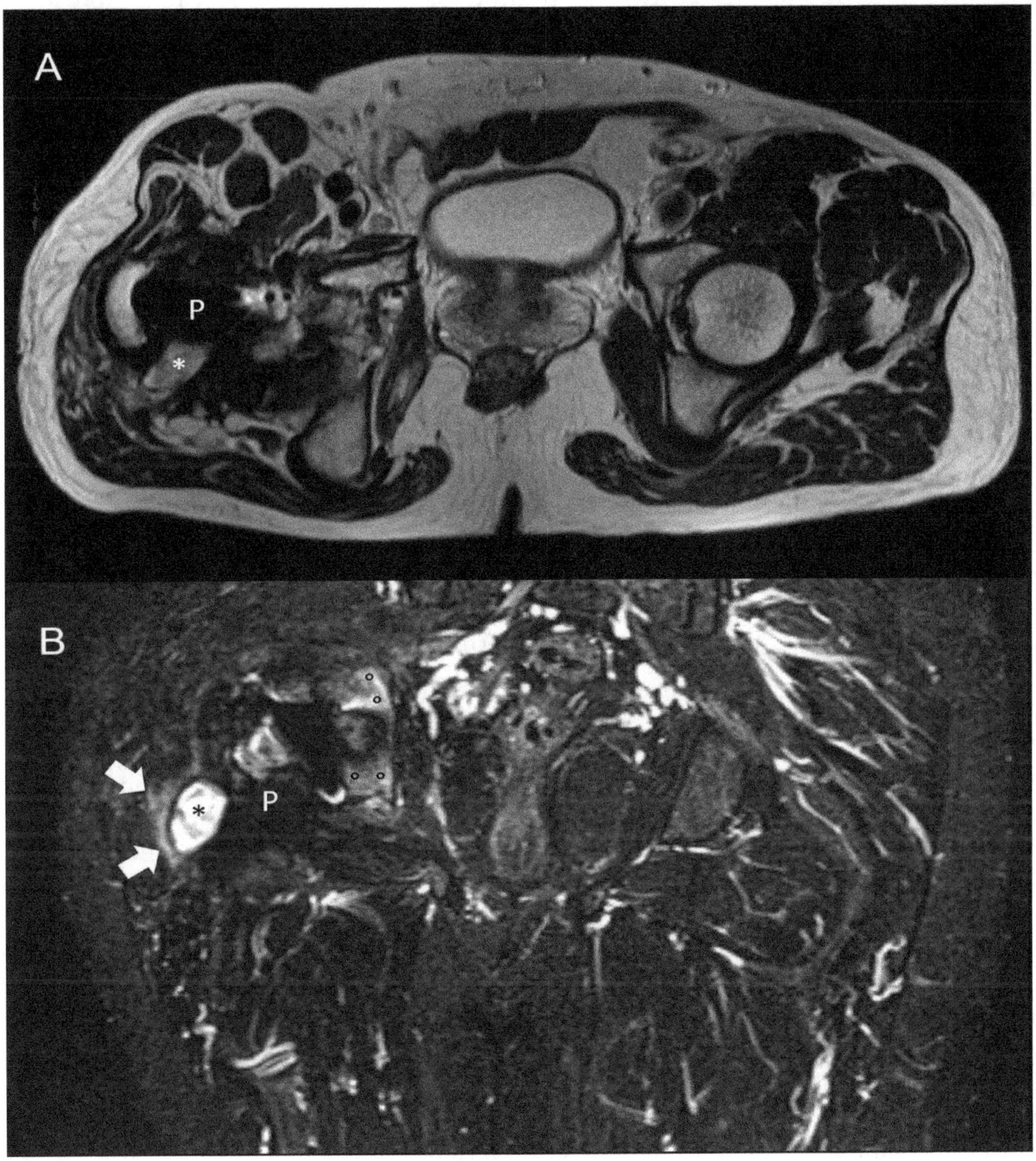

Figure 2. Magnetic resonance imaging (MRI) of a 58-year-old patient with culture-proven infected right hip prosthesis. (**A**) T2-weighted axial and (**B**) short-tau inversion recovery coronal scan show hyperintense synovitis (asterisks), extra-capsular edema (arrows), and bone edema (circles). Metallic artefact is limited to the implant only (P) and does not obscure the findings of infection.

Both CT and MRI may be useful to document the extent of bone lesions as well as abnormalities in the articular space and, therefore, they may help the surgeon in planning the most appropriate strategy. Moreover, US and CT are extremely useful for performing (when feasible) fluid aspirations, thus representing an important tool in the diagnostic work-up of PJI.

4. Nuclear Medicine Techniques for Diagnosis of PJI

Several imaging techniques can be used to evaluate PJI including bone scintigraphy, radio-labelled white blood cell (WBC) scintigraphy (with or without combined bone marrow scintigraphy), anti-granulocyte antibody scintigraphy, and fluorodeoxyglucose positron emission tomography ([^{18}F]-FDG-PET).

Both planar and tomographic acquisitions, with single photon emission tomography (SPECT), can be performed and the use of hybrid modalities such as SPECT/CT or PET/CT increases the diagnostic accuracy in terms of the exact location and extent of the infectious process. Importantly, scintigraphic techniques by gamma camera are not affected by metallic hardware; PET/CT may present some artefacts.

4.1. Bone Scintigraphy

Bone scintigraphy is usually performed after the injection of ^{99m}Tc-labelled diphosphonates and a three-phase bone scintigraphy can be performed to assess early perfusion, diffusion, and late bone uptake. The uptake of these tracers is usually related to bone remodelling. After a prosthetic implant, the periprosthetic bone is obviously damaged and a remodelling process will occur in the months following surgery.

This remodelling process is more evident for bio-inductive prostheses compared to cemented prostheses. The main advantage of bone scintigraphy is its very high sensitivity (when negative, it rules out an infection with high certainty), but this method is accompanied by a low specificity for PJI.

Conversely, this method may be able to detect bone abnormalities in case of prosthetic mobilization, particularly if a hybrid SPECT/CT technique is used. Recently, the EANM Bone and Joint Committee has published procedural guidelines on how to perform this modality best for each pathology [27].

4.2. White Blood Cell Scintigraphy

WBCs can be labelled with ^{99m}Tc- hexamethylene-propyleneamine oxime (HMPAO) (Figure 3) or ^{111}In-oxine (Figure 4). The labelling method, image acquisition and interpretation are regulated by several national rules and guidelines [28–30].

Taking into account the different biodistribution and kinetics of radio-labelled WBCs in blood, bone-marrow, infection and sterile inflammation, images should be acquired at three different time points with decay time-corrected acquisition: "early images" (within 30 min and 1 h after radiopharmaceutical injection), "delayed images" (between 2 h and 4 h after radiopharmaceutical injection) and "late images" (between 20 h and 24 h after radiopharmaceutical injection). Even though the diagnosis of a PJI is made on planar images (increase in uptake or size between the delayed images at 3–4 h and the late images at 20–24 h), tomographic images are recommended in case of positive planar images to assess the exact location and extent of the infectious process. Using these image acquisition parameters and interpretation criteria, this technique reaches a high sensitivity and specificity, as a recent multicenter study has shown [31]. The overall diagnostic accuracy of this technique exceeds 90% for PJI and this method constitutes the gold standard imaging technique for diagnosing PJI.

4.3. Anti-Granulocyte Antibody Scintigraphy

^{99m}Tc-labelled monoclonal antibodies (mAbs) may be used as an alternative to WBC scintigraphy to evaluate PJI. Besilesomab is a full size anti-granulocyte mAb produced in murine cells and designed to attach to the non-specific cross reacting antigen (NCA)-95 antigen localized on the surface of granulocytes. Sulesomab is an antigen-binding mAb fragment designed to target the NCA-90 antigen on the surface of granulocytes. For radio-labelled mAbs, imaging protocols differ between complete and fragmented antibodies [32]. The acquisition protocol for full length antibodies (Besilesomab) is similar to WBC scintigraphy. The best time point for SPECT images is at 16–24 h post injection, similarly to WBC, but an early scan can also be performed if required.

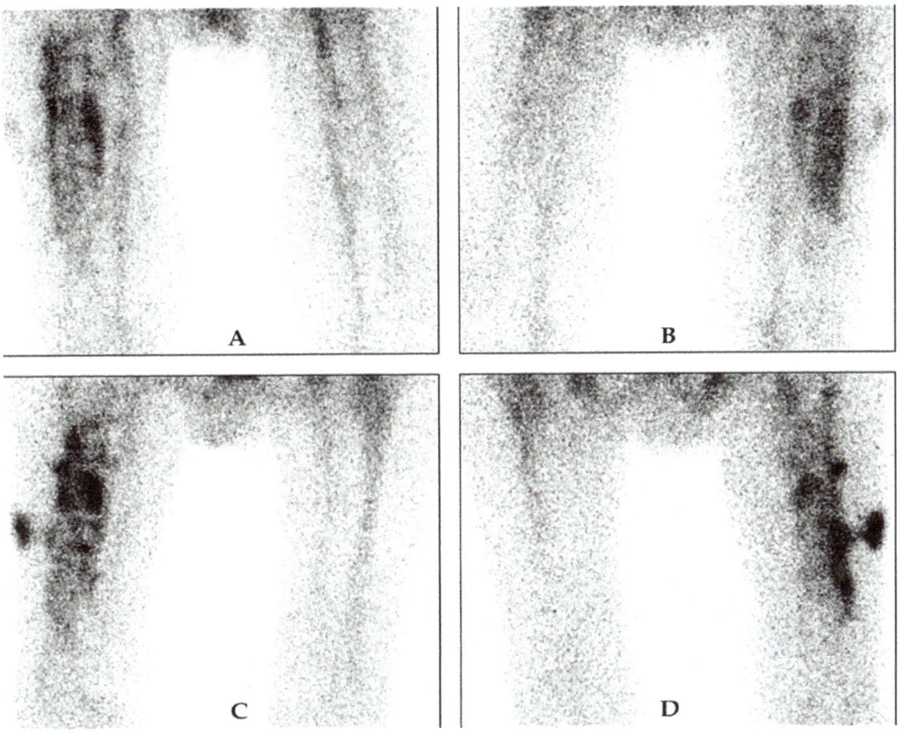

Figure 3. Example of ^{99m}Tc- hexamethylene-propyleneamine oxime (HMPAO)-WBC scintigraphy in a patient with suspected PJI. Upper row: delayed images, (**A**) anterior and (**B**) posterior view, and lower row: late images, (**C**) anterior and (**D**) posterior view. There is increase in intensity and in size between the delayed and late images, which is very suspicious of a PJI. There is also extension of the infection to the peri-prosthetic soft tissue at the lateral side.

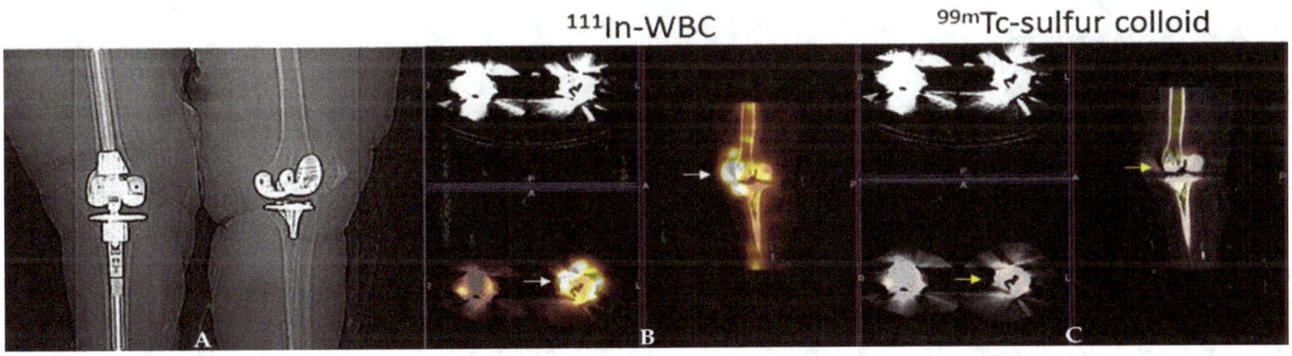

Figure 4. Periprosthetic infection left knee arthroplasty. Scout radiograph (**A**) demonstrates bilateral knee arthroplasties. The right is a revision arthroplasty and the left is a primary implant. On the ^{111}In-WBC single photon emission computed tomography/computed tomography (SPECT)/CT) (**B**) there is abnormal labeled leukocyte activity along the anterior aspect of the left knee arthroplasty (white arrows). On the ^{99m}Tc-sulfur colloid SPECT/CT (**C**), there is no corresponding activity in this region (yellow arrows) and therefore the study is positive for infection.

In contrast, with ^{99m}Tc-sulesomab, planar images should be performed 1 h and 4–6 h post injection due to the faster clearance of the fragmented antibody [30].

4.4. Bone Marrow Scintigraphy

Bone marrow scintigraphy is usually recommended in addition to WBC scintigraphy in equivocal cases. The radiopharmaceutical used is ^{99m}Tc-colloids (colloids greater than 500 nm) that enables visualization of the bone marrow (thus distinguishing expanded bone marrow from sites of leukocyte accumulation). About 185 MBq of ^{99m}Tc-colloids are intravenously injected and planar scintigraphic images of the region of interest are usually acquired after a minimum of 20–30 min and a maximum of 6 h post injection [30]. Concordant findings between both techniques rule out an infectious process while discordant findings (uptake on WBC scintigraphy without corresponding uptake on bone marrow scintigraphy) are highly suggestive of an infection.

4.5. FDG PET/CT

Although [^{18}F]-FDG-PET/CT offers several advantages over WBC scintigraphy (more convenient for the patient, no need for cell labeling, whole procedure takes less than 2 h), looking at the available published data so far, it is unclear whether [^{18}F]-FDG-PET may offer significant advantages over radio-labelled WBC or anti-granulocyte monoclonal antibodies for the evaluation of PJI [33,34]. Different interpretation criteria for PJI have been proposed by Reinartz et al. [35], Chacko et al. [36], Love et al. [37], Familiari et al. [38] and Stumpe et al. [39], but all these studies led to an overall accuracy of <90% with conflicting results amongst studies [40,41]. In any case, visual interpretation is generally more reliable than quantitative (SUV) analysis, which is currently not recommended (Figure 5).

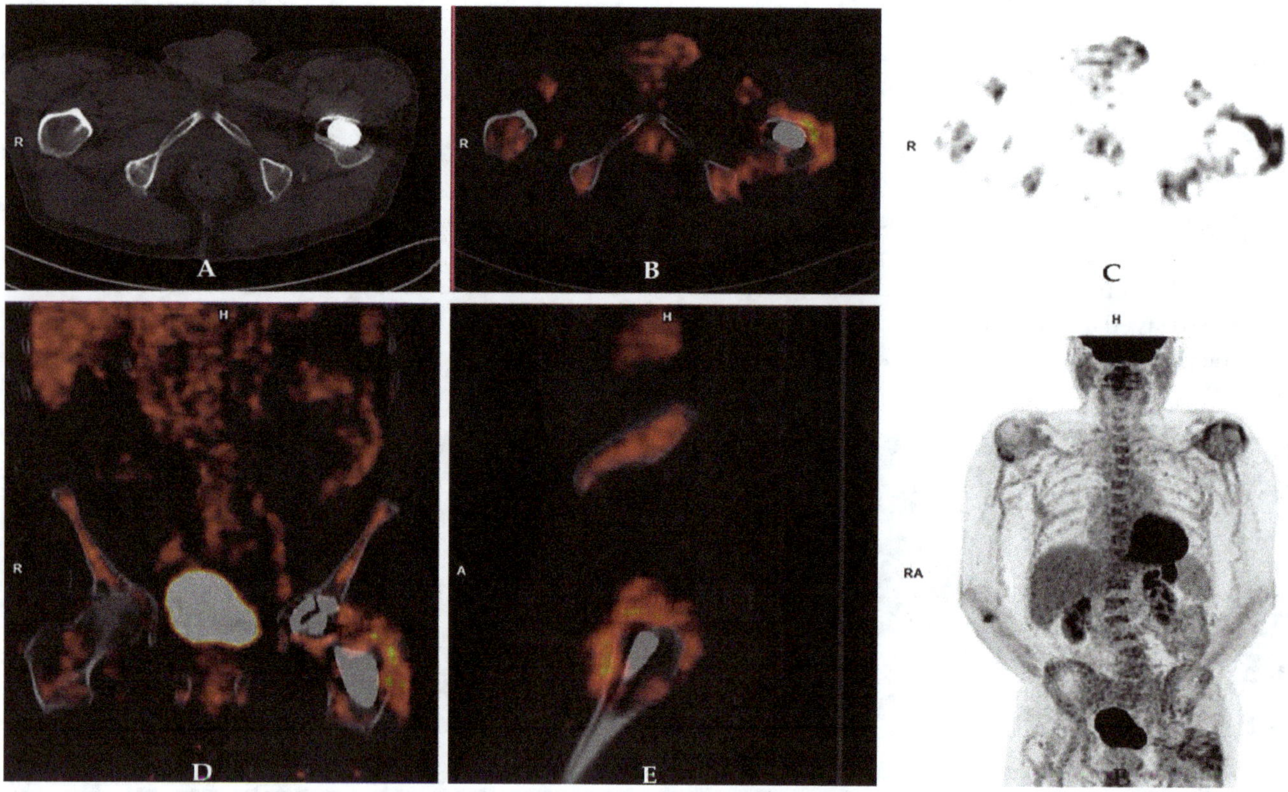

Figure 5. Prosthetic joint infection detected by 18Fluorine-fluorodeoxyglucose positron emission tomography/computed tomography ([^{18}F]-FDG-PET/CT) in a 72-year-old male patient who underwent left hip arthroplasty four years before the PET/CT scan. [^{18}F]-FDG-PET/CT images (**A**: axial view of CT scan; **B**: axail fused images; **C**: axial PET images; **D**: coronal [^{18}F]-FDG-PET/CT view; **E**: sagittal [^{18}F]-FDG-PET/CT view; **F**: maximum intensity projection [^{18}F]-FDG-PET images) showed increased radiopharmaceutical uptake in the periprosthetic bone and soft tissues at the level of the femoral component of the prosthesis. These findings were indicative of prosthetic joint infection, which was confirmed by further examinations including microbiological culture.

4.6. Hybrid Imaging Techniques

Hybrid imaging modalities combining functional and anatomical data have significantly increased the accuracy of conventional nuclear medicine modalities by reducing the number of doubtful cases.

The hybrid imaging approach leads to a more accurate assessment of both localization (soft tissue vs. bone vs. both) and disease extent.

SPECT/CT is nowadays often performed as an integral part of a conventional WBC/mAb scintigraphy in order to better localize the uptake into bone or soft tissues and to accurately assess the extent of the infection [42–46]. [^{18}F]-FDG-PET/CT can be considered as a first-line diagnostic tool for evaluating patients with inflammatory diseases and/or fever of unknown origin, according to evidence-based data [41]; in cases of spondylodiscitis and fungal infections, its role has also been well described.

More recently, the introduction of PET/MRI has emerged as a powerful diagnostic tool, but its value in PJI has not been systematically addressed. The general advantages of MRI compared to CT include a better evaluation of soft tissue and a lack of radiation burden. In addition, MRI sequences that avoid artefacts from metallic implants are now widely available [23–26,47–51].

Finally, it is worth mentioning that one should always keep in mind that the final decision for a particular imaging technique will be highly dependent on the local availability, time, cost and expertise.

5. Clinical Questions and Consensus Answers

At the Third European Congress on Inflammation/Infection Imaging, held in Rome on December 2019, there were several sessions dedicated to radiological and nuclear medicine imaging of prosthetic joint infections. The round table discussions, with clinicians and specialists in infective disease, were very much animated in particular with regard to the role of CT vs. MRI and FDG-PET/CT vs. radio-labelled WBC. Below are the main points raised by orthopedic surgeons and the answers provided by radiologists and nuclear medicine physicians.

5.1. What Is the Role of Conventional X-ray to Diagnose a PJI?

There is no role of plain films for differential diagnosis of PJI. Nevertheless, an X-ray image can be very useful to evaluate other concomitant problems, the degree of loosening, bone reabsorption, fractures, etc. that may all help for the interpretation of images obtained by other modalities, particularly non-radiological modalities [52]. For this reason, conventional radiography remains the first imaging modality in patients with suspected PJI and for their follow-up [14].

5.2. What Is the Role of Ultrasound to Diagnose a PJI?

Data on the use of US to diagnose PJI are scarce and conflicting [14]. At present, US is mostly used to guide joint aspiration or biopsy to perform microbial culture [21].

5.3. What Is the Role of CT to Diagnose a PJI?

Whenever CT is used to diagnose a PJI, artefacts caused by the interaction between X-ray beams and metallic hardware should be reduced by suitable software and techniques [16]. Joint capsule distension and the presence of fluid collections in the soft tissues surrounding a hip implant showed 100% sensitivity, 87% specificity, and 89% accuracy when at least one soft tissue abnormality was used as an infection criterion, and 83% sensitivity, 96% specificity, and 94% accuracy when joint distension was used as infection criterion [22]. CT may be used to more effectively diagnose bone resorption and bone lucency around the implant compared to plain films, however this may not be considered a reliable parameter to differentiate between infection and other reasons for implant failure [22]. CT is useful for guiding biopsies and fluid aspiration.

5.4. What Is the Role of MRI to Diagnose a PJI?

The advent of prostheses made with less ferromagnetic alloy materials and the introduction of metal artefact reduction sequences (MARS), slice encoding for metal artefact correction (SEMAC), and multi-acquisition with variable-resonance image combination (MAVRIC) has pave the way for the use of MRI in patients with joint prosthesis, limiting the artefacts to the area of the implant itself. However, published data about the role of MRI to diagnose PJI are still very limited. In knee implants, the sensitivity and specificity of MRI in diagnosing PJI range from 65% to 92% and 85% to 99%, respectively [14]. Similarly, in the hip, the presence of periosteal reaction, capsule edema, and intramuscular edema demonstrated a sensitivity ranging from 78% to 95% and a specificity from 86% to 97%, depending on the signs that are considered for the diagnosis [23,50]. MRI also has the great advantage of not using ionizing radiation or contrast agents [24–26]. MRI may be limited by patient claustrophobia or the presence of an implanted non-MR compatible device.

5.5. What Is the Role of Three-Phase Bone Scan to Diagnose a PJI (Is a Negative Scan Sufficient to Exclude a PJI)?

Three-phases (perfusion, blood pool, osteometabolic phase) are necessary to perform a ^{99m}Tc bone scan in suspected PJI. A positive bone scan may be observed in many conditions characterized by increased osteoblast activity, and therefore it is not specific for infection; a negative scan in all three phases means that there is no increased perfusion and no increased osteoblastic activity. Given its high negative predictive value (NPV), a negative three-phase bone scan is sufficient to rule out infection [14,53].

5.6. What Is the Minimum Time Window between the Date of Surgery and a Three-Phase Bone Scan to Diagnose a PJI?

Within the first year after hip arthroplasty, periprosthetic uptake patterns are variable depending on the type of surgery and device [54]. For cemented hip arthroplasties, the majority of asymptomatic patients have a normal bone scan, but up to 10% will have persistent periprosthetic uptake after one year from implantation. For porous-coated hip arthroplasties, persistent uptake beyond one year is even more frequent. Furthermore, few data are available about the longitudinal evolution of normal periprosthetic uptake patterns around hybrid, bipolar, and hydroxyapatite-coated devices. Periprosthetic activity around knee arthroplasties in asymptomatic patients is present in more than 50% of femoral components and nearly 90% of tibial components more than one year following implantation. Although periprosthetic activity usually becomes milder over time, there is considerable variation among patients and therefore serial scans should be performed [55]. Since it is not possible to clearly define a date, it has been suggested that positive bone scans should be interpreted with caution for a period of two years from surgery for hip and shoulder prosthesis and a period of five years for knee prosthesis. On the other hand, it can be postulated that a negative bone scan virtually excludes a PJI even within the above reported time windows [53].

5.7. What Is the Role of a WBC Scan to Diagnose a PJI (Is a Negative Scan Sufficient to Exclude a PJI)?

Several systematic reviews and meta-analyses have been published indicating that WBC scans—if necessary, combined with a bone marrow scan—have very high specificity for identifying peri-prosthetic joint infection versus aseptic loosening [55–60], thus representing the most reliable imaging tool able to achieve this differentiation. The reported accuracy of the use of combined WBC scintigraphy (using either ^{99m}Tc-HMPAO-WBC or ^{111}In-oxine-WBC) and bone marrow scintigraphy ranges from 83% to 98% for both hip and knee prosthesis infections [34].

Expert opinions and most research studies indicate a high NPV for WBC scintigraphy. This could be even higher if the correct acquisition protocols and interpretation criteria are applied [30]. In fact, NPVs ranging from 92% to 100% have been reported in the largest and most recent studies. [31,56]. Therefore, we can conclude that a negative WBC is sufficient to exclude a PJI.

5.8. What Is the Role of [^{18}F]-FDG-PET/CT to Diagnose a PJI (Is a Negative Scan Sufficient to Exclude a PJI)?

While there is considerable debate about the specificity of [^{18}F]-FDG, most investigators agree that the test is very sensitive and therefore the negative predictive value is high [54,61,62]. In an investigation of 21 patients with suspected PJI of the knee, [^{18}F]-FDG-PET was 100% sensitive, but only 73% specific for infection [63]. In a recent investigation in 130 patients with suspected PJI of the hip, with final diagnosis based on the criteria recommended by the MSIS, [^{18}F]-FDG-PET/CT yielded a sensitivity and specificity of 95% and 39%, respectively, for infection [64]. Based on the available literature, it seems reasonable to conclude that a negative result effectively excludes PJI. Whether or not [^{18}F]-FDG is superior to bone scintigraphy for excluding infection is not answerable with currently available data.

5.9. What Is the Spatial Resolution of Currently Available Imaging Techniques in Order to Describe the Extent of a PJI?

The spatial resolution of a planar WBC scan is approximately 0.8–1 cm and by SPECT, the spatial resolution is 0.5–0.6 cm. The newest digital PET/CT scanners can reach resolutions as low as 2–3 mm.

Morphological examinations such as CT and MRI have much higher special resolution as compared to nuclear medicine modalities.

However, available imaging techniques only reflect the extent of the host's response, i.e., the inflammatory process, or describe morphological changes due to the interaction between the pathogen and the host. This does not necessarily reflect the extent of the infection. Accurate delineation of the extent of the infection around an implant would require an infection-specific imaging technique, which is currently lacking.

5.10. Can Clinicians Rely on a Scan to Decide to Maintain a Component of an Implant If Infection Is Ruled Out by Imaging Investigations?

If imaging modalities (radiological and/or nuclear medicine) exclude the presence of infection, clinicians can decide to maintain one or all components of the prosthesis mainly because all imaging modalities have very high sensitivity. In these cases, a component should be removed based on the degree of loosening and patient compliance. On the other hand, if an infection is suspected by imaging, to the best of our knowledge, there are no published data suggesting that infection can be limited to an individual component of an arthroplasty and that this can be reliably assessed by an imaging modality.

5.11. Is There Any Evidence That Imaging Techniques May Have Different Accuracy or Thresholds to Diagnose High-Grade and Low-Grade Peri-Prosthetic Joint Infections?

There are no comparative studies investigating the accuracy of imaging techniques in patients with high-grade, acute peri-prosthetic infections versus low-grade, sub-acute or chronic clinical presentations.

Nuclear imaging has been shown to be effective at differentiating chronic low-grade infection in painful knee prostheses with a sensitivity and specificity of 71% and 95%, respectively, for combined WBC/bone marrow scintigraphy [53].

However, the sensitivity of nuclear imaging techniques can be significantly reduced in low-grade, chronic PJI of the shoulder. In fact, remarkably poor sensitivity of both [^{18}F]-FDG and combined labelled leukocyte/marrow imaging to diagnose chronic, low-grade periprosthetic shoulder infection has been reported, with respective values of 14% and 18% [65,66]. Since there are no data on "high grade" shoulder arthroplasty infections, it is impossible to determine if these results are related to the chronic/low grade presentation of PJI or if it is just a specific feature of shoulder PJI.

5.12. Are There Any Studies Comparing Intra-Operative Histological Findings and/or Microbiological Examination with Imaging Investigations?

In most investigations, final diagnoses are based on histopathology/microbiology. Overall, these studies have been summarized in several systematic reviews and were considered for preparing "evidence based guidelines" by EANM [14,16,30].

5.13. Is It Necessary to Stop Antibiotic Treatment before Performing a Scan to Diagnose a PJI?

It is not necessary to discontinue antibiotic treatment for a CT or MRI scan, neither for a bone scintigraphy or FDG-PET/CT. In contrast, it is believed that antimicrobial treatment may reduce the diagnostic accuracy of WBC scintigraphy, probably because of decreased number and activity of bacteria, which reduces the release of chemotactic factors, hence the accumulation of WBC at the site of infection over time. This accumulation over time is the physio-pathological principle on which the interpretation of WBC images is based.

However, there are only two studies in PJI [67,68] and one study in fracture-related infections using radio-labelled WBC [69] that show no differences in diagnostic accuracy between patients under antibiotics vs. antibiotic discontinuation. To the best of our knowledge, there is currently no data available on the impact of antibiotic treatment on the diagnostic performance of FDG-PET/CT in PJI.

5.14. What Are the Most Promising Technologies Currently under Investigation to Diagnose PJI and Other Implant-Related Infections?

Given the challenges in diagnosing PJI, an infection-specific agent would be very valuable. To achieve this aim, several attempts have been made using a variety of approaches including radio-labelled antibiotics, vitamins, sugars and peptides [70,71].

5.15. Should Nuclear Medicine Imaging Techniques Be Included in the Definition of Peri-Prosthetic Joint Infection and, in Case of a Positive Answer, Which One Would You Recommend?

Nuclear medicine imaging techniques should be included in the modern definition of PJI. In fact, these diagnostic tools, if adequately performed, provide an overall accuracy that can be considered similar to that of other commonly accepted examinations, or even better.

Unfortunately, despite several systematic reviews, meta-analyses and single studies, some clearly indicate that WBC scans—combined or not with bone marrow scans—are the most reliable imaging tool for identifying peri-prosthetic joint infection. Others suggest the use of FDG-PET or radio-labelled anti-granulocyte antibodies, or even bone scans [34,53,56,61,65,67,72–84]. This needs to be clarified. There is a considerable variation in results when looking at individual studies due to different labelling methods, image acquisition protocols, image interpretation, patient selection, etc. Furthermore, most systematic reviews do not include all published studies, nor a set time interval for paper selection. As a result, in some "systematic reviews" we find as little as three, or even two or just one, paper(s) on nuclear medicine modalities. In other meta-analyses, there are often a mixture of very old papers with very recent ones using completely different methodologies. Unfortunately, no recent large multicenter prospective multimodal comparative studies with standardized image acquisition and interpretation parameters exist, and therefore we cannot provide a firm evidence-based conclusion with regard to the imaging modality of choice for PJI.

Despite this, some practical considerations can be made. Indeed, in clinical practice, the choice of imaging modality will highly depend on local availability, waiting lists, patient claustrophobia, metal devices, operator experience and cost (which is country dependent). FDG costs approximately 150 €, takes approximately 2 h to perform, the waiting list is approximately 1–2 weeks, costs for the National Health Service (NHS) are approximately 1200 €, the radiation dose for the patient is approximately 6–8 mSv and the overall diagnostic accuracy for PJI ranges from 65% to 90%. A WBC scan (or anti-granulocyte antibodies) costs approximately 150 €, takes approximately 2 h for labelling (the patient is busy from 8:00 am to 3:00 pm on the first day and from 8:00 am to 9:00 am the following day), the waiting list is approximately 1–3 weeks, the cost for the NHS is approximately 450–1000 €, the radiation dose for the patient is approximately 5 mSv and the overall diagnostic accuracy for PJI ranges from 70% to 95%.

It emerges that there are pros and cons for both modalities. If we require a very urgent screening test, particularly in patients with a low pre-test probability of infection, we can perform a bone scan or FDG (both able to effectively rule-out a PJI when negative, but could show residual inflammation for a long time after surgery) [53,54,85–87]. If we know upfront that there is a high suspicion of infection, or if we do not know if there is an infection or an aseptic loosening, it is preferable to perform a WBC scan [14,16,30,88,89].

6. Conclusions

Several definitions of PJI exist, but the use of imaging modalities is lacking in most of these scoring systems.

In this manuscript, we focused on the current role of several different imaging techniques in order to understand if this exclusion is justified in light of their possible contribution to diagnose a peri-prosthetic infection.

The panel highlighted how several imaging techniques, their limits notwithstanding, may play a key role in PJI definition.

While X-ray examinations may currently be regarded as a general screening for patients with joint replacement, MRI and nuclear imaging techniques are much more specifically concerned with the differential diagnostic work-up of PJI.

Based on available data in the literature, three-phase bone scans, WBC scans and FDG-PET scans are all highly sensitive investigations; whenever negative, they can all be reliably considered as a criteria to exclude a PJI. Furthermore, a positive WBC scan (if necessary, combined with a bone marrow scan), is to be considered a confirmative criteria of PJI.

Concerning FDG-PET/CT, there is a need to establish clear and standardized interpretation criteria to differentiate infection from non-infectious pathologies, especially aseptic loosening.

Finally, although very promising and attractive for its preliminary results, easy accessibility and lack of ionizing radiation, MRI appears to be a potential important player; if further studies confirm its accuracy in diagnosing PJI, it may be another imaging modality that will need to be included in the upcoming PJI definitions.

Author Contributions: Conceptualization, C.L.R. and A.S.; methodology, C.L.R.; writing, C.L.R., N.P., G.A., L.M.S., G.T., A.A., A.W.J.M.G., O.G., A.M., C.L., C.J.P. and A.S. All authors have read and agreed to the published version of the manuscript.

References

1. Renz, N.; Yermak, K.; Perka, C.; Trampuz, A. Alpha Defensin Lateral Flow Test for Diagnosis of Periprosthetic Joint Infection: Not a Screening but a Confirmatory Test. *J. Bone Jt. Surg. Am.* **2018**, *100*, 742–750. [CrossRef] [PubMed]
2. Pérez-Prieto, D.; Portillo, M.E.; Puig-Verdié, L.; Alier, A.; Martínez, S.; Sorlí, L.; Horcajada, J.P.; Monllau, J.C. C-reactive protein may misdiagnose prosthetic joint infections, particularly chronic and low-grade infections. *Int. Orthop.* **2017**, *41*, 1315–1319. [CrossRef] [PubMed]
3. Romanò, C.L.; Romanò, D.; Morelli, I.; Drago, L. The Concept of Biofilm-Related Implant Malfunction and "Low-Grade Infection". *Adv. Exp. Med. Biol.* **2017**, *971*, 1–13. [CrossRef]
4. Baumbach, S.F.; Prall, W.C.; Scharpf, A.M.; Hererich, V.; Schmidt, M.; Suedkamp, N.P.; Stoehr, A.; Mayr, H.O. Significant increase of pathogen detection rate by dry arthroscopic biopsies at suspected low-grade infection following total knee arthroplasty: A prospective observational study. *Arch. Orthop. Trauma Surg.* **2018**, *138*, 1583–1590. [CrossRef] [PubMed]
5. Morgenstern, C.; Cabric, S.; Perka, C.; Trampuz, A.; Renz, N. Synovial fluid multiplex PCR is superior to culture for detection of low-virulent pathogens causing periprosthetic joint infection. *Diagn. Microbiol. Infect. Dis.* **2018**, *90*, 115–119. [CrossRef] [PubMed]
6. Goswami, K.; Parvizi, J.; Maxwell Courtney, P. Current Recommendations for the Diagnosis of Acute and Chronic PJI for Hip and Knee-Cell Counts, Alpha-Defensin, Leukocyte Esterase, Next-generation Sequencing. *Curr. Rev. Musculoskelet. Med.* **2018**, *11*, 428–438. [CrossRef]

7. Parvizi, J.; Zmistowski, B.; Berbari, E.F.; Bauer, T.W.; Springer, B.D.; Della Valle, C.J.; Garvin, K.L.; Mont, M.A.; Wongworawat, M.D.; Zalavras, C.G. New definition for periprosthetic joint infection: From the workgroup of the Musculoskeletal infection Society. *Clin. Orthop. Relat. Res.* **2011**, *469*, 2992e4. [CrossRef]
8. Osmon, D.R.; Berbari, E.F.; Berendt, A.R.; Lew, D.; Zimmerli, W.; Steckelberg, J.M.; Rao, N.; Hanssen, A.; Wilson, W.R. Infectious Diseases Society of America. Diagnosis and management of prosthetic joint infection: Clinical practice guidelines by the Infectious Diseases Society of America. *Clin. Infect. Dis.* **2013**, *56*, e1–e25. [CrossRef]
9. Parvizi, J.; Gehrke, T.; International Consensus Group on Periprosthetic Joint Infection. Definition of periprosthetic joint infection. *J. Arthroplast.* **2014**, *29*, 1331. [CrossRef]
10. Parvizi, J.; Tan, T.L.; Goswami, K.; Higuera, C.; Della Valle, C.; Chen, A.F.; Shohat, N. The 2018 Definition of Periprosthetic Hip and Knee Infection: An Evidence-Based and Validated Criteria. *J. Arthroplast.* **2018**, *33*, 1309–1314. [CrossRef]
11. Parvizi, J.; Gehrke, T. *Proceedings of the Second International Consensus Meeting on Musculoskeletal Infection*; Hip and Knee Section Data Trace Publishing Company: Brooklandville, MD, USA, 2018; ISBN 978-1-57400-157-0.
12. Romanò, C.L.; Khawashki, H.A.; Benzakour, T.; Bozhkova, S.; Del Sel, H.; Hafez, M.; Johari, A.; Lob, G.; Sharma, H.K.; Tsuchiya, H.; et al. The W.A.I.O.T. Definition of High-Grade and Low-Grade Peri-Prosthetic Joint Infection. *J. Clin. Med.* **2019**, *8*, 650. [CrossRef]
13. Bozhkova, S.; Suardi, V.; Sharma, H.K.; Tsuchiya, H.; Del Sel, H.; Hafez, M.A.; Benzakour, T.; Drago, L.; Romanò, C.L. The, W.A.I.O.T. Definition of Peri-Prosthetic Joint Infection: A Multi-center, Retrospective Validation Study. *J. Clin. Med.* **2020**, *9*, 1965. [CrossRef]
14. Signore, A.; Sconfienza, L.M.; Borens, O.; Glaudemans, A.W.J.M.; Cassar-Pullicino, V.; Trampuz, A.; Winkler, H.; Gheysens, O.; Vanhoenacker, F.M.H.M.; Petrosillo, N.; et al. Consensus document for the diagnosis of prosthetic joint infections: A joint paper by the EANM, EBJIS, and ESR (with ESCMID endorsement). *Eur. J. Nucl. Med. Mol. Imaging* **2019**, *46*, 971–988. [CrossRef]
15. Sessa, G.; Romanò, C.L. Linea guida SIOT diagnosi di infezione peri-protesica articolare ritardata o tardiva (tempo trascorso dall'intervento > 90 giorni). *G. Ital. Ortop. Traumatol.* **2019**, *45*, 187–213. [CrossRef]
16. Sconfienza, L.M.; Signore, A.; Cassar-Pullicino, V.; Cataldo, M.A.; Gheysens, O.; Borens, O.; Trampuz, A.; Wörtler, K.; Petrosillo, N.; Winkler, H.; et al. Diagnosis of peripheral bone and prosthetic joint infections: Overview on the consensus documents by the EANM, EBJIS, and ESR (with ESCMID endorsement). *Eur. Radiol.* **2019**, *29*, 6425–6438. [CrossRef]
17. Li, C.; Renz, N.; Trampuz, A. Management of Periprosthetic Joint Infection. *Hip Pelvis.* **2018**, *30*, 138–146. [CrossRef]
18. Yoon, H.K.; Cho, S.H.; Lee, D.Y.; Kang, B.H.; Lee, S.H.; Moon, D.G.; Kim, D.H.; Nam, D.C.; Hwang, S.C. A Review of the Literature on Culture-Negative Periprosthetic Joint Infection: Epidemiology, Diagnosis and Treatment. *Knee Surg. Relat. Res.* **2017**, *29*, 155–164. [CrossRef]
19. Drago, L.; Clerici, P.; Morelli, I.; Ashok, J.; Benzakour, T.; Bozhkova, S.; Alizadeh, C.; Del Sel, H.; Sharma, H.K.; Peel, T.; et al. The World Association against Infection in Orthopaedics and Trauma (WAIOT) procedures for Microbiological Sampling and Processing for Periprosthetic Joint Infections (PJIs) and other Implant-Related Infections. *J. Clin. Med.* **2019**, *8*, 933. [CrossRef]
20. Boettner, F.; Koehler, G.; Wegner, A.; Schmidt-Braekling, T.; Gosheger, G.; Goetze, C. The Rule of Histology in the Diagnosis of Periprosthetic Infection: Specific Granulocyte Counting Methods and New Immunohistologic Staining Techniques may Increase the Diagnostic Value. *Open Orthop. J.* **2016**, *10*, 457–465. [CrossRef]
21. Klauser, A.S.; Tagliafico, A.; Allen, G.M.; Boutry, N.; Campbell, R.; Grainger, A.; Guerini, H.; McNally, E.; O'Connor, P.J. Clinical indications for musculoskeletal ultrasound: A Delphi-based consensus paper of the European Society of Musculoskeletal Radiology. *Eur. Radiol.* **2012**, *22*, 1140–1148. [CrossRef]
22. Cyteval, C.; Hamm, V.; Sarrabère, M.P.; Lopez, F.M.; Maury, P.; Taourel, P. Painful infection at the site of hip prosthesis: CT imaging. *Radiology* **2002**, *224*, 477–483. [CrossRef] [PubMed]
23. Galley, J.; Sutter, R.; Stern, C.; Filli, L.; Rahm, S.; Pfirrmann, C.W.A. Diagnosis of Periprosthetic Hip Joint Infection Using MRI with Metal Artifact Reduction at 1.5 T. *Radiology* **2020**, *12*, 191901. [CrossRef] [PubMed]
24. Lee, Y.H.; Lim, D.; Kim, E.; Kim, S.; Song, H.T.; Suh, J.S. Usefulness of slice encoding for metal artifact correction (SEMAC) for reducing metallic artifacts in 3-T MRI. *Magn. Reson. Imaging* **2013**, *31*, 703–706. [CrossRef]

25. Li, A.E.; Sneag, D.; Greditzer, H.G., 4th; Johnson, C.C.; Miller, T.T.; Potter, H.G. Total Knee Arthroplasty: Diagnostic Accuracy of Patterns of Synovitis at MR Imaging. *Radiology* **2016**, *27*, 152828. [CrossRef]
26. Plodkowski, A.J.; Hayter, C.L.; Miller, T.T.; Nguyen, J.T.; Potter, H.G. Lamellated hyperintense synovitis: Potential MR imaging sign of an infected knee arthroplasty. *Radiology* **2013**, *266*, 256–260. [CrossRef]
27. Van den Wyngaert, T.; Strobel, K.; Kampen, W.U.; Kuwert, T.; van der Bruggen, W.; Mohan, H.K.; Gnanasegaran, G.; Delgado-Bolton, R.; Weber, W.A.; Beheshti, M.; et al. EANM Bone & Joint Committee and the Oncology Committee. The EANM practice guidelines for bone scintigraphy. *Eur. J. Nucl. Med. Mol. Imaging* **2016**, *43*, 1723–1738. [CrossRef]
28. De Vries, E.F.; Roca, M.; Jamar, F.; Israel, O.; Signore, A. Guidelines fort the labelling of leucocytes with (99m)Tc-HMPAO. Inflammation/Infection Taskgroup of the European Association of Nuclear Medicine. *Eur. J. Nucl. Med. Mol. Imaging* **2010**, *37*, 842–848. [CrossRef]
29. Roca, M.; De Vries, E.F.J.; Jamar, F.; Israel, O.; Signore, A. Guidelines for the labelling of leucocytes with 111In-oxine. *Eur. J. Nucl. Med. Mol. Imaging* **2010**, *37*, 835–841. [CrossRef]
30. Signore, A.; Jamar, F.; Israel, O.; Buscombe, J.; Martin-Comin, J.; Lazzeri, E. Clinical indications, image acquisition and data interpretation for white blood cells and anti-granulocyte monoclonal antibody scintigraphy: An EANM procedural guideline. *Eur. J. Nucl. Med. Mol. Imaging* **2018**, *45*, 1816–1831. [CrossRef]
31. Erba, P.A.; Glaudemans, A.W.; Veltman, N.C.; Sollini, M.; Pacilio, M.; Galli, F.; Dierckx, R.A.; Signore, A. Image acquisition and interpretation criteria for 99mTc-HMPAO-labelled white blood cell scintigraphy: Results of a multicentre study. *Eur. J. Nucl. Med. Mol. Imaging* **2014**, *41*, 615–623. [CrossRef]
32. Gratz, S.; Reize, P.; Kemke, B.; Kampen, W.U.; Luster, M.; Höffken, H. Targeting osteomyelitis with complete [^{99m}Tc]besilesomab and fragmented [^{99m}Tc]sulesomab antibodies: Kinetic evaluations. *Q. J. Nucl. Med. Mol. Imaging* **2016**, *60*, 413–423. [PubMed]
33. Jin, H.; Yuan, L.; Li, C.; Kan, Y.; Hao, R.; Yang, J. Diagnostic performance of FDG PET or PET/CT in prosthetic infection after arthroplasty: A meta-analysis. *Q. J. Nucl. Med. Mol. Imaging* **2014**, *58*, 85–93. [PubMed]
34. Gemmel, F.; van den Wyngaert, H.; Love, C.; Welling, M.M.; Gemmel, P.; Palestro, C.J. Prosthetic joint infections: Radionuclide state-of-the-art imaging. *Eur. J. Nucl. Med. Mol. Imaging* **2012**, *39*, 892–909. [CrossRef] [PubMed]
35. Reinartz, P. FDG-PET in patients with painful hip and knee arthroplasty: Technical breakthrough or just more of the same. *Q. J. Nucl. Med. Mol. Imaging* **2009**, *53*, 41–50.
36. Chacko, T.K.; Zhuang, H.; Stevenson, K.; Moussavia, B.; Alavi, A. The importance of the location of fluorodeoxyglucose uptake in periprosthetic infection in painful hip prostheses. *Nucl. Med. Commun.* **2002**, *23*, 851–855. [CrossRef]
37. Love, C.; Marwin, S.E.; Tomas, M.B.; Krauss, E.S.; Tronco, G.G.; Bhargava, K.K.; Nichols, K.J.; Palestro, C.J. Diagnosing infection in the failed joint replacement: A comparison of coincidence detection ^{18}F-FDG and ^{111}In-labeled leukocyte/^{99m}Tc-sulfur colloid marrow imaging. *J. Nucl. Med.* **2004**, *45*, 1864–1871.
38. Familiari, D.; Glaudemans, A.W.; Vitale, V.; Prosperi, D.; Bagni, O.; Lenza, A.; Cavallini, M.; Scopinaro, F.; Signore, A. Can sequential ^{18}F-FDG PET/CT replace WBC imaging in the diabetic foot? *J. Nucl. Med.* **2011**, *52*, 1012–1019. [CrossRef]
39. Stumpe, K.D.; Nötzli, H.P.; Zanetti, M.; Kamel, E.M.; Hany, T.F.; Görres, G.W.; von Schulthess, G.K.; Hodler, J. FDG PET for differentiation of infection and aseptic loosening in total hip replacements: Comparison with conventional radiography and three-phase bone scintigraphy. *Radiology* **2004**, *231*, 333–341. [CrossRef]
40. Wenter, V.; Müller, J.P.; Albert, N.L.; Lehner, S.; Fendler, W.P.; Bartenstein, P.; Cyran, C.C.; Friederichs, J.; Militz, M.; Hacker, M.; et al. The diagnostic value of [(18)F]FDG PET for the detection of chronic osteomyelitis and implant-associated infection. *Eur. J. Nucl. Med. Mol. Imaging* **2016**, *43*, 749–761. [CrossRef]
41. Treglia, G. Diagnostic Performance of (18)F-FDG PET/CT in Infectious and Inflammatory Diseases according to Published Meta-Analyses. *Contrast Media Mol. Imaging* **2019**, 3018349. [CrossRef]
42. Thang, S.P.; Tong, A.K.; Lam, W.W.; Ng, D.C. SPECT/CT in musculoskeletal infections. *Semin. Musculoskelet. Radiol.* **2014**, *18*, 194–202. [CrossRef]
43. Tam, H.H.; Bhaludin, B.; Rahman, F.; Weller, A.; Ejindu, V.; Parthipun, A. SPECT-CT in total hip arthroplasty. *Clin. Radiol.* **2014**, *69*, 82–95. [CrossRef]
44. Mariani, G.; Bruselli, L.; Kuwert, T.; Kim, E.E.; Flotats, A.; Israel, O.; Dondi, M.; Watanabe, N. A review on the clinical uses of SPECT/CT. *Eur. J. Nucl Med. Mol. Imaging* **2010**, *37*, 1959–1985. [CrossRef]

45. Scharf, S. SPECT/CT imaging in general orthopedic practice. *Semin. Nucl. Med.* **2009**, *39*, 293–307. [CrossRef]
46. van der Bruggen, W.; Bleeker-Rovers, C.P.; Boerman, O.C.; Gotthardt, M.; Oyen, W.J. PET and SPECT in osteomyelitis and prosthetic bone and joint infections: A systematic review. *Semin. Nucl. Med.* **2010**, *40*, 3–15. [CrossRef]
47. Aliprandi, A.; Sconfienza, L.M.; Randelli, P.; Bandirali, M.; Tritella, S.; Di Leo, G.; Sardanelli, F. Magnetic resonance imaging of the knee after medial unicompartmental arthroplasty. *Eur. J. Radiol.* **2011**, *80*, e416–e421. [CrossRef]
48. White, L.M.; Kim, J.K.; Mehta, M.; Merchant, N.; Schweitzer, M.E.; Morrison, W.B.; Hutchison, C.R.; Gross, A.E. Complications of total hiparthroplasty: MR imaging-initial experience. *Radiology* **2000**, *215*, 254–262. [CrossRef]
49. Hayter, C.L.; Koff, M.F.; Shah, P.; Koch, K.M.; Miller, T.T.; Potter, H.G. MRI after arthroplasty: Comparison of MAVRIC and conventional fast spin-echo techniques. *Am. J. Roentgenol.* **2011**, *197*, W405–W411. [CrossRef]
50. He, C.; Lu, Y.; Jiang, M.; Feng, J.; Wang, Y.; Liu, Z. Clinical value of optimized magnetic resonance imaging for evaluation of patients with painful hip arthroplasty. *Chin. Med. J.* **2014**, *127*, 3876–3880.
51. Gille, J.; Ince, A.; González, O.; Katzer, A.; Loehr, J.F. Single-stage revision of peri-prosthetic infection following total elbow replacement. *J. Bone Joint Surg. Br.* **2006**, *88*, 1341–1346. [CrossRef]
52. Zajonz, D.; Wuthe, L.; Tiepolt, S.; Brandmeier, P.; Prietzel, T.; von Salis-Soglio, G.F.; Roth, A.; Josten, C.; Heyde, C.E.; Zajonz, M.G. Diagnostic Work-Up Strategy for Periprosthetic Joint Infections After Total Hip and Knee Arthroplasty: A 12-year Experience on 320 Consecutive Cases. *Patient Saf. Surg.* **2015**, *16*, 20. [CrossRef]
53. Niccoli, G.; Mercurio, D.; Cortese, F. Bone scan in painful knee arthroplasty: Obsolete or actual examination? *Acta Biomed.* **2017**, *88*, 68–77. [CrossRef] [PubMed]
54. Zhuang, H.; Chacko, T.K.; Hickeson, M.; Stevenson, K.; Feng, Q.; Ponzo, F.; Garino, J.P.; Alavi, A. Persistent non-specific FDG uptake on PET imaging following hip arthroplasty. *Eur. J. Nucl. Med.* **2002**, *29*, 1328–1333. [CrossRef] [PubMed]
55. Palestro, C.J. Nuclear medicine and the failed joint replacement: Past, present, and future. *World J. Radiol.* **2014**, *6*, 446–458. [CrossRef] [PubMed]
56. Auletta, S.; Riolo, D.; Varani, M.; Lauri, C.; Galli, F.; Signore, A. Labelling and clinical performance of human leukocytes with 99mTc-HMPAO using Leukokit® with gelofusine versus Leukokit® with HES as sedimentation agent. *Contrast Media Mol. Imaging* **2019**, 4368342. [CrossRef] [PubMed]
57. Kim, H.O.; Na, S.J.; Oh, S.J.; Jung, B.S.; Lee, S.H.; Chang, J.S.; Bin, S., II; Ryu, J.S. Usefulness of Adding SPECT/CT to 99mTc-Hexamethylpropylene Amine Oxime (HMPAO)-labeled Leukocyte Imaging for Diagnosing Prosthetic Joint Infections. *J. Comput. Assist. Tomogr.* **2014**, *38*, 313–319. [CrossRef]
58. El Espera, I.; Blondet, C.; Moullart, V.; Saïdi, L.; Havet, E.; Mertl, P.; Canarelli, B.; Schmit, J.-L.; Meyer, M.-E. The Usefulness of 99mTc Sulfur Colloid Bone Marrow Scintigraphy Combined With 111In Leucocyte Scintigraphy in Prosthetic Joint Infection. *Nucl. Med. Commun.* **2004**, *25*, 171–175. [CrossRef]
59. Aksoy, S.Y.; Asa, S.; Ozhan, M.; Ocak, M.; Sager, M.S.; Erkan, M.E.; Halac, M.; Kabasakal, L.; Sönmezoglu, K.; Kanmaz, B. FDG and FDG-labelled leucocyte PET/CT in the imaging of prosthetic joint infection. *Eur. J. Nucl. Med. Mol. Imaging* **2014**, *41*, 556–564. [CrossRef]
60. Teiler, J.; Ahl, M.; Åkerlund, B.; Wird, S.; Brismar, H.; Bjäreback, A.; Hedlund, H.; Holstensson, M.; Axelsson, R. Is 99mTc-HMPAO-leukocyte Imaging an Accurate Method in Evaluating Therapy Result in Prosthetic Joint Infection and Diagnosing Suspected Chronic Prosthetic Joint Infection? *Q. J. Nucl. Med. Mol. Imaging* **2020**, *64*, 85–95. [CrossRef]
61. Kwee, T.C.; Kwee, R.M.; Alavi, A. FDG-PET for diagnosing prosthetic joint infection: Systematic review and metaanalysis. *Eur. J. Nucl. Med. Mol. Imaging* **2008**, *35*, 2122–2132. [CrossRef]
62. Basu, S.; Kwee, T.C.; Saboury, B.; Garino, J.P.; Nelson, C.N.; Zhuang, H.; Parsons, M.; Chen, W.; Kumar, R.; Salavati, A.; et al. FDG-PET for diagnosing infection in hip and knee prostheses: Prospective study in 221 prostheses and subgroup comparison with combined 111In-labeled leukocyte/99mTc- sulfur colloid bone marrow imaging in 88 prostheses. *Clin. Nucl. Med.* **2014**, *39*, 609–615. [CrossRef] [PubMed]
63. Van Acker, F.; Nuyts, J.; Maes, A.; Vanquickenborne, B.; Stuyck, J.; Bellemans, J.; Vleugels, S.; Bormans, G.; Mortelmans, L. FDG-PET, ^{99m}Tc-HMPAO white blood cell SPET and bone scintigraphy in the evaluation of painful total knee arthroplasties. *Eur. J. Nucl. Med.* **2001**, *28*, 1496–1504. [CrossRef] [PubMed]

64. Kiran, M.; Donnelly, T.D.; Armstrong, C.; Kapoor, B.; Kumar, G.; Peter, V. Diagnostic utility of fluorodeoxyglucose positron emission tomography in prosthetic joint infection based on MSIS criteria. *Bone Jt. J.* **2019**, *101-B*, 910–914. [CrossRef] [PubMed]
65. Falstie-Jensen, T.; Lange, J.; Daugaard, H.; Vendelbo, M.H.; Sørensen, A.K.; Zerahn, B.; Ovesen, J.; Søballe, K.; Gormsen, L.C.; ROSA study-group. 18F FDG-PET/CT has poor diagnostic accuracy in diagnosing shoulder PJI. *Eur. J. Nucl. Med. Mol. Imaging* **2019**, *46*, 2013–2022. [CrossRef] [PubMed]
66. Falstie-Jensen, T.; Daugaard, H.; Søballe, K.; Ovesen, J.; Arveschoug, A.K.; Lange, J.; ROSA study group. Labeled white blood cell/bone marrow single-photon emission computed tomography with computed tomography fails in diagnosing chronic periprosthetic shoulder joint infection. *J. Shoulder Elbow Surg.* **2019**, *28*, 1040–1048. [CrossRef]
67. Blanc, P.; Bonnet, E.; Giordano, G.; Monteil, J.; Salabert, A.-S.; Payou, P. The use of labelled leucocyte scintigraphy to evaluate chronic periprosthetic joint infections: A retrospective multicentre study on 168 patients. *Eur. J. Clin. Microbiol. Infect. Dis.* **2019**, *38*, 1625–1631. [CrossRef]
68. Liberatore, M.; AL-Nahhas, A.; Rubello, D. White blood cell scan in the follow-up of infectious diseases: Is the withdrawal of antibiotic therapy necessary? Nucl. *Med. Commun.* **2007**, *28*, 151–153. [CrossRef]
69. Govaert, G.A.M.; Bosch, P.; IJpma, F.F.A.; Glauche, J.; Jutte, P.C.; Lemans, J.V.C.; Wendt, K.W.; Reininga, I.H.F.; Glaudemans, A.W.J.M. High diagnostic accuracy of white blood cell scintigraphy for fracture related infections: Results of a large retrospective single-center study. *Injury* **2018**, *49*, 1085–1090. [CrossRef]
70. Auletta, S.; Galli, F.; Lauri, C.; Martinelli, D.; Santino, I.; Signore, A. Imaging bacteria with radiolabelled quinolones, cephalosporins and siderophores for imaging infection: A systematic review. *Clin. Transl. Imaging* **2016**, *4*, 229–252. [CrossRef]
71. Auletta, S.; Varani, M.; Horvat, R.; Galli, F.; Signore, A.; Hess, S. PET Radiopharmaceuticals for Specific Bacteria Imaging: A Systematic Review. *J. Clin. Med.* **2019**, *8*, 197. [CrossRef]
72. Xing, D.; Ma, X.; Ma, J.; Wang, J.; Chen, Y.; Yang, Y. Use of Anti-Granulocyte Scintigraphy With 99mTc-labeled Monoclonal Antibodies for the Diagnosis of Periprosthetic Infection in Patients After Total Joint Arthroplasty: A Diagnostic Meta-Analysis. *PLoS ONE* **2013**, *26*, e69857. [CrossRef] [PubMed]
73. Trevail, C.; Ravindranath-Reddy, P.; Sulkin, T.; Bartlett, G. An evaluation of the role of nuclear medicine imaging in the diagnosis of periprosthetic infections of the hip. *Clin Radiol.* **2016**, *71*, 211–219. [CrossRef] [PubMed]
74. Ahmad, S.S.; Shaker, A.; Saffarini, M.; Chen, A.F.; Hirschmann, M.T.; Kohl, S. Accuracy of diagnostic tests for prosthetic joint infection: A systematic review. *Knee Surg. Sports Traumatol. Arthrosc.* **2016**, *24*, 3064–3074. [CrossRef] [PubMed]
75. Diaz-Ledezma, C.; Lamberton, C.; Lichstein, P.; Parvizi, J. Diagnosis of Periprosthetic Joint Infection: The Role of Nuclear Medicine May Be Overestimated. *J. Arthroplasty.* **2015**, *30*, 1044–1049. [CrossRef]
76. Sousa, R.; Massada, M.; Pereira, A.; Fontes, F.; Amorim, I.; Oliveira, A. Diagnostic Accuracy of Combined 99mTc-sulesomab and 99mTc-nanocolloid Bone Marrow Imaging in Detecting Prosthetic Joint Infection. *Nucl. Med. Commun.* **2011**, *32*, 834–839. [CrossRef]
77. Gratz, S.; Reize, P.; Pfestroff, A.; Höffken, H. Intact Versus Fragmented 99mTc-monoclonal Antibody Imaging of Infection in Patients With Septically Loosened Total Knee Arthroplasty. *J. Int. Med. Res.* **2012**, *40*, 1335–1342. [CrossRef]
78. Bhoil, A.; Caw, H.; Vinjamuri, S. Role of 18F-flurodeoxyglucose in orthopaedic implant-related infection: Review of literature and experience. *Nucl. Med. Commun.* **2019**, *40*, 875–887. [CrossRef]
79. Zoccali, C.; Teori, G.; Salducca, N. The Role of FDG-PET in Distinguishing Between Septic and Aseptic Loosening in Hip Prosthesis: A Review of Literature. *Int. Orthop.* **2009**, *33*, 1–5. [CrossRef]
80. Khalid, V.; Schønheyder, H.C.; Larsen, L.H.; Nielsen, P.T.; Kappel, A.; Thomsen, T.R.; Aleksyniene, R.; Lorenzen, J.; Ørsted, I.; Simonsen, O.; et al. Multidisciplinary Diagnostic Algorithm for Evaluation of Patients Presenting with a Prosthetic Problem in the Hip or Knee: A Prospective Study. *Diagnostics* **2020**, *11*, 98. [CrossRef]
81. Savarino, L.; Tigani, D.; Baldini, N.; Bochicchio, V.; Giunti, A. Pre-operative diagnosis of infection in total knee arthroplasty: An algorithm. *Knee Surg. Sports Traumatol. Arthrosc.* **2009**, *17*, 667–675. [CrossRef]
82. Volpe, L.; Indelli, P.F.; Latella, L.; Poli, P.; Yakupoglu, J.; Marcucci, M. Periprosthetic joint infections: A clinical practice algorithm. *Joints* **2015**, *13*, 169–174. [CrossRef]

83. Plate, A.; Weichselbaumer, V.; Schüpbach, R.; Fucentese, S.F.; Berli, M.; Hüllner, M.; Achermann, Y. Diagnostic Accuracy of 99 m Tc-antigranulocyte SPECT/CT in Patients With Osteomyelitis and Orthopaedic Device-Related Infections: A Retrospective Analysis. *Int. J. Infect. Dis.* **2020**, *91*, 79–86. [CrossRef] [PubMed]
84. Graute, V.; Feist, M.; Lehner, S.; Haug, A.; Müller, P.E.; Bartenstein, P.; Hacker, M. Detection of Low-Grade Prosthetic Joint Infections Using 99mTc-antigranulocyte SPECT/CT: Initial Clinical Results. *Eur. J. Nucl. Med. Mol. Imaging* **2010**, *37*, 1751–1759. [CrossRef]
85. Delank, K.-S.; Schmidt, M.; Michael, J.W.-P.; Dietlein, M.; Schicha, H.; Eysel, P. The Implications of 18F-FDG PET for the Diagnosis of Endoprosthetic Loosening and Infection in Hip and Knee Arthroplasty: Results from a Prospective, Blinded Study. *BMC Musculoskelet Disord.* **2006**, *3*, 7–20. [CrossRef]
86. Stumpe, K.D.; Romero, J.; Ziegler, O.; Kamel, E.M.; von Schulthess, G.K.; Strobel, K.; Hodler, J. The value of FDG-PET in patients with painful total knee arthroplasty. *Eur. J. Nucl. Med. Mol. Imaging* **2006**, *33*, 1218–1225. [CrossRef] [PubMed]
87. Pill, S.G.; Parvizi, J.; Tang, P.H.; Garino, J.P.; Nelson, C.; Zhuang, H.; Alavi, A. Comparison of Fluorodeoxyglucose Positron Emission Tomography and (111)indium-white Blood Cell Imaging in the Diagnosis of Periprosthetic Infection of the Hip. *J. Arthroplast.* **2006**, *21*, 91–97. [CrossRef] [PubMed]
88. Verberne, S.J.; Raijmakers, P.G.; Temmerman, O.P. The Accuracy of Imaging Techniques in the Assessment of Periprosthetic Hip Infection: A Systematic Review and Meta-Analysis. *J. Bone Jt. Surg. Am.* **2016**, *5*, 1638–1645. [CrossRef]
89. Filippi, L.; Schillaci, O. Usefulness of Hybrid SPECT/CT in 99mTc-HMPAO-labeled Leukocyte Scintigraphy for Bone and Joint Infections. *J. Nucl. Med.* **2006**, *47*, 1908–1913.

13

Usefulness of ^{18}F-FDG PET/CT in Patients with Cardiac Implantable Electronic Device Suspected of Late Infection

Giuseppe Rubini [1], Cristina Ferrari [1], Domenico Carretta [2], Luigi Santacroce [3], Rossella Ruta [1], Francesca Iuele [1], Valentina Lavelli [1], Nunzio Merenda [1], Carlo D'Agostino [2], Angela Sardaro [4,*] and Artor Niccoli Asabella [5]

1 Nuclear Medicine Unit, Interdisciplinary Department of Medicine – University of Bari "Aldo Moro", Piazza Giulio Cesare, 11, 70124 Bari, Italy; giuseppe.rubini@uniba.it (G.R.); ferrari_cristina@inwind.it (C.F.); rossella.ruta@yahoo.it (R.R.); francescaiuele@hotmail.com (F.I.); valentina.lavelli@gmail.com (V.L.); nu.me@hotmail.it (N.M.)

2 CardioThoracic Department – Policlinic of Bari, Piazza Giulio Cesare, 11, 70124, Bari, Italy; carrettacardiologia@gmail.com (D.C.); carlo.dagostino@policlinico.ba.it (C.D.)

3 Ionian Department, Microbiology and Virology Lab – University of Bari "Aldo Moro", Piazza Giulio Cesare, 11, 70124 Bari, Italy; luigi.santacroce@uniba.it

4 Radiation Oncology Unit, Interdisciplinary Department of Medicine – University of Bari "Aldo Moro", Piazza Giulio Cesare, 11, 70124 Bari, Italy

5 Nuclear Medicine Unit, A. O. Policlinic "A. Perrino", Strada Statale 7 per Mesagne, 72100 Brindisi, Italy; artor.niccoliasabella@asl.brindisi.it

* Correspondence: angela.sardaro@uniba.it

Abstract: The presence of a cardiovascular implantable electronic device (CIED) can be burdened by complications such as late infections that are associated with significant morbidity and mortality and require immediate and effective treatment. The aim of this study was to evaluate the role of ^{18}F-fluorodeoxyglucose positron-emission tomography/computed tomography (^{18}F-FDG PET/CT) in patients with suspected CIED infection. Fifteen patients who performed a ^{18}F-FDG PET/CT for suspicion of CIED infection were retrospectively analyzed; 15 patients, with CIED, that underwent ^{18}F-FDG PET/CT for oncological reasons, were also evaluated. Visual qualitative analysis and semi-quantitative analysis were performed. All patients underwent standard clinical management regardless ^{18}F-FDG PET/CT results. Sensitivity, specificity, accuracy, positive predictive value (PPV) and negative predictive value (NPV) resulted as 90.91%, 75%, 86.67%, 90.91% and 75% respectively. Maximum standardized uptake values (SUV_{max}) and semi-quantitative ratio (SQR) were collected and showed differences statistically significant between CIED infected patients and those who were not. Exploratory cut-off values were derived from receiver operating characteristic (ROC) curves for SUV_{max} (2.56) and SQR (4.15). This study suggests the clinical usefulness of ^{18}F-FDG PET/CT in patients with CIED infection due to its high sensitivity, repeatability and non-invasiveness. It can help the clinicians in decision making, especially in patients with doubtful clinical presentation. Future large-scale and multicentric studies should be conducted to establish precise protocols about ^{18}F-FDG PET/CT performance.

Keywords: ^{18}F-FDG PET/CT; infection; cardiac implantable electronic device

---

1. Introduction

Implantations of cardiac implantable electronic devices (CIEDs) have increased significantly over recent years, due to growing evidence of improved quality of life, population growth and increased life expectancy [1–3]. Despite the many benefits of this surgical practice, it can be burdened by complications such as infections that are associated with significant morbidity and mortality and require immediate and effective treatment [4–7]. CIED infections (CIEDIs) can onset late after placement and in these cases the diagnosis is more difficult because presentation is highly variable; a significant number of late infections presents with more indolent manifestation [8–10]. Delays in diagnosing and treating can result in progression to infectious endocarditis or sever sepsis with worse clinical outcomes [9,11]. CIED consists on both intravascular and extravascular components and any part of it can be involved by infection. Once any segment of the device gets involved by infection, the entire system is considered infected [12,13]. The main therapeutic option is complete device removal, which is complex, expensive and potentially accompanied by complications [13]. For this reason it is important to have as much information as possible to help clinicians choosing the most appropriate treatment [14]. ^{18}F-fluorodeoxyglucose positron-emission tomography/computed tomography (^{18}F-FDG PET/CT) is a validated multimodality whole-body technique that can identify invective foci because ^{18}F-FDG uptake increases due to the high concentration of neutrophils and monocyte/macrophages, which overexpress glucose transporters, and hexokinase activity. For this reason ^{18}F-FDG PET/CT has been recently proposed also in the diagnostic workflow of numerous infectious conditions [15–19].

The aim of this study was to investigate the possible role of ^{18}F-FDG PET/CT in the diagnosis of suspected CIED infection.

2. Materials and Methods

2.1. Design and Patients

This observational and retrospective analysis included 30 patients with CIED implanted at least 6 months before the performance of ^{18}F-FDG PET/CT. Written informed consent for collecting data for clinical research was obtained from all patients at the moment of the first hospital admission. ^{18}F-FDG PET/CT were performed from November 2017 to December 2018. Our institutional review board did not require ethical committee approval for the review of patients' files and data. 15/30 patients (14 men and 1 woman, mean age 69 years, range: 46–84 years) performed ^{18}F-FDG PET/CT for suspected CIED infection (group CIEDIsusp) [12]. The suspicion of CIED infection was postulated according to the presence of at least 2 of the following signs: (1) clinical signs: fever >38 °C, local signs of generator pocket infection (erythema and/or localized cellulitis and/or swelling and/or discharge and/or dehiscence and/or pain over the pocket and/or fluid collection and/or CIED exposure); (2) laboratory signs: increased values of inflammatory index: erythrosedimentation rate (ESR) and/or C-reactive protein (CRP) and/or procalcitonin (PCT) and/or white blood cells (WBC), blood culture positivity; (3) instrumental signs: trans-thoracic echocardiography (TTE) positivity, trans-esophageal echocardiography (TEE) positivity. 15/30 patients (13 men and 2 women, mean age 76 years, range: 59–93 years) were selected as control group among patients with CIED who underwent ^{18}F-FDG PET/CT for oncological surveillance without clinical suspicion of CIED infection (group ONCOctrl).

2.2. ^{18}F-Fluorodeoxyglucose Positron-Emission Tomography/Computed Tomography (^{18}F-FGD PET/CT) Technique

All patients were instructed to fast for 8 h before the exam; CIEDIsusp patients also underwent a fat-enriched and lacking carbohydrates diet for 24 h before the 8-h fast, in order to reduce the physiological uptake of the ^{18}F-FDG by myocardium [20]. Patients' blood glucose level was evaluated before ^{18}F-FDG administration and all patients had a capillary level lower than 150 mg/dL. Images were acquired with a combined modality PET/CT Discovery LSA (GE Healthcare, Waukesha, Wisconsin, USA), integrating a PET with a 16-slice low-dose CT scanner, in order to perform PET images' correction for attenuation and anatomical reconstruction. The image acquisition was obtained 45–60 min after the intravenous injection of a dose of 2.5–3.0 MBq/kg of ^{18}F-FDG. Patients were hydrated by drinking 500 mL of water and instructed to empty the bladder before image acquisition. The PET acquisition was obtained in cranial-caudal direction, carried out from the external acoustic meatus to the root of the thigh; PET was reconstructed with a matrix of 128 × 128, ordered subset expectation maximum iterative reconstruction algorithm (two iterations, 28 subset), 8 mm Gaussian filter and 50 cm field of view. The CT acquisition parameters were the following: slice thickness 3.75 mm; 350 mA; 120 kV; tube rotation time 0.8 ms and collimation field of view (FOV) 50 cm. The CT images were reconstructed with a filtered back-projection. No iodate intravenous contrast was administered to patients.

2.3. ^{18}F-FGD PET/CT Imaging Interpretation

^{18}F-FDG PET/CT images were blindly reviewed by 2 nuclear physicians with more than 5 years of experience (C.F., N.M.) by using MultiVol PET/CT program (Volume Share 4.7 with Volume Viewer Software) of Advantage Workstation (GE Healthcare, Waukesha, Wisconsin, USA). Qualitative and semi-quantitative analysis were assessed both with and without the attenuation correction; non-attenuation corrected images were reviewed for final interpretation, in order to avoid artifacts induced by metallic components of CIED [21–24]. The visual qualitative analysis defined whether the ^{18}F-FDG PET/CT was positive or negative for CIED infection. Positive ^{18}F-FDG PET/CT was defined by increased ^{18}F-FDG uptake around the device (generator pocket and/or leads) greater than mediastinal blood pool activity. Negative ^{18}F-FDG PET/CT was defined if no increased ^{18}F-FDG uptake around the device relative to surrounding tissues or mediastinal blood pool was detected [21–23]. Discordant analysis interpretation was discussed and resolved by consensus [23]. Semi-quantitative parameters were collected by volumes of interest (VOIs) semi-automatically drawn nearby the generator pocket and along the leads' pathway. Maximum standardized uptake values (SUV_{max}), normalized basing on the patient's injected dose and weight, were collected from the VOI with the highest value. Semi-quantitative ratios (SQRs) were also calculated: SQR was defined as the maximum count rate in the region surrounding CIED over a mean count rate between normal left and right lung parenchyma; areas of abnormal lung parenchyma were avoided in the analysis.

2.4. Assessment of Patients' Outcome

Management of patients and treatment decisions were made by the same cardiologists (D.C., C.D.A.) in all cases and established on the basis of the current clinical guidelines [12,25]. ^{18}F-FDG PET/CT results were not used to guide the management decision. In patients who underwent surgery and whose CIED was removed, the final diagnosis was reached by the microbiological analysis. In the remnant patients, the final diagnosis was reached by clinical and instrumental follow-up, according to modified Duke's criteria [25]. All patients were followed by the same cardiologists (D.C., C.D.A.) for 6 months after the performance of ^{18}F-FDG PET/CT, both in case surgical CIED removal was performed and not.

2.5. Statistical Analysis

Sensitivity (Se), specificity (Sp), accuracy (Acc), positive predictive value (PPV) and negative predictive value (NPV) were calculated for CIEDIsusp patients. Reliability of ^{18}F-FDG PET/CT qualitative analysis among the observers was evaluated with Cohen's K. Semi-quantitative parameters were compared by Student's *t*-test; *p* value lower than 0.05 was considered statistically significant. Ninety-five percent confidence intervals (95% CI) were added for all diagnostic accuracy parameters (Se, Sp, Acc, PPV, NPV). Receiver operating characteristic (ROC) curve analysis were performed to derive exploratory cut-off values. All statistical analysis was carried out using MedCalc® Statistical Software version 2020 (MedCalc Software Ltd., Ostend, Belgium).

3. Results

3.1. Patients' Baseline Characteristics

Demographic, clinical and instrumental characteristics about CIEDIsusp patients are reported in Table 1.

Table 1. Demographic, clinical and instrumental characteristics of cardiac implantable electronic devices infection group (CIEDIsusp) patients.

Patients				Clinical Signs		Laboratory Signs					Instrumental Signs	
ID	Age	Sex	Type of CIED Implanted	Fever	Local Signs of CIED Infection	ESR (v.n. <20 mm/h)	CRP (v.n. <2.9 mg/L)	PCT (v.n. <0.5 ng/mL)	WBC (v.n. 3.7-9.7 x10^3 uL)	Blood Culture	TTE	TEE
1	75	M	ICD	Yes	Yes	48	18.4	16	5.6	0	Negative	/
2	74	M	PM	Yes	No	8	3.1	3.7	5.5	0	Negative	/
3	73	M	PM	Yes	No	18	35	0.02	10.05	0	Negative	/
4	83	M	PM	Yes	Yes	25	1	0.03	7.65	*Staphyl. Aureus*	Negative	Negative
5	83	M	ICD	Yes	Yes	48	3	0.04	6.57	*Staphyl. Epiderm.*	Negative	/
6	59	F	PM	No	Yes	38	0	0.02	6.7	0	Negative	/
7	46	M	PM	Yes	Yes	52	42.7	0.07	7.77	0	Negative	Positive
8	84	M	ICD	Yes	No	50	70.6	11	6.2	0	Negative	/
9	56	M	PM	No	No	31	99	0.13	8.91	0	Positive	Positive
10	63	M	PM	Yes	No	50	3.1	3.4	4.35	0	Negative	/
11	71	M	PM	Yes	Yes	0	1	0.02	5.48	0	Negative	Positive
12	53	M	ICD	No	No	16	1.7	0.03	6.31	0	Negative	/
13	73	M	ICD	Yes	No	37	38	0.07	7.04	0	Negative	Positive
14	62	M	ICD	No	Yes	0	0	0	4.5	0	Negative	/
15	78	M	ICD	No	No	1	1	0.03	5.93	*Staphyl. Epiderm.*	Negative	/

CIED: cardiac implantable electronic device; ESR: erythrosedimentation rate; CRP: C-reactive protein; PCT: procalcitonin; WBC: white blood cells; TTE: trans-thoracic echocardiography; TEE: trans-esophageal echocardiography; ICD: implantable cardioverter defibrillators; PM: pacemakers.

As regards the kinds of device implanted, 7/15 (47%) patients had implantable cardioverter defibrillators (ICDs) and 8/15 (53%) had pacemakers (PMs). Fever was present in 10/15 (67%) patients and local signs of pocket infection was found in 7/15 (47%) patients. Values of ESR and CRP were increased in 9/15 (60%) patients, while values of PCT and WBC were altered respectively in 4/15 (27%) and 1/15 (7%) patients. Blood cultures resulted positive in 3/15 (20%) patients and negative in the remnant 12/15 (80%). The bacteria identified were *Staphylococcus epidermidis* (n. 2) and *Staphylococcus aureus* (n. 1). TTE resulted positive in 1/15 (7%) patient (also confirmed by TEE); TEE was performed in 5/15 (33%) patients and it resulted positive in 4/5 patients; TEE was not performed in the remnants patients because of their clinical conditions.

The 15 ONCOctrl patients performed ^{18}F-FDG PET/CT for oncological surveillance and they had no clinical suspicion of CIED infection. The devices implanted were ICDs in 5/15 (33%) and PMs in 10/15 (67%). They were affected by lung carcinoma (3/15), chronic lymphatic leukemia (2/15), non-Hodgkin lymphoma (2/15), kidney carcinoma (2/15), melanoma (3/15), intestinal carcinoma (2/15) and gastric cancer (1/15).

The mean time elapsing between the statement of possible CIED infection and the ^{18}F-FDG PET/CT execution was 2 days (range: 1–3 days). During this time empirical antibiotic therapies were started: 4 patients assumed cefazolin, 2 amoxicillin + clavulanic acid, 3 amoxicillin + clavulanic acid and levoxacin, 1 daptomycin, 1 cefazolin and teicoplanin, one amoxicillin + clavulanic acid and daptomycin, 1 teicoplanin + ceftriaxone, 1 daptomycin and piperacillin tazobactam and 1 azithromycin and daptomycin and piperacillin tazobactam. The therapies did not interfere with the microbiological study of samples and did not invalidate ^{18}F-FDG PET/CT results, because the short interval of time elapsing between the start of the therapy and the instrumental exam execution was not sufficient to obtain a complete bacterial count reduction so it did not influence ^{18}F-FDG uptake.

The mean time elapsing between the CIED implantation and the ^{18}F-FDG PET/CT execution was 3.2 years (range: 6 months–7 years) and the mean time elapsing between the ^{18}F-FDG PET/CT execution and the surgical device removal was 5 days (range: 3–7 days). In the control group, the mean time elapsing between the CIED implantation and the ^{18}F-FDG PET/CT execution was 3.5 years (range: 10 months–8 years).

3.2. ^{18}F-FGD PET/CT Analysis Results

According to visual qualitative analysis, ^{18}F-FDG PET/CT resulted positive in 11/15 (73%) CIEDIsusp patients; in the remnants 4/15 (27%) patients, the exam was considered negative [Figure 1, Figure 2].

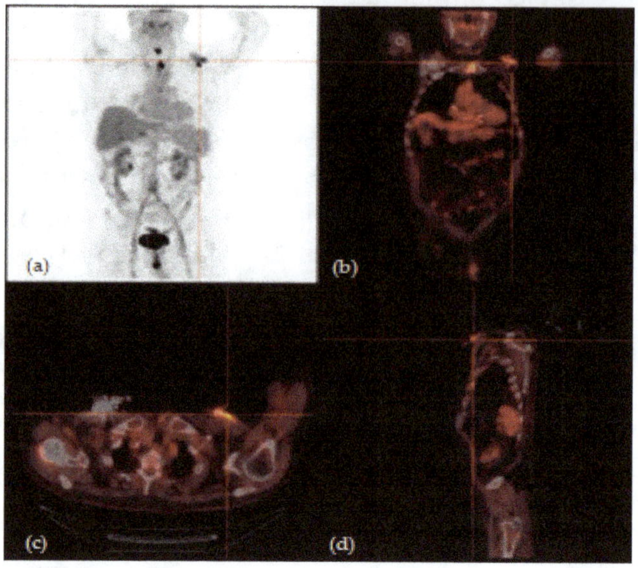

Figure 1. ^{18}F-fluorodeoxyglucose positron-emission tomography/computed tomography (^{18}F-FDG PET/CT) of a 78-year-old man with suspicion of cardiac implantable electronic device (CIED) infection because of bacterial blood culture positive for *Staphylococcus epidermidis*. (**a**) Maximum intensity projection (MIP), (**b**) coronal fusion, (**c**) axial fusion and (**d**) sagittal fusion images showed increased ^{18}F-FDG uptake involving the CIED pocket. After surgical CIED removal, microbiological analysis of explanted materials confirmed *Staphylococcus epidermidis* infection.

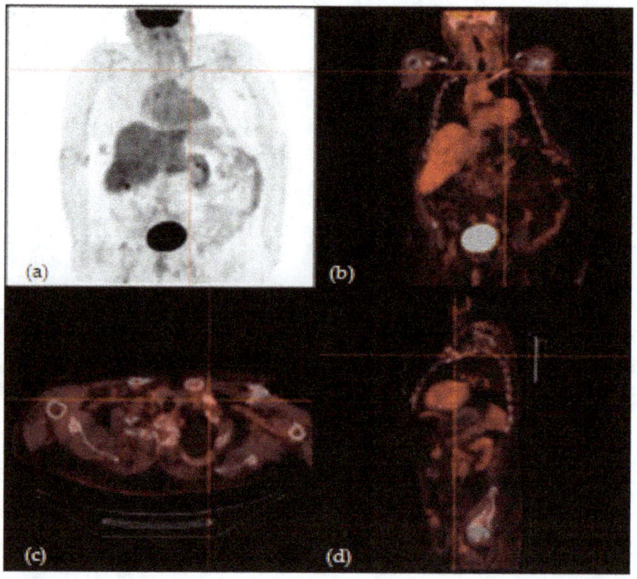

Figure 2. ^{18}F-FDG PET/CT of a 56-year-old man with suspicion of CIED infection; both TTE and TEE were positive, but bacterial blood culture was negative. (**a**) Maximum intensity projection (MIP), (**b**) coronal fusion, (**c**) axial fusion and (**d**) sagittal fusion images showed increased ^{18}F-FDG uptake involving the leads. After surgical CIED removal, microbiological analysis of explanted materials showed *Staphylococcus epidermidis* infection.

Sites of infection were generator pocket in 9/11 and leads' extracardiac pathway in the remnant 2/11 patients. No other pathological areas of ^{18}F-FDG uptake were found even in the endocardium in any patient. All ONCOctrl patients did not show any abnormal ^{18}F-FDG uptake area in proximity of the generator pocket or leads, so none of them was considered positive. The description of ^{18}F-FDG PET/CT results is reported in Table 2.

Table 2. ^{18}F-FDG PET/CT and final results in CIEDIsusp patients.

18F-FDG PET/CT Analysis Results					Final Results	
ID	Result	Site	SUVmax	SQR	Microbiological Analysis	Clinical Follow-Up
1	Positive	Pocket	3.65	3.80	*Staphyl. haemolyticus*	/
2	Positive	Pocket	4.96	9.54	/	Negative
3	Negative	Pocket	2.19	3.37	Negative	/
4	Positive	Pocket	3.32	4.61	*Staphyl. aureus*	/
5	Positive	Pocket	4.31	8.71	*Staphyl. epidermidis*	/
6	Negative	Pocket	2.56	3.24	/	Negative
7	Positive	Lead	2.80	4.41	*Staphyl. epidermidis*	/
8	Negative	Pocket	1.96	3.24	*Staphyl. epidermidis*	/
9	Positive	Lead	2.69	2.88	*Staphyl. epidermidis*	/
10	Positive	Pocket	6.55	9.63	*Staphyl. epidermidis*	/
11	Positive	Pocket	6.75	10.38	*Staphyl. epidermidis*	/
12	Negative	Pocket	1.82	1.43	/	Negative
13	Positive	Pocket	2.20	4.58	*Staphyl. epidermidis*	/
14	Positive	Pocket	4.61	8.46	*Staphyl. epidermidis*	/
15	Positive	Pocket	7.33	11.63	*Staphyl. epidermidis*	/

SUV_{max}: maximum standardized uptake values; SQR: semi-quantitative ratio.

3.3. Patients' Outcome

The cardiac device was surgically removed in 12/15 (80%) CIEDIsusp patients; the entire pacing system was extracted intravenously. In these patients the final diagnosis was reached by the microbiological analysis: it was positive in 11/12 and negative in 1/12. In the remnant 3/15 (20%) patients who did not remove CIED the clinical and instrumental follow-up resulted negative for infection. The description of microbiological and clinical follow-up results is reported in Table 2. All ONCOctrl patients resulted negative during clinical follow-up.

3.4. Statistical Analysis Results

As regards the CIEDIsusp patients, 10/15 resulted as true positives (TPs), 3/15 true negatives (TNs) 1/15 false positive (FP) and 1/15 false negative (FN). As regards the ONCOctrl patients, agreement between ^{18}F-FDG PET/CT and outcome was complete: all patients showed negativity in ^{18}F-FDG PET/CT and resulted negative during clinical follow-up. In CIEDIsusp patients, Se, Sp, Acc, PPV and NPV of ^{18}F-FDG PET/CT resulted 90.91% (95% CI: 58.72% to 99.77%), 75% (95% CI: 19.41% to 99.37%), 86.67% (95% CI: 59.54% to 98.34%), 90.91% (95% CI: 64.45% to 98.22%) and 75% (95% CI: 29.86% to 95.48%) respectively. Reproducibility among nuclear medicine physicians as regards qualitative analysis resulted as excellent (K value = 0.89).

In CIEDIsusp patients positive at ^{18}F-FDG PET/CT, the mean value of SUV_{max} was 4.47 (range: 2.20–7.33; SD = 1.76) and the mean value of SQR was 7.15 (range: 2.88–11.63; SD = 3.11). In CIEDIsusp patients negative at ^{18}F-FDG PET/CT, the mean value of SUV_{max} was 2.13 (range: 1.82–2.56; SD = 0.32) and the mean value of SQR was 2.82 (range: 1.43–3.37; SD = 0.93). In ONCOctrl patients, the mean value of SUV_{max} was 1.98 (range: 1.29–2.96; SD = 0.50) and the mean value of SQR was 3.48 (range: 1.90–5.38; SD = 0.93) [Figure 3].

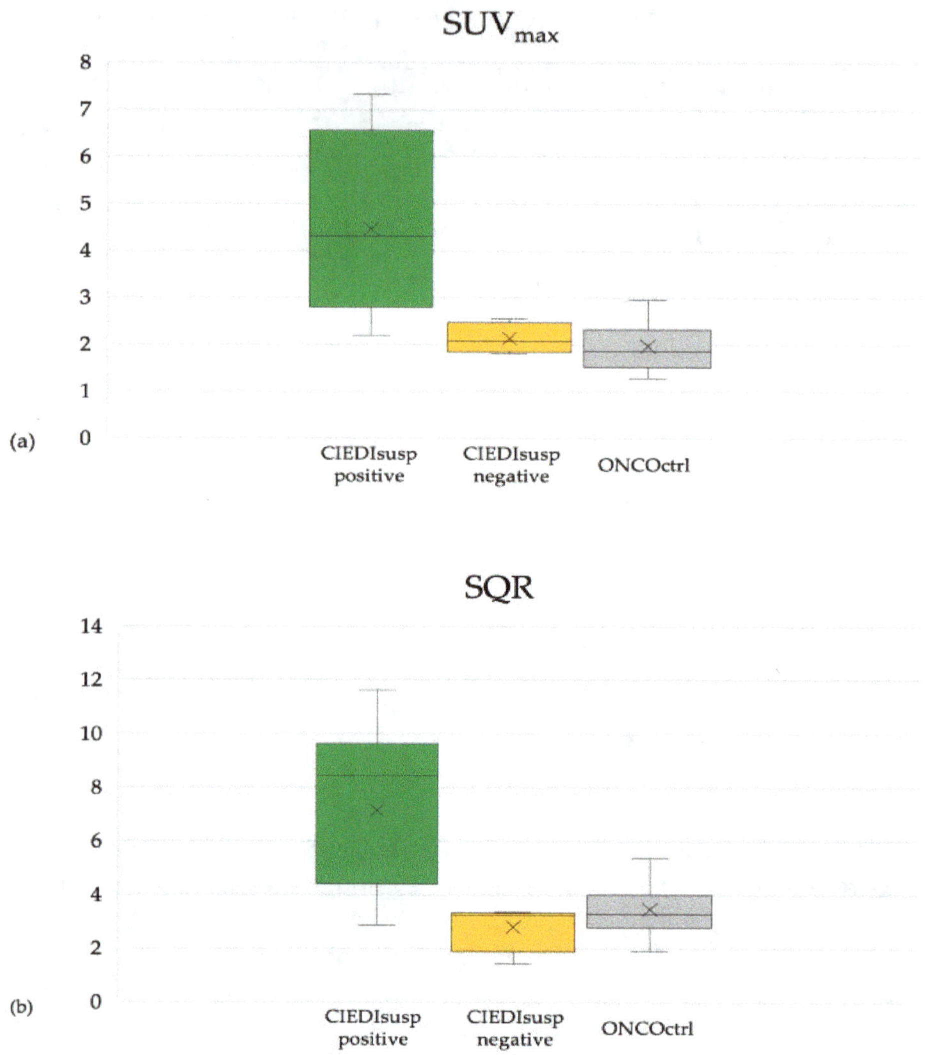

Figure 3. (**a**) SUV_{max} distribution in CIEDIsusp patients positive at ^{18}F-FDG PET/CT, CIEDIsusp patients negative at ^{18}F-FDG PET/CT and oncological surveillance without clinical suspicion of CIED infection group (ONCOctrl) patients. (**b**) SQR distribution in CIEDIsusp patients positive at ^{18}F-FDG PET/CT, CIEDIsusp patients negative at ^{18}F-FDG PET/CT and ONCOctrl patients.

In patients with diagnosis of CIED infection, the mean value of SUV_{max} was 3.91 (range: 1.96–7.33; SD = 1.87). In patients without CIED infection, the mean value of SUV_{max} was 2.14 (range: 1.29–4.96; SD = 0.86). The difference between them was statistically significant ($t = 3.35$; 95% CI: 0.68% to 2.85%; $p < 0.05$) [Figure 4a]. The mean value of SQR was 6.07 (range: 2.88–11.63; SD = 3.17) in patients positive for CIED infection and 3.72 (range: 1.43–9.54; SD = 1.8) in negative ones. The difference was statistically significant ($t = 2.57$; 95% CI: 0.40% to 4.29%; $p < 0.05$) [Figure 4b].

Exploratory SUV_{max} cut-off value resulted as 2.56 (area under the curve (AUC) = 0.957; ES = 0.032; 95% CI: 0.395% to 0.519%) while exploratory SQR cut-off value resulted as 4.15 (AUC = 0.878; ES = 0.071; 95% CI: 0.239% to 0.517%).

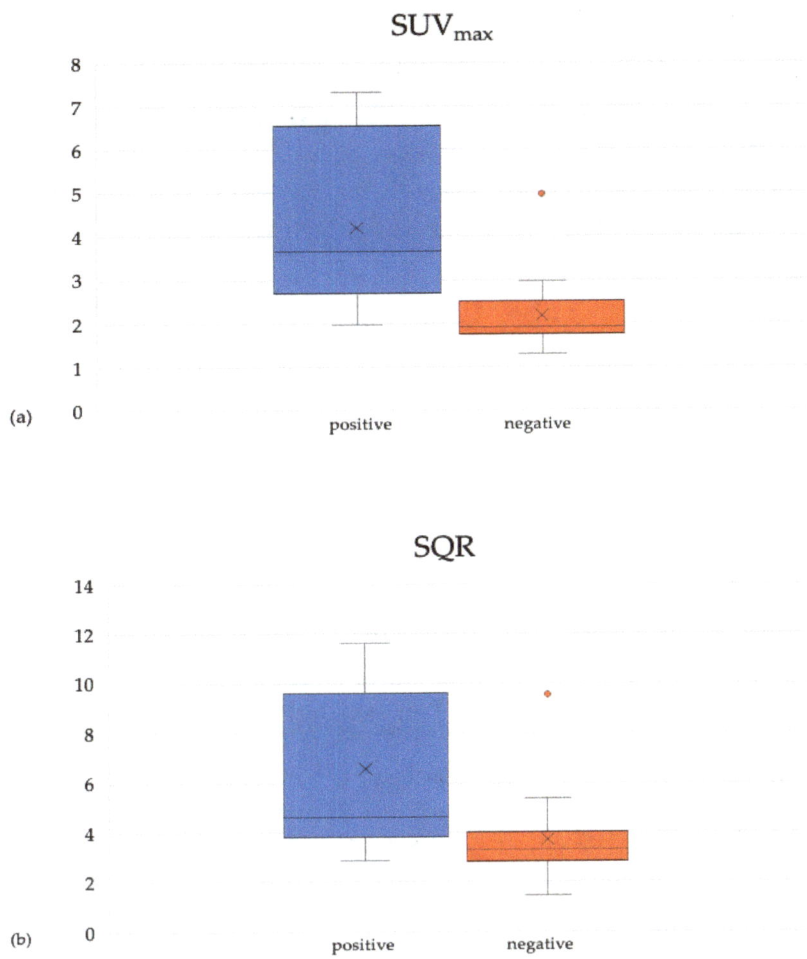

Figure 4. (**a**) SUV$_{max}$ distribution in patients with CIED infection (positive) and patients without CIED infection (negative). (**b**) SQR distribution in patients with CIED infection (positive) and patients without CIED infection (negative).

4. Discussion

Our study aims to assess the value of ^{18}F-FDG PET/CT in patients who referred to cardiologist for suspected CIED infection. Previous studies already evaluated the role of ^{18}F-FDG PET/CT in these patients, but there was not homogeneity in methodological criteria [22,24,26–28]. In our study all patients with suspicion of CIED infection were instructed to follow a high-fat/low-carbohydrate (HFLC) diet that allowed an optimal suppression of physiological myocardial glucose utilization, facilitating the evaluation of intracardiac sites of elevated ^{18}F-FDG uptake. A correct diet before ^{18}F-FDG PET/CT was useful to reduce the physiological myocardial uptake avoiding either false-positive (physiological uptake interpreted as infection) or false-negative results (infectious uptake unrecognized because of predominant diffuse physiological uptake) [21,25,29,30]. Although a precise protocol for ^{18}F-FDG PET/CT is not completely standardized for cardiac infection imaging, it is highly recommended a dietary preparation with 1 or 2 meals of high fat and low carbohydrates followed by a fasting period of at 8 h [14].

Furthermore, in all patients with suspicion of CIED infection the timing of ^{18}F-FDG PET/CT was accurately defined in order not to be influenced by antibiotic therapy. According to the current guidelines, empirical antimicrobial therapies have to be commenced as soon as possible in patients with suspected CIED infection [12] and in our study, ^{18}F-FDG PET/CT was performed no more than 2 days after the beginning of them; this period of time was not sufficient to interfere with ^{18}F-FDG uptake. Previous studies with the same aim as ours, even if analyzed in a larger population, presented a bias of the lack of dietary preparation and duration of antibiotic therapy that resulted from being performed for weeks before ^{18}F-FDG PET/CT, influencing the results [26–28].

In our study all patients were evaluated by the same cardiologist and ^{18}F-FDG PET/CT results were not used to guide the management of patients; treatment decisions were established on the basis of the current guidelines [12,25,31]. In the majority of patients (12/15) CIED was removed and the microbiological analysis was performed while in the remnants (3/15), for whom cardiologist did not remove the device, patients' outcome was assessed by follow-up according to modified Duke's criteria [25,32].

About patients with CIED infection, even if ^{18}F-FDG PET/CT is not recommended for routine performance, it is mentioned as a potential useful additive tool in selected cases, in particular when there is uncertainty about generator pocket infection [14,20,25,26,33].

Our study revealed a good reliability of ^{18}F-FDG PET/CT thanks to the good agreement with final outcomes. Discordance was observed only in two patients. In one patient ^{18}F-FDG PET/CT was considered positive for CIED infection, but the clinical follow-up resulted in being negative; this false positive result has been ascribed to the presence of a foreign-body inflammation reaction nearby the pocket. In this patient the suspicion of CIED infection was postulated on the basis of the presence of fever and increased values of inflammatory indexes, without local signs of generator pocket infection. The cardiologist decided not to surgically remove the device, because the patient was in a good general health state and both fever and inflammatory indexes were slightly increased. The patient underwent close clinical monitoring, showing rapid temperature decrease and laboratory indexes normalization. These findings supported the hypothesis of high ^{18}F-FDG PET/CT uptake due to tissue's inflammatory reaction as also reported in literature [21]. In one patient ^{18}F-FDG PET/CT resulted negative, but the microbiological analysis after CIED removal showed *Staphylococcus epidermidis* infection; the false negative result can be explained by the small site of the infection near the electrocatheter, less than the resolution of the technique [13,26_28,34].

Our results from the diagnostic performance of ^{18}F-FDG PET/CT were also encouraging, revealing better results for sensitivity and PPV (both 90.91%) in line with those reported in literature (80–97%) [21,23,35,36]. In our analysis these good results, such as 86.67% accuracy, can be at least in part attributed to the high number of pocket infection of our patients' cohort. The specificity and NPV resulted lower (both 75%) because of the ^{18}F-FDG uptake also in unspecific inflammatory conditions; other factors that can influence the cardiac glucose uptake of ^{18}F-FDG are sugar blood level, insulin blood level, left vs right ventricle blood shunt, vasculitis and ateromatous arteries [4,7].

In our study the reliability of visual qualitative analysis of ^{18}F-FDG PET/CT images by the 2 nuclear medicine physicians resulted in being excellent (K = 0.89). It was thanks to the high quality of images both corrected and non-corrected for attenuation that artifacts related to the metallic components of the device were avoided [22,23]. Our results confirmed those of Granados et al. and Bensimhon et al.; in their studies, K values for presence of CIED infection were, respectively, 0.81 and 0.80 [22,36].

In addition to visual qualitative assessment, semi-quantitative parameters were also collected in order to investigate their usefulness in the diagnosis of CIED infection. In literature there is no consensus about the choice of them and their evaluation; we have chosen the SUV_{max} because it is the most validated parameter and SQR because it allows any error in the radiotracer uptake detection during the attenuation correction process to be avoided [21–24].

In our study, the differences of mean values of SUV_{max} and SQR between patients with confirmed and unconfirmed CIED infection were statistically significant ($p < 0.05$) suggesting that these values could further contribute to the correct interpretation of ^{18}F-FDG PET/CT images; however, it is opportune to underline that these results must be interpreted with caution due to the small size of our sample and the overlap of the ranges of values collected.

Besides these limitations, it was possible to propose exploratory cut-off values of SUV_{max} and SQR, which are useful to discriminate patients with CIED infection from negative ones. In our study SUV_{max} cut-off value resulted 2.56 and SQR cut-off value 4.15, obtained by ROC analysis. Also, Bensimhon et al.

proposed a SUV_{max} cut-off value of 2.2; Ahmed et al. and Sarrazin et al. proposed SQR cut-off values of 2.00 and 1.87 respectively [21,23,36]. Our results are similar to those reported in literature about SUV_{max} and different about SQR, but it is important to consider that differences in methodological statistical analysis and in the population samples analyzed can interfere with the comparison.

^{18}F-FDG PET/CT is whole-body multimodality imaging; its most relevant advantages are the evaluation of extracardiac components of the device, which are beyond the echocardiographic field of view, the detection of unexpected sources of primary infection, and the identification of embolic consequences of endocarditis [14,23,35,37]. In our study no sites of infection different from those of CIED were detected, excluding more complicated diseases. Otherwise ^{18}F-FDG PET/CT uses ionizing radiation, but current technologies reduce considerably the radiation exposure; it should be also remembered that CIED patients are generally of high age and for them the risks of CIED infection are more serious than those potentially of ionizing radiation [14].

Although our study showed promising results, it is not devoid of limitations such as the retrospective and monocentric nature of our analysis; our sample was small, but homogeneous and in line with samples reported in literature; conventional instrumental exams such as TEE and CIED removal were not always performed, but this reflects the real situations that clinicians have to face.

5. Conclusions

This study suggests the clinical usefulness of ^{18}F-FDG PET/CT in patients with CIED infection due to its high sensitivity, repeatability and non-invasiveness. It can help the clinicians in decision making, especially in patients with doubtful clinical presentation, and it should be considered as a possible methodological step into the flowchart of management of patients with suspected CIED infection. Future large-scale and multicentric studies should be conducted to establish precise protocols about ^{18}F-FDG PET/CT performance.

Author Contributions: G.R.: project administration; C.F.: conceptualization and imaging interpretation; D.C.: resources and assessment of patients' outcome; L.S.: resources; R.R.: writing—original draft preparation; F.I.: writing—review and editing; V.L.: data curation; N.M.: methodology and imaging interpretation; C.D.: conceptualization and assessment of patients' outcome; A.S.: supervision; A.N.A.: visualization. All authors have read and agreed to the published version of the manuscript.

Acknowledgments: None.

References

1. Polewczyk, A.; Jacheć, W.; Polewczyk, A.M.; Tomasik, A.; Janion, M.; Kutarski, A. Infectious complications in patients with cardiac implantable electronic devices: Risk factors, prevention, and prognosis. *Pol. Arch. Intern. Med.* **2017**, *127*, 597–607. [CrossRef] [PubMed]
2. Chrispin, J.; Love, C.J. Cardiac Implantable Electronic Device Infections and Lead Extraction: Are Patients with Renal Insufficiency Special? *Circ. Arrhythmia Electrophysiol.* **2018**, *11*, 1–3. [CrossRef] [PubMed]
3. Bongiorni, M.G.; Burri, H.; Deharo, J.C.; Starck, C.; Kennergren, C.; Saghy, L.; Rao, A.; Tascini, C.; Lever, N.; Kutarski, A.; et al. 2018 EHRA expert consensus statement on lead extraction: Recommendations on definitions, endpoints, research trial design, and data collection requirements for clinical scientific studies and registries: Endorsed by APHRS/HRS/LAHRS. *Europace* **2018**, *20*, 1217. [CrossRef] [PubMed]
4. Juneau, D.; Golfam, M.; Hazra, S.; Zuckier, L.S.; Garas, S.; Redpath, C.; Bernick, J.; Leung, E.; Chih, S.; Wells, G.; et al. Positron Emission Tomography and Single-Photon Emission Computed Tomography Imaging in the Diagnosis of Cardiac Implantable Electronic Device Infection. *Circ. Cardiovasc. Imaging* **2017**, *10*, e005772. [CrossRef] [PubMed]
5. Voigt, A.; Shalaby, A.; Saba, S. Continued rise in rates of cardiovascular implantable electronic device infections in the United States: Temporal trends and causative insights. *PACE-Pacing Clin. Electrophysiol.* **2010**, *33*, 414–419. [CrossRef] [PubMed]

6. Baddour, L.M.; Cha, Y.M.; Wilson, W.R. Infections of cardiovascular implantable electronic devices. *N. Engl. J. Med.* **2012**, *367*, 842–849. [CrossRef]
7. Nery, P.B.; Fernandes, R.; Nair, G.M.; Sumner, G.L.; Ribas, C.S.; Menon, S.M.D.; Wang, X.; Krahn, A.D.; Morillo, C.A.; Connolly, S.J.; et al. Device-related infection among patients with pacemakers and implantable defibrillators: Incidence, risk factors, and consequences. *J. Cardiovasc. Electrophysiol.* **2010**, *21*, 786–790. [CrossRef]
8. Baddour, L.M.; Epstein, A.E.; Erickson, C.C.; Knight, B.P.; Levison, M.E.; Lockhart, P.B.; Masoudi, F.A.; Okum, E.J.; Wilson, W.R.; Beerman, L.B.; et al. Update on cardiovascular implantable electronic device infections and their management: A scientific statement from the american heart association. *Circulation* **2010**, *121*, 458–477. [CrossRef]
9. Maytin, M.; Jones, S.O.; Epstein, L.M. Long-term mortality after transvenous lead extraction. *Circ. Arrhythmia Electrophysiol.* **2012**, *5*, 252–257. [CrossRef]
10. Welch, M.; Uslan, D.Z.; Greenspon, A.J.; Sohail, M.R.; Baddour, L.M.; Blank, E.; Carrillo, R.G.; Danik, S.B.; Del Rio, A.; Hellinger, W.; et al. Variability in clinical features of early versus late cardiovascular implantable electronic device pocket infections. *PACE-Pacing Clin. Electrophysiol.* **2014**, *37*, 955–962. [CrossRef]
11. Singer, M.; Deutschman, C.S.; Seymour, C.; Shankar-Hari, M.; Annane, D.; Bauer, M.; Bellomo, R.; Bernard, G.R.; Chiche, J.D.; Coopersmith, C.M.; et al. The third international consensus definitions for sepsis and septic shock (sepsis-3). *JAMA-J. Am. Med. Assoc.* **2016**, *315*, 801–810. [CrossRef]
12. Sandoe, J.A.T.; Barlow, G.; Chambers, J.B.; Gammage, M.; Guleri, A.; Howard, P.; Olson, E.; Perry, J.D.; Prendergast, B.D.; Spry, M.J.; et al. Guidelines for the diagnosis, prevention and management of implantable cardiac electronic device infection. report of a joint working party project on behalf of the british society for antimicrobial chemotherapy (BSAC, host organization), british heart rh. *J. Antimicrob. Chemother.* **2015**, *70*, 325–359. [CrossRef] [PubMed]
13. DeSimone, D.C.; Sohail, M.R. Approach to diagnosis of cardiovascular implantable-electronic-device infection. *J. Clin. Microbiol.* **2018**, *56*. [CrossRef] [PubMed]
14. Chen, W.; Sajadi, M.M.; Dilsizian, V. Merits of FDG PET/CT and Functional Molecular Imaging Over Anatomic Imaging With Echocardiography and CT Angiography for the Diagnosis of Cardiac Device Infections. *JACC Cardiovasc. Imaging* **2018**, *11*, 1679–1691. [CrossRef] [PubMed]
15. Asabella, A.N.; Di Palo, A.; Altini, C.; Ferrari, C.; Rubini, G. Multimodality imaging in tumor angiogenesis: Present status and perspectives. *Int. J. Mol. Sci.* **2017**, *18*, 1864. [CrossRef]
16. Niccoli Asabella, A.; Simone, M.; Ballini, A.; Altini, C.; Ferrari, C.; Lavelli, V.; Luca, R.D.E.; Inchingolo, F.; Rubini, G. Predictive value of 18F-FDG PET/CT on survival in locally advanced rectal cancer after neoadjuvant chemoradiation. *Eur. Rev. Med. Pharmacol. Sci.* **2018**, *22*, 8227–8236. [CrossRef]
17. Ferrari, C.; Niccoli Asabella, A.; Merenda, N.; Altini, C.; Fanelli, M.; Muggeo, P.; De Leonardis, F.; Perillo, T.; Santoro, N.; Rubini, G. Pediatric Hodgkin lymphoma: Predictive value of interim 18 F-FDG PET/CT in therapy response assessment. *Medicine* **2017**, *96*, e5973. [CrossRef]
18. Alavi, A.; Hess, S.; Werner, T.J.; Høilund-Carlsen, P.F. An update on the unparalleled impact of FDG-PET imaging on the day-to-day practice of medicine with emphasis on management of infectious/inflammatory disorders. *Eur. J. Nucl. Med. Mol. Imaging* **2020**, *47*, 18–27. [CrossRef]
19. Gormsen, L.C.; Hess, S. Challenging but Clinically Useful: Fluorodeoxyglucose PET/Computed Tomography in Inflammatory and Infectious Diseases. *PET Clin.* **2020**, *15*, xi–xii. [CrossRef]
20. Sarrazin, J.-F.; Philippon, F.; Trottier, M.; Tessier, M. Role of radionuclide imaging for diagnosis of device and prosthetic valve infections. *World J. Cardiol.* **2016**, *8*, 534. [CrossRef]
21. Ahmed, F.Z.; James, J.; Cunnington, C.; Motwani, M.; Fullwood, C.; Hooper, J.; Burns, P.; Qamruddin, A.; Al-Bahrani, G.; Armstrong, I.; et al. Early diagnosis of cardiac implantable electronic device generator pocket infection using 18F-FDG-PET/CT. *Eur. Heart J. Cardiovasc. Imaging* **2015**, *16*, 521–530. [CrossRef] [PubMed]
22. Granados, U.; Fuster, D.; Pericas, J.M.; Llopis, J.L.; Ninot, S.; Quintana, E.; Almela, M., Paré, C.; Tolosana, J.M.; Falces, C.; et al. Diagnostic accuracy of 18F-FDG PET/CT in infective endocarditis and implantable cardiac electronic device infection: A cross-sectional study. *J. Nucl. Med.* **2016**, *57*, 1726–1732. [CrossRef]
23. Sarrazin, J.F.; Philippon, F.; Tessier, M.; Guimond, J.; Molin, F.; Champagne, J.; Nault, I.; Blier, L.; Nadeau, M.; Charbonneau, L.; et al. Usefulness of fluorine-18 positron emission tomography/computed tomography for identification of cardiovascular implantable electronic device infections. *J. Am. Coll. Cardiol.* **2012**, *59*, 1616–1625. [CrossRef] [PubMed]

24. Diemberger, I.; Bonfiglioli, R.; Martignani, C.; Graziosi, M.; Biffi, M.; Lorenzetti, S.; Ziacchi, M.; Nanni, C.; Fanti, S.; Boriani, G. Contribution of PET imaging to mortality risk stratification in candidates to lead extraction for pacemaker or defibrillator infection: A prospective single center study. *Eur. J. Nucl. Med. Mol. Imaging* **2019**, *46*, 194–205. [CrossRef] [PubMed]
25. Erba, P.A.; Lancellotti, P.; Vilacosta, I.; Gaemperli, O.; Rouzet, F.; Hacker, M.; Signore, A.; Slart, R.H.J.A.; Habib, G. Recommendations on nuclear and multimodality imaging in IE and CIED infections. *Eur. J. Nucl. Med. Mol. Imaging* **2018**, *45*, 1795–1815. [CrossRef]
26. Tlili, G.; Amroui, S.; Mesguich, C.; Rivière, A.; Bordachar, P.; Hindié, E.; Bordenave, L. High performances of 18F-fluorodeoxyglucose PET-CT in cardiac implantable device infections: A study of 40 patients. *J. Nucl. Cardiol.* **2015**, *22*, 787–798. [CrossRef]
27. Cautela, J.; Alessandrini, S.; Cammilleri, S.; Giorgi, R.; Richet, H.; Casalta, J.P.; Habib, G.; Raoult, D.; Mundler, O.; Deharo, J.C. Diagnostic yield of FDG positron-emission tomography/computed tomography in patients with CEID infection: A pilot study. *Europace* **2013**, *15*, 252–257. [CrossRef]
28. Graziosi, M.; Nanni, C.; Lorenzini, M.; Diemberger, I.; Bonfiglioli, R.; Pasquale, F.; Ziacchi, M.; Biffi, M.; Martignani, C.; Bartoletti, M.; et al. Role of 18F-FDG PET/CT in the diagnosis of infective endocarditis in patients with an implanted cardiac device: A prospective study. *Eur. J. Nucl. Med. Mol. Imaging* **2014**, *41*, 1617–1623. [CrossRef]
29. Osborne, M.T.; Hulten, E.A.; Murthy, V.L.; Skali, H.; Taqueti, V.R.; Dorbala, S.; DiCarli, M.F.; Blankstein, R. Patient preparation for cardiac fluorine-18 fluorodeoxyglucose positron emission tomography imaging of inflammation. *J. Nucl. Cardiol.* **2017**, *24*, 86–99. [CrossRef]
30. Niccoli-Asabella, A.; Iuele, F.; Merenda, N.; Pisani, A.R.; Notaristefano, A.; Rubini, G. 18F-FDGPET/CT: Diabetes and hyperglycaemia. *Nucl. Med. Rev.* **2013**, *16*, 57–61. [CrossRef]
31. Habib, G.; Lancellotti, P.; Antunes, M.J.; Grazia Bongiorni, M.; Casalta, J.-P.; Del Zotti, F.; Dulgheru, R.; El Khoury, G.; Anna Erba, P.; Iung, B.; et al. ESC GUIDELINES 2015 ESC Guidelines for the management of infective endocarditis The Task Force for the Management of Infective Endocarditis of the European Society of Cardiology (ESC) Endorsed by: European Association for Cardio-Thoracic Surgery (EACTS), the European Association of Nuclear Medicine (EANM). *Eur. Heart J.* **2015**, *36*, 3075–3128. [CrossRef] [PubMed]
32. Erba, P.A.; Pizzi, M.N.; Roque, A.; Salaun, E.; Lancellotti, P.; Tornos, P.; Habib, G. Multimodality Imaging in Infective Endocarditis: An Imaging Team Within the Endocarditis Team. *Circulation* **2019**, *140*, 1753–1765. [CrossRef] [PubMed]
33. Marciniak-Emmons, M.B.; Sterliński, M.; Syska, P.; Maciąg, A.; Farkowski, M.M.; Firek, B.; Dziuk, M.; Zając, D.; Pytkowski, M.; Szwed, H. New diagnostic pathways urgently needed. Protocol of PET Guidance i pilot study: Positron emission tomography in suspected cardiac implantable electronic device-related infection. *Kardiol. Pol.* **2016**, *74*, 47–52. [CrossRef] [PubMed]
34. Dy Chua, J.; Abdul-Karim, A.; Mawhorter, S.; Procop, G.W.; Tchou, P.; Niebauer, M.; Saliba, W.; Schweikert, R.; Wilkoff, B.L. The role of swab and tissue culture in the diagnosis of implantable cardiac device infection. *PACE-Pacing Clin. Electrophysiol.* **2005**, *28*, 1276–1281. [CrossRef]
35. Saby, L.; Laas, O.; Habib, G.; Cammilleri, S.; Mancini, J.; Tessonnier, L.; Casalta, J.P.; Gouriet, F.; Riberi, A.; Avierinos, J.F.; et al. Positron emission tomography/computed tomography for diagnosis of prosthetic valve endocarditis: Increased valvular 18F- fluorodeoxyglucose uptake as a novel major criterion. *J. Am. Coll. Cardiol.* **2013**, *61*, 2374–2382. [CrossRef] [PubMed]
36. Bensimhon, L.; Lavergne, T.; Hugonnet, F.; Mainardi, J.L.; Latremouille, C.; Maunoury, C.; Lepillier, A.; Le Heuzey, J.Y.; Faraggi, M. Whole body [^{18}F]fluorodeoxyglucose positron emission tomography imaging for the diagnosis of pacemaker or implantable cardioverter defibrillator infection: A preliminary prospective study. *Clin. Microbiol. Infect.* **2011**, *17*, 836–844. [CrossRef] [PubMed]
37. Bertagna, F.; Bisleri, G.; Motta, F.; Merli, G.; Cossalter, E.; Lucchini, S.; Biasiotto, G.; Bosio, G.; Terzi, A.; Muneretto, C.; et al. Possible role of F18-FDG-PET/CT in the diagnosis of endocarditis: Preliminary evidence from a review of the literature. *Int. J. Cardiovasc. Imaging* **2012**, *28*, 1417–1425. [CrossRef]

14

Diabetic Foot Infections: The Diagnostic Challenges

Chiara Lauri [1,2,*], Antonio Leone [3], Marco Cavallini [4], Alberto Signore [1,2], Laura Giurato [5] and Luigi Uccioli [5]

1 Nuclear Medicine Unit, Department of Medical-Surgical Sciences and of Translational Medicine, "Sapienza" University of Rome, 00161 Rome, Italy; alberto.signore@uniroma1.it
2 Department of Nuclear Medicine and Molecular Imaging, University of Groningen, University Medical Center Groningen, 9700 Groningen, The Netherlands
3 Department of Radiological and Haematological Sciences, Fondazione Policlinico Universitario A. Gemelli, ISCSS—Università Cattolica del Sacro Cuore, 00168 Rome, Italy; antonio.leonemd@gmail.com
4 Wound Care Department of Medical-Surgical Sciences and of Translational Medicine, "Sapienza" University of Rome, 00161 Rome, Italy; marco.cavallini@uniroma1.it
5 Diabetic Foot Unit, Department of Systems Medicine, University of Rome Tor Vergata, 00133 Rome, Italy; lauragiurato@yahoo.it (L.G.); luccioli@yahoo.com (L.U.)
* Correspondence: chialau84@hotmail.it

Abstract: Diabetic foot infections (DFIs) are severe complications of long-standing diabetes, and they represent a diagnostic challenge, since the differentiation between osteomyelitis (OM), soft tissue infection (STI), and Charcot's osteoarthropathy is very difficult to achieve. Nevertheless, such differential diagnosis is mandatory in order to plan the most appropriate treatment for the patient. The isolation of the pathogen from bone or soft tissues is still the gold standard for diagnosis; however, it would be desirable to have a non-invasive test that is able to detect, localize, and evaluate the extent of the infection with high accuracy. A multidisciplinary approach is the key for the correct management of diabetic patients dealing with infective complications, but at the moment, no definite diagnostic flow charts still exist. This review aims at providing an overview on multimodality imaging for the diagnosis of DFI and to address evidence-based answers to the clinicians when they appeal to radiologists or nuclear medicine (NM) physicians for studying their patients.

Keywords: infection; diabetic foot; imaging; WBC scintigraphy; [^{18}F]FDG PET/CT; MRI

---

1. Introduction

Diabetic foot infection (DFI) is a common complication of longstanding diabetes, and it is associated with considerable morbidity, the increased risk of lower extremity amputation, and a high mortality rate [1]. The development of DFI derives from a complex interplay among peripheral neuropathy, peripheral arterial disease (PAD), and the immune system.

Neuropathy is the most prominent risk factor for diabetic foot ulcerations (DFU). Motor neurons damage results in foot deformities that contribute to the injury of foot tissues and bones. Sensory neurons damage leads to a loss of protective sensation. Therefore, neuropathic patients could develop skin ulcers that might remain unrecognized for a long time, thus exposing the adjacent soft tissues to the colonization of pathogens and causing a soft tissue infection (STI). If not promptly identified and treated, the infection could spread to the underlying bone and cause osteomyelitis (OM).

PAD further facilitates micro-organisms invasion and rapid progression to infection, since insufficient tissues oxygenation might impair the healing of ulcers, creating an optimal substratum for the colonization of pathogen. In addition to this, PAD reduces granulocytes migration and antibiotic penetration into infected site, thus contributing to the spread of infection and complicating its therapeutic management. Moreover, patients with severe PAD are prone to sudden ischemia resulting from arterial thrombosis with consequent critical limb ischemia and an increased risk of amputation [2,3]. Indeed, both ischemia and infection are the most important factors in determining the prognosis of foot ulcerations, since patients with PAD and infection show more severe comorbidities and worst clinical outcomes compared with the classic "neuropathic foot patients" [4]. Uncontrolled hyperglycaemia represents another pivotal aspect in the pathogenesis of DFI being responsible of an impairment of both cell-mediated and humoral immune response mainly characterized by altered leukocyte's functions, reduced chemotaxis, and phagocytosis proprieties [5,6].

A prompt identification of foot ulcers, STI, and OM and an accurate evaluation of the extent of the infective process is crucial for prognostication of the patients and for planning the most appropriate treatment that usually requires a combination of metabolic control, medical treatment with specific antibiotic regimen, and surgical approach. The International Working Group (IWGDF) and the Infectious Diseases Society (IDSA) proposed a single scheme to assess the presence and the severity of infection [7,8], and this classification is currently applied for predicting the need for hospitalization, the likelihood of undergoing lower extremity amputation, and other adverse outcomes [9]. However, in the latest update of these guidelines, OM and STI have been addressed separately, since they are two distintict conditions, although they may coexist in the same patient, with different diagnostic, therapeutic, and prognostic implications [10].

Clinical suspicion through a comprehensive history and physical exam are the starting points for the diagnosis of DFI, which is validated by a complete laboratory evaluation, microbiologic assessment, and imaging.

Clinical diagnosis of superficial STI is based on the presence of at least two local signs of inflammation: rubor, calor, dolor, tumour, or purulent secretion. Other secondary features suggestive of infection may be present, such as friable or discolored granulation tissue, necrosis, and failure of the wound to heal [11]. Clinical manifestations of acute deep infection include abscess, necrotizing fasciitis, and gangrene. In those cases, the infection process may involve one or more foot compartments and may require a first urgent surgical treatment and eventually distal revascularization to reduce the amputation level [12].

The development of an OM is one of the most serious and disabling complications of diabetes, being associated with prolonged antibiotic therapy and hospitalization, as well as higher re-infection rates and risk of amputations compared with patients with STI, resulting in high social costs [13].

Diagnosing OM is sometimes a challenge for the clinicians, since it may occur in the absence of local or systemic signs of infection and inflammation, especially in chronic infections. Several wound characteristics, in particular the width and depth of the lesion, may be helpful in predicting the presence of bone infection. A lesion's surface greater than 2 cm^2 has a sensitivity of 56% and a specificity of 92% for the diagnosis of OM. Similarly a deep ulcer over 3 mm is significantly associated with an underlying OM in comparison with a more superficial one (82% versus 33%) [14].

Another diagnostic criterion is represented by the possibility to reach the bone with a blunt at the base of the lesion, the "probe-to-bone test". Combining the results of the probe-to-bone test with those of plain radiography improves the overall diagnostic accuracy of OM [15,16].

However, the gold standard for the definitive diagnosis of OM still remains the bone biopsy that provides histological and microbiological information and, at the same time, it is useful to determine the susceptibility to various antibiotics [7]. Although bone biopsy is the more accurate technique in identifying the pathogenic germs, it is an invasive procedure, and it is not always feasible. However, a culture of deep soft tissue that is in direct contact with the bone shows a good correlation with bone biopsy in identifying the responsible pathogen and, therefore, this approach may be useful in alternative to bone biopsy [17].

Imaging offers the possibility to diagnose DFI by using a less invasive approach that is complementary to physical examination, laboratory, and microbiological evaluations. A wide panel of modalities may be very helpful for the clinicians to better understand whether the patient has a STI, OM, or sterile inflammation that is a hallmark of Charcot osteoarthropathy, for example (Table 1). To achieve an accurate differential diagnosis is mandatory in the optic of promptly starting an appropriate treatment reducing the need for hospitalization and the risk of major amputations, but univocal consensus on diagnostic criteria for imaging modalities still does not exist.

This review aims at providing an overview of radiologic and nuclear medicine (NM) modalities able to achieve an accurate differential diagnosis between the different kinds of DFI and to guide therapeutic strategies.

Table 1. Common interpretation criteria of different imaging modalities in diabetic foot infections.

	OM	STI	Charcot	Pitfalls
Radiography	Anatomical overview of the area of interest and any preexisting conditions that might influence the interpretation of subsequent procedures	Soft-tissue gas, and calcifications	Bony fragmentation, debris formation, subluxation/dislocation, bony fragments fusion, sclerosis of bone ends, fractures, osteophytosis, and deformity	Very poor sensitivity in the early stages of the diseases. BM edema cannot be detected
CT	Cortical erosions, periosteal reaction, small sequestra	Soft-tissue gas, and calcifications	No potential in acute condition. In chronic condition, CT may be acquired for a preoperative bone assessment	Very limited role in the imaging of DFI. BM oedema can not be detected
MRI	Diffuse BM involvement: decreased marrow signal intensity on T1-w images, increased marrow signal intensity on fluid-sensitive, fat-suppressed sequences, and post-contrast enhancement. Ghost sign	Identification of subtending skin ulcer, sinus tract, abscess, tenosynovitis	BM involvement is limited to periarticular locations	Poor discrimination between infection and sterile inflammation in Charcot
Radiolabelled WBC	Planar images: focal activity at 20–24 h that is often increased compared with the uptake at 3–4 h; SPECT/CT: uptake clearly associated with bone at CT	Planar images: focal/diffuse activity at 20–24 h that is often stable or decreased compared with the uptake at 3–4 h; SPECT/CT: uptake clearly associated with soft tissues at CT	Planar images: diffuse activity at 20–24 h that is stable or decreased compared with the uptake at 3–4 h; positive match with BMS; SPECT/CT: uptake clearly associated with bone destruction	Possible FN during antibiotic treatment or severe vascular disease
[^{18}F]FDG PET/CT	Focal or diffuse uptake clearly associated with bone at CT	Focal or diffuse uptake clearly associated with soft tissues at CT without bone involvement	Diffuse uptake involving tarsal/metatarsal joints and bone destruction at CT	Poor discrimination between infection and sterile inflammation. FP in Charcot and. after foot surgery

BMS: bone marrow scintigraphy; CT: computer tomography; OM: osteomyelitis; STI: soft tissue infection; DFI: diabetic foot infection; WBC: white blood cells; BM: bone marrow; BMS: bone marrow scan; SPECT: single photon emission computed tomography; T1-w: T1-weighted; FN: false negative; FP: false positive.

2. Surgical Management of DFI: How Can Imaging Be Useful?

Surgical management for diabetic foot (DF) deformities and complications is a critical aspect in dealing with these patients. Understanding of the DF 'syndrome' has improved the approach to diabetic patients affected by a complicated foot. In the last decades, we observed an increasing interest in developing less invasive surgical procedures as alternatives to major lower extremity amputation. They are focused on local resections and the drainage of infected underlying soft tissue, toes, and metatarsal heads for neuropathic or neuroischemic complicated DF [18,19]. In this optic, imaging plays a crucial role in diagnosing the infection and defining its extent, aiming at selecting those cases candidate to more conservative approaches.

Structural deformities and high plantar pressures are a predisposing risk factor to diabetic foot ulceration (DFU) [20–23]. Common deformities include hammertoes, prominent metatarsal heads, hallux limitus, Charcot foot, and previous toe or partial foot amputations [24]. Each leads to high pressures that contribute, in the case of an insensitive DF, to tissue inflammation and ulceration. Ameliorating these high pressures by structurally realigning or removing bony prominences is the rationale for foot surgery. In the presence of infection, phlegmon, and/or OM, surgery becomes a critical urgent component of care [25]. A proposed scheme for classifying the types of foot surgery in diabetic patients refers to the presence of open wounds and their acuity [26]:

- Prophylactic procedures are those performed in neuropathic patients to reduce the risk of ulceration or recurrent ulceration in the absence of open wounds;
- Curative surgery when cutaneous ulcers are present is often performed to provide a cure by joint resection, removing underlying bony prominences (surgical decompression), osteomyelitis, or by draining underlying abscesses or phlegmons;
- Urgent procedures are performed for severe deep or ascending infections (infectious gangrene, necrotizing fasciitis, etc.) to control the progression of infection. These procedures are performed emergently and usually consist in wide open drainages or minor amputations at the foot level.

In daily clinical practice, curative and urgent procedures are most frequent, since usually patients arrive to a surgical referral with an active more or less complicated DFU.

When dealing with deep infected cutaneous ulcers, the primary principle in treating surgical infection is source control. Most infected DFUs respond well to local debridement, the administration of culture-specific antibiotics, and offloading of the foot with specific footwear. Some develop a rapid spread of infection along the tissue planes and tendon sheaths and present with local tissue necrosis, spreading cellulitis and systemic inflammatory response [27].

According to the T.I.M.E. (Tissue, Infection, Moisture and Edges) procedure, source control includes the resection and/or debridement of any dead/infected tissue/bone and avoid fluid stasis by draining any hidden infected site [28]. However, Time stands also for "do not waste Time" in referral the patient to specialists who can better deal with the patient's need and also stands for "Timing", indicating untimely or adequate choice of procedure (for example, limb revascularization) to treat the patient at its presentation. Since deep foot infection can potentially be limb threatening without timely intervention, delay will lead to further tissue loss. In this case, we can state that "Time is Tissue".

The endpoints of curative approach to deep foot ulcer and osteomyelitis are:

- Treat and cure the infection;
- Reduce pain (not always present because of neuropathy);
- Retain foot and allow best function (rehabilitation);
- Reduce recurrency.

Radical surgical resection, including healthy bone and soft tissue, is sometimes required and must follow an "oncologic approach" in the case of deep foot infections and OM [29,30], since they are difficult to treat and they could relapse.

Our understanding of the pathophysiology has been greatly improved by the biofilm model, which explains the wide variety of symptoms, courses, and the complex therapeutic management. The pathogens first form the surface layer of colonies, which then multiply into a three-dimensional structure. This biofilm structure offers the bacteria protection from mechanical influences and makes it harder for antibiotics, the body's own defensive cells, and antibodies to penetrate, functioning as a diffusion barrier. The pathogens pass from a planktonic, free-floating phase with a high metabolic rate and rapid multiplication into a sessile form with greatly reduced metabolism and slowed biological reactions. This phenotypic change makes them more resistant to antibiotics compared to planktonic counterparts, since cellular growth within biofilms produces a matrix that protects the pathogens from the immune system and antimicrobial drugs. In OM and prosthesis-related infections, it has been calculated that this particular type of growth can reduce their sensitivity to antibiotics by a factor of 10^3 [31]. The time required for a mature biofilm formation is about 24–48 h [32]. Mechanical forces of surgical debridement are effective in disrupting that matrix, exposing bacteria to the effects of antibiotics and body's immune response. Therefore, with a surgical medication, we can realize a therapeutic window of 1–2 days where a sharp debridement should be repeated in order to remove all instable tissues and biofilm covering the wound bed.

All foreign bodies including screws and stitches must be removed, since they might be biofilm carriers. Any infected tendons and bone should be cleaned and irrigated in order to remove necrotic and/or infected tissues. The remaining tissues must be viable and well-perfused. There are no objective criteria for defining bone resection limits; therefore, it remains an individual decision of the surgeon, but generally, it should be up to when a hard bone is touched with the surgical instrument [33]. In some cases, non-infected bones must be removed or reduced in order to relieve the pressure to the underlying ulcerated cutaneous plane. The size of the defect produced by the procedure is not a primary consideration; only the vascular supply should be evaluated and preserved. What happens next depends on how radical the débridement and resection has been. Thereafter, the most important aspect is the management of dead space, which, if not treated properly, may lead to the early recurrence of infection and inadequate rehabilitation, especially if it involves the foot plantar surface. Surgical drainage is mandatory for the prevention of any fluid or exudate stasis that might be responsible for persistent bacterial contamination, biofilm, or infection and wound-healing impairment and delay [34] (Figure 1).

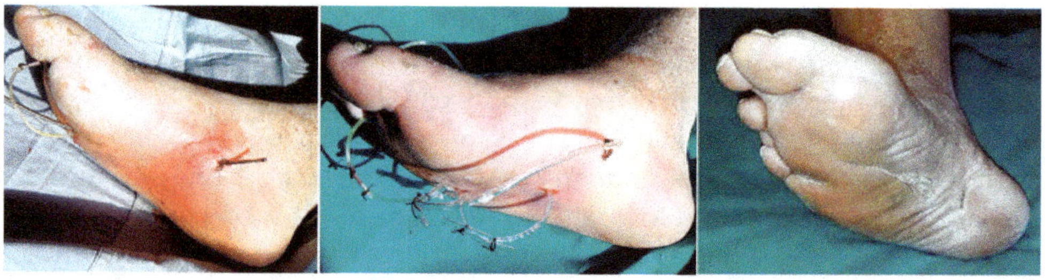

Figure 1. Extended plantar phlegmon. Left: With a probe, it is possible to follow the real spaces produced by the phlegmon spread along tissue plans. Where the end of the tract becomes superficial toward the skin, interposed tissues and the skin are pierced and incised in order to pass through the probe. Middle: A silastic tube is, thereafter, anchored to the probe in order to pass it backward along the fistula tract. Once this drainage is passed, the two ends are tied together with two silk stitches in order to construct the ulcer piercing ring (UP ring). Right: A diabetic foot ulceration (DFU) completely healed after 8 months in an out patient facility with daily medications and irrigations and with occasional antibiotic therapy and resulting with a small plantar scar. (Courtesy of Marco Cavallini).

Concluding, the surgical management of DF complications is challenging and it requires an appropriate diagnosis in order to correctly identify the problem and to promptly start an adequate and a personalized treatment for the single patient. An interdisciplinary approach derived from close collaboration between clinicians, surgeons, radiologists, NM physicians, microbiologists, podiatrists, and nurses is mandatory.

3. Radiological Modalities for Imaging DFI

Although the reference standard for the diagnosis of diabetes-related OM still remains bone biopsy, the diagnosis is largely based on the presence of clinical and laboratory findings such as an erythrocyte sedimentation rate (ESR) >70 mm/h, and a positive result of a probe-to-bone test (palpation of bone in the depths of infected pedal ulcers) [10,11]. However, it should be kept in mind that (1) an ESR of more than 70 mm/h is highly specific for OM, but has a sensitivity of only 28% [35], and (2) the reliability of the probe-to-bone test may vary with the performing clinician's experience and ulcer location [10,11,35]. In addition, the benefit of this test is substantially influenced by the pre-test probability of the patient having an OM or not. A positive probe-to-bone test suggests the diagnosis in a high-risk patient. A negative test indicates a low probability of OM in a low-risk patient [36,37]. Hence, the diagnosis of DFI may be difficult when based on clinical and laboratory findings alone. Advanced imaging of the foot has improved our ability to evaluate the possibility of OM, and it may be helpful for the diagnosis and definition of deep or soft-tissue purulent collections.

Radiography and magnetic resonance imaging (MRI) are the most commonly used radiological modalities to evaluate the DF infective complications. Ultrasounds can be employed for guiding the aspiration of suspect fluid collections or removing foreign bodies; however, it is not currently recommended by the IWGDF [10] and the diabetic foot guidelines of the American College of Radiology [38]. Computed tomography (CT), despite its higher sensitivity compared with radiography and MRI in detecting cortical erosions, periosteal reaction, small sequestra, soft tissue gas, and calcifications within sites of chronic osteomyelitis, plays a limited role in the imaging of diabetic patients with suspected OM or STI of the foot [38]. The main disadvantages of CT are the low soft tissue contrast resolution and the inability to detect the bone marrow edema seen in the early stages of infection. If MRI is contraindicated or unavailable, post-contrast CT may be used to detect soft-tissue and osseous abscess formation. However, the risk of use of iodinated contrast in diabetic patients should be taken into account, as diabetic nephropathy progressing to end-stage renal disease is commonly a comorbidity in patients with diabetes [39].

3.1. *Radiography*

The sensitivity of radiography is rather low in this setting, since radiographic findings of DF infective complications can be undetected for up to four weeks after the onset of infection, and these changes can be caused by Charcot osteoarthropathy and other disorders such as gout [40,41]. However, radiography should be the first-line imaging modality in any patient with suspected infection. It is cheap, widely available, and when radiographic findings such as demineralization, bone resorption, cortical destruction, periosteal reaction, bowing, or the obliteration of fat stripes and fascial planes, arthropathic changes, and the presence of soft tissue gas and foreign bodies are interpreted by an experienced radiologist, they are highly suggestive of DF infective complications [10].

3.2. *Magnetic Resonance Imaging*

After initial radiography, MRI with fluid-sensitive, fat-suppressed sequences (i.e., short-tau inversion recovery [STIR] or fat-saturated T2-weighted images) is the modality of choice for investigating OM and associated soft-tissue complications [42,43] with high sensitivity and high specificity (90% and 83%, respectively) in the diagnosis of OM [38,44]. Post-contrast images improve the evaluation of soft tissue pathology, as they help in detecting abscesses and sinus tracts more easily [43]. Moreover, its radiation-free assessment becomes particularly important in the young population and when repeated follow-up imaging is likely to be necessary. However, standard MRI is typically based only on morphologic sequences, which provide only structural information. In the last years, technical improvements have allowed the capability to add functional quantitative information to structural information. The application of Dixon sequences improves image quality and increases the detection of sinus tracts and intraosseus sequestrums [45]. Diffusion-weighted imaging and the apparent diffusion coefficient value can help in the differentiation of diabetic neuropathic osteoarthropathy from OM with excellent inter-observer agreement [45].

Bone marrow (BM) with normal signal intensity excludes the diagnosis of OM in diabetic patients with STIs. Early OM is characterized by BM edema with low marrow signal intensity on T1-weighted images, high marrow signal intensity on fluid-sensitive fat-suppressed sequences, and post-contrast enhancement (Figure 2).

However, there are several mimickers of diabetes-related OM that may present problems to making a correct MRI diagnosis by showing BM edema and post-contrast enhancement. Furthermore, these conditions, including biomechanical stress changes related to altered weight bearing, recent post-operative surgery, inflammatory arthritis, and primarily neuropathic osteoarthropathy, may coexist with OM, further complicating the ability to make an accurate diagnosis. Consequently, if marrow edema is used as the primary diagnostic criterion, MRI may not be very specific.

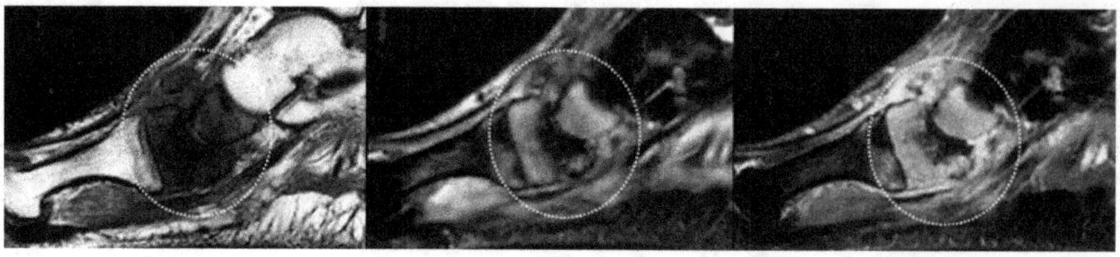

Figure 2. OM of the scaphoid and medial cuneiform. (From left to right) Sagittal T1-weighted, T2-fat-suppressed, and post-contrast T1-weighted fat-suppressed MRI clearly show that the marrow in the scaphoid and medial cuneiform has a low signal on a T1-weighted image (circle in left panel), increased signal on a fluid-sensitive fat-suppressed image (circle in middle panel), and post-gadolinium enhancement (circle in panel). These findings are indicative of OM.

Several secondary features such as subtending skin ulcer, sinus tract, abscess, tenosynovitis, or septic arthritis tend to be associated with OM. Their presence strongly suggests that osteomyelitis is present and can improve diagnostic accuracy [42,46].

- Skin ulcer: Skin ulceration is typified by focal interruption of the cutaneous line, with raised margins (secondary to preexisting callus formation). Acute ulcer appears hyperintense on fluid-sensitive fat-suppressed images, with marked peripheral post-contrast enhancement, which is a finding that is indicative of granulation tissue at the base of the ulcer. Chronic ulcer may be associated with fibrous healing and thus appears as a mass with low signal intensity on T1-weighted images and low to intermediate signal intensity on fluid-sensitive fat-suppressed images [42,43,46].
- Sinus tract and abscess: Sinus tracts and abscesses are some of the major findings in osteomyelitis. Morrison et al. determined the usefulness of primary and secondary MRI signs of OM and found that the identification of a sinus tract showed high specificity (average, 85%) for the diagnosis of osteomyelitis in the adjacent bone [47]. Sinus tracts typically extend from skin ulcers to tendon sheaths, bones, or joints, and they represent a route for the subsequent spread of infection leading to abscesses, septic tenosynovitis, and/or osteomyelitis [47]. Sinus tracts appear as linear fluid signal intensity on fluid-sensitive fat-suppressed images and display a characteristic "tram-track" pattern of the enhancement on contrast-enhanced images. The latter are the most sensitive MRI feature for detecting sinus tracts (Figure 3). Abscess is seen as a focal fluid collection that is hypointense on T1-weighted images and hyperintense on fluid-sensitive fat-suppressed images, with a thick rim post-contrast enhancement, due to the presence of granulation tissue (Figure 3). The presence of rim enhancement is essential in distinguishing abscesses from cellulitis or phlegmons, which present diffuse post-contrast enhancement [42,43,46].
- Septic tenosynovitis: Septic tenosynovitis generally results from the contiguous spread of infection from an adjacent ulcer, abscess, or sinus tract. On MRI, it is characterized by an abnormal increase in fluid within the tendon sheath, and post-contrast images may show a thick rim enhancement around the tendon, due to inflamed synovium. The tendon loses its constant low signal intensity and becomes thickened and indistinct [42,43,46].
- Septic arthritis: Similar to OM and tenosynovitis, septic arthritis occurs also as a result of contiguous spread from an adjacent ulcer, abscess, or sinus tract. No single MRI feature can differentiate septic from nonseptic arthritis; increased joint fluid and synovial thickening with contrast enhancement may also be seen in non-infectious inflammatory arthropathies. However, in pedal infections, the diagnosis of septic arthritis may be more specific if an ulcer and adjacent soft-tissue infection directly abut the joint, or, a sinus tract extends into the joint. Septic arthritis may demonstrate edema with post-contrast enhancement in adjacent soft tissue and on both sides of the joint. Reactive BM oedema, secondary to septic arthritis, should be differentiated from a superimposed OM. A low signal intensity on T1-weighted images, and proximal extension of subchondral edema beyond the subchondral bone usually indicate OM [42,48].

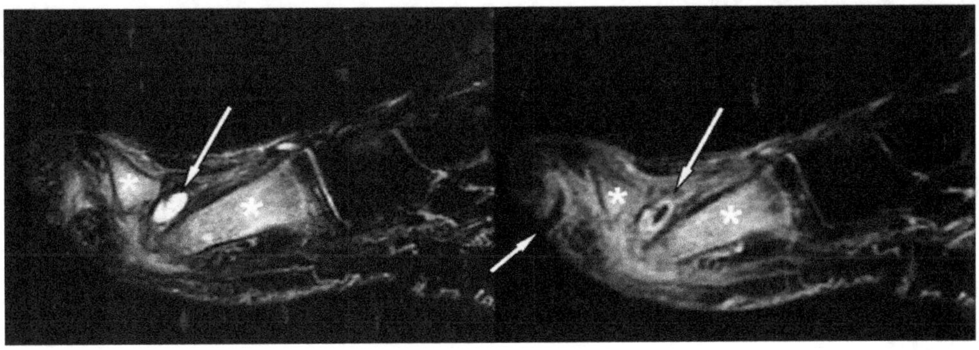

Figure 3. Forefoot ulcer, sinus track, and abscess associated with OM in a 57-year-old diabetic man with a 16-year history of insulin-dependent diabetes. Sagittal T2 fat-suppressed (left panel), and post-contrast T1-weighted fat-suppressed MRI (right panel) shows a dorsal thick rim-enhancing abscess adjacent to the first metatarsal head (arrows). Note a plantar ulcer appearing as a focal skin interruption and a sinus tract with rim-like enhancement (small arrow in right panel) extending near the first proximal interphalangeal joint. Given these findings, the hyperintensity (** in left panel), and post-contrast enhancement (** in right panel) in the first metatarsal, and proximal phalanx respectively, are indicative of OM.

Distinguishing OM from neuropathic osteoarthropathy, in the absence of secondary signs of infection, is a common and difficult clinical and radiological problem. An accurate differentiation is mandatory, because the early detection of OM is essential to initiate prompt medical and/or surgical treatment. The location and distribution of anatomical changes may be helpful. Indeed, neuropathic osteoarthropathy usually involves the tarsometatarsal and metatarsophalangeal joints, while OM mostly involves the calcaneum, malleoli, and forefoot [49]. The biggest diagnostic problem arises in the midfoot. In this region, MRI findings may be inconclusive, and secondary signs of infection are invaluable in determining the presence of OM. Furthermore, neuropathic osteoarthropathy is primarily an articular disease; thus, BM oedema is limited to juxta-articular locations, whereas OM, which almost invariably results from an ulcer or abscess in contiguous soft tissue, shows diffuse marrow changes (Figure 3) [38,50].

The differentiation of infected from non-infected neuropathic osteoarthropathy remains extremely challenging, as the clinical and radiological findings may overlap. However, several MRI findings may be useful for distinguishing between these two conditions. Sinus tract formation, the replacement of soft tissue fat, fluid collections and diffuse marrow abnormality, diffuse joint fluid enhancement, and joint erosion support superimposed infection [43,51]. Thin rim enhancement of effusion, the presence of subchondral cysts, or intraarticular bodies indicate the absence of infection [19]. Bones that "disappear" on T1-weighted images and then "reappear" on contrast-enhanced or T2-weighted images (the "ghost sign") is another MRI feature that indicates the presence of a superimposed infection. In uncomplicated neuropathic osteoarthropathy, the "ghost sign" is absent because there is bone destruction, but there is no infiltration of the marrow by inflammatory cells resulting in absence of the "ghost sign" [42,43,46].

4. Nuclear Medicine Imaging for DFI

NM techniques offer the possibility to image a process from a functional point of view, and they allow the identification of pathophysiological changes even before they become clinically detectable. Several radiopharmaceuticals are available for imaging infection and inflammation for both single photon emission computed tomography (SPECT) and positron emission tomography (PET) modalities, and most of them are currently applied for the diagnosis and follow-up of DFI.

4.1. Gamma-Camera Imaging for DFI

Radiolabelled white blood cells (WBC) scintigraphy using both ^{111}In or ^{99m}Tc represent the NM cornerstone for the diagnosis of infection, since it specifically targets activated granulocytes, thus representing a surrogate marker of bacterial infections [52]. Several guidelines have been published by the European Society of Nuclear Medicine (EANM) with the aim to standardize labeling procedures, acquisition protocols, and interpretation criteria in all the centers [53–55]. In particular, to provide an in vivo imaging of the physiologic dynamic process of migration of granulocytes into the infective site, it is recommended to acquire images with times corrected for isotope decay at three time points after the reinjection of autologous cells. Once correctly acquired and displayed, the correct interpretation derives from the comparison of uptake extent and intensity between late images, acquired 20 h (h) post injection (p.i.) and delayed images (3 h p.i.). By following these recommendations, we can easily differentiate between a bone infection from a sterile inflammation. Indeed, in the first situation, the uptake increases over time in terms of extent and/or intensity, whereas in inflammation, the uptake decreases or remains stable over time [55–57]. By using these recommendations, and when combined with SPECT/CT acquisitions for the evaluation of the extent of the process and for the precise localization of the uptake, this modality reaches a very high accuracy in diagnosing an infection [58] (Figure 4). In a recently published meta-analysis and systematic review comparing the diagnostic performance of WBC scan, Fluorine-18 Fluorodeoxyglucose positron emission tomography ([^{18}F]FDG PET/CT) and MRI for the detection of DF osteomyelitis (DFO), the pooled sensitivity and specificity of radiolabelled WBC were respectively 91% and 92% for ^{99m}Tc hexamethylpropylene amine oxine (HMPAO) and 92% and 75% for ^{111}In-oxine. In particular, ^{99m}Tc-HMPAO WBC scintigraphy, followed by [^{18}F]FDG PET/CT, showed higher specificity than other imaging modalities in the diagnosis of DFO, whereas the sensitivities were similar (approximately 90% for all) [59].

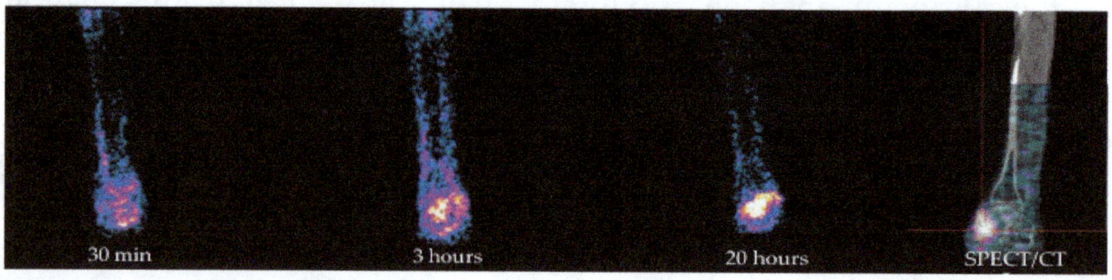

Figure 4. Example of ^{99m}Tc-HMPAO WBC scintigraphy in a patient with a skin ulcer in the medial right malleolus region, previous amputations of left leg, and of all metatarsal heads of the right foot. From left to right: Planar images acquired after 30 min, 3 h, and 20 h p.i. of radiolabelled autologous leukocytes show an increased amount of activity over time in terms of intensity and extent, being consistent with OM with an involvement of adjacent soft tissues. Further SPECT/CT acquisition (right panel) correctly localized the uptake in the right talus and accurately evaluated its extent into surrounding soft tissues. HMPAO: hexamethylpropylene amine oxine, WBC: white blood cell.

However, data regarding the use of radiolabelled WBC scintigraphy in DF are very discordant in the literature [60]. The sensitivity and specificity of this modality range from 75% [61] to 100% [62–64] and from 67% [64] to 100% [65] respectively, depending on deviation from the suggested labeling procedure, interpretation criteria adopted and, of course, different acquisitions protocols. In particular, several papers adopted only one-time point images, while others adopted outdated protocols of acquisition using fixed times or a fixed count, thus reflecting a wide heterogeneity of approach and results [64,66–69]. Hybrid imaging with SPECT/CT has also a great role in determining the accuracy of radiolabelled WBC scintigraphy, especially in discriminating superficial STIs from deeper infections. This differentiation is not easy achievable by using only planar images, but it is crucial for the correct management of the patient. Indeed, the primary goal for a correct therapeutic intervention derives from an accurate diagnosis of foot complications and, in particular, from the differentiation between sterile inflammation, STI, OM, and Charcot foot with or without a superimposed infection.

In this optic, radiolabelled WBC scintigraphy is the most accurate NM imaging modality able to achieve this differential diagnosis, since it provides an in vivo demonstration of the pathophysiology that underlies inflammatory and infective processes. However, the accuracy of radiolabelled WBC in differentiating OM from STI also depends on the district of the foot [60]. Despite previous considerations may be applied for a correct discrimination between these two conditions in forefoot disorders, in mid- and hindfoot, the presence of Charcot osteoarthropaty may also be considered. In this situation, radiolabelled WBC uptake could also be related to physiological BM expansion secondary to chronic inflammation, thus resulting in a lower specificity of this modality [70–72]. Therefore, in order to overcome this limitation and to improve the accuracy of WBC scintigraphy, it is suggested to perform an additional bone marrow scintigraphy (BMS) using nanocolloids. Indeed, both radiopharmaceuticals accumulate in BM but only WBC accumulate in infective foci, so if the images of these two modalities are congruent (match), the diagnosis of Charcot is the most probable; conversely, in case of mismatch (positive at WBC scintigraphy and negative at colloids), the diagnosis of OM may be done.

Despite radiolabelled WBC scintigraphy still representing the NM gold standard for the diagnosis of infections, some practical and technical issues, unfortunately, limit its use in all the centers. Indeed, this modality requires qualified personnel, adequate laboratories, and equipment. Moreover, it is a time-consuming procedure for both labeling and images acquisition, since acquisition at three time points is necessary. However, its accuracy has no peers in this field, and the availability of closed and single use kits has simplified the separation and labeling procedures, making all the steps safer for the operator [73].

The use of monoclonal antibodies (MoAbs) or antibodies fragments (Fab′) direct against specific antigens expressed by activated granulocytes has been proposed as an alternative to radiolabelled WBC scintigraphy, but they also have several cons mainly related to the high molecular weight of the entire antibodies that constitutes a limiting factor for their diffusion into the infective focus, their long plasma half-life, and their non-specific accumulation into inflamed sites. Furthermore, MoAbs induce human murine antibodies (HAMA) in the host, thus limiting their use at only one time in the life. Moreover, the role of MoAbs or Fab′ fragments has not been extensively investigated in DF, and data in the literature are mainly based on small groups of patients [74–76]. Moreover, at the moment, there are no standardized protocols for the acquisition and interpretation, and the few data in literature are not sufficient to conclude that MoAbs or their fragments have to be preferred to radiolabelled WBC scintigraphy in the assessment of DF disorders.

4.2. PET/CT Imaging for DFI

In the last decades, [^{18}F]FDG PET/CT has gained an important role also for several indications in the field of infection and inflammation as specifically summarized in the guidelines published in 2013 by EANM and Society of Nuclear Medicine and molecular Imaging (SNMMI) [77].

[^{18}F]FDG offers several advantages over conventional scintigraphy. First of all, it avoids the manipulation of potentially infected blood; secondly, the acquisition time is considerably shorter than radiolabelled WBC, and thirdly, the images' quality resolution is better than those obtained with planar scintigraphy. Moreover, in the presence of CT co-registration, it is possible to have a precise definition of the anatomical landmarks, therefore evaluating the extent of the infective process into soft tissues or bone. However, [^{18}F]FDG accumulates in infections, inflammations, malignancies, reparative processes, and in all the other conditions in which the glucose is metabolized as a source of energy.

In a meta-analysis published in 2013, the per-patients-based analysis showed a pooled sensitivity of 74% and a specificity of 91% [78]. Nevertheless, this meta-analysis was conducted only on 4 studies. Another more recent meta-analysis including 6 studies on 254 patients, in which the sensitivity and specificity of [^{18}F]FDG PET/CT were 89% and 92%, respectively [59]. CT co-registration, of course, has a great influence on the accuracy of this imaging modality, but it also relies on correct interpretation criteria for a [^{18}F]FDG PET/CT scan that, unfortunately, are not still well defined and standardized.

In a large cohort of 110 diabetic patients with suspected pedal OM, Nawaz et al. compared [^{18}F]FDG PET and MRI. In this series, the first modality was less sensitive (81% versus 91%) but more specific (93% versus 78%) and accurate (90% versus 81%) than the second [79]. In this study, the diagnosis of OM was based on visual assessment of [^{18}F]FDG uptake on bony structures without any semi-quantitative analysis of maximum Standardized Uptake Value (SUVmax). Furthermore, no CT co-registration was performed in this study, which may be influencing the relative low sensitivity compared to MRI.

Basu et al. explored the role of semi-quantitative analysis with SUVmax on 63 patients with DF disorders [80]. Patients with OM showed higher SUVmax values than patients with Charcot and uncomplicated DF, thus concluding that SUVmax could be a good parameter for differentiating these conditions. Although these findings were confirmed by other groups, some others did not find any correlation between SUVmax values and the different DF complications [81].

So, concluding, at present, well-defined interpretation criteria for differentiating infection, inflammation, STI, OM, and Charcot do not exist yet for [^{18}F]FDG, thus representing a great limiting factor for this specific clinical indication. CT co-registration, although useful for localizing the uptake into bone rather than in soft tissue, does not solve the problem of discriminating an infection from inflammation/degeneration [82] (Figure 5).

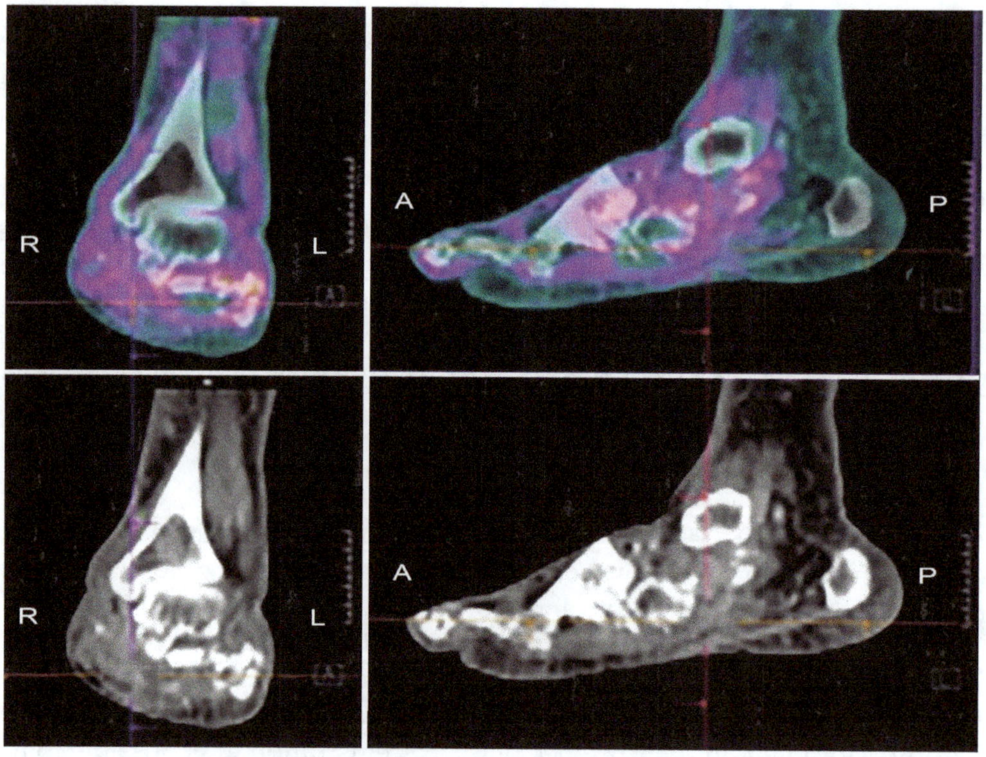

Figure 5. Example of [^{18}F]FDG PET/CT in a patient with Charcot osteoarthropathy. Fused images (upper panels) show moderate and diffuse uptake, which is interesting in particular bones and joints of the mid and hind-foot. Co-registered low-dose CT images (lower panels) show the evident destruction of bony architecture. These findings are consistent with the diagnosis of Charcot foot, but they do not allow discriminating a pan-inflammation from a possible superimposed infection.

Aiming to develop a more specific radiopharmaceutical for PET imaging, WBC have also been labeled with [^{18}F]FDG, but published studies on DF still do not exist in literature.

5. Consensus Statements Emerged from Round Table of 3rd European Congress of Infection and Inflammation

During the 3rd European Congress of Infection and Inflammation organized in Rome in December 2019, several specialists evaluating patients with DF complications gave their lectures on this topic from different points of view. Here, we summarize several statements that emerged from the following round table, aiming to provide evidence-based answers to the most frequent clinical questions.

5.1. Is Radiography Useful in a Patient with Suspected OM?

Radiography should be the first-line imaging modality when evaluating for bone involvement in the DF. This approach is cheap, widely available, and associated with minimal harm. It provides an anatomic overview of the area of interest and any preexisting conditions that could influence the selection and interpretation of subsequent imaging modalities. Although we are not aware of any studies of the role of serial radiographs to diagnose OM, useful information can be obtained by performing serial radiographs to detect progressive bony changes.

5.2. Is a Negative Radiographic Examination Enough to Rule Out OM?

From a radiological point of view, a negative radiographic examination is not enough to rule out OM, since it is not sensitive in the detection of early stages of acute OM [10]. Radiographs may remain unremarkable for up to four weeks after the onset of infection. Furthermore, when radiographic changes of OM such as demineralization, bone resorption, and periosteal reaction become detectable, they may be difficult to be correctly interpreted because similar abnormalities may occur with Charcot osteoarthropathy and other disorders such as gout [40]. Therefore, the appeal to advanced imaging is madatory in order to achieve an accurate diagnosis.

5.3. Is MRI Indicated Since the First Diagnostic Steps?

MRI is not appropriate as first line imaging modality to diagnose OM; however, it is strongly recommended as an additional modality after initial radiography, when OM is suspected. MRI provides excellent spatial resolution and precise anatomical details; it allows preoperative mapping of the extent of infection, thus being helpful in minimizing the area of resection. Moreover, its radiation-free assessment becomes particularly important in the young population and when repeated follow-up imaging is necessary, and it is now widely available and less expensive than other imaging modalities [38].

5.4. Is MRI Indicated for Therapy Evaluation?

There is no relevant literature to support the use of MRI in the follow-up of DFO. However, this imaging modality can be very appropriate for determining whether the patients healed from the infection after treatment. Given that normal marrow signal reliably excludes OM [42], this condition should not be considered "cured" until there has been no evidence of recurrence for at least a year [83]. The radiation-free assessment as well as the high sensitivity and specificity for determining the presence or absence of pedal OM and STI [44] makes MRI imaging very suitable as a follow-up imaging modality, especially in young people.

5.5. Is WBC Scintigraphy Able to Differentiate between Superficial or Deep Infection?

The main disadvantage of planar NM imaging techniques is the limited spatial resolution and the lack of anatomic landmarks, which is especially a problem in the foot, where all the bony structures are very small and close each other. Indeed, an uptake on the soft tissues at planar images may overlap the underlying bone and vice versa, leading to a wrong interpretation of the scan and consequently to a wrong treatment. Therefore, as previously mentioned, the appeal to hybrid images is mandatory in order to improve the diagnostic accuracy of planar images.

Several authors explored the added value of SPECT/CT in the diagnosis [66,67,84–86] and therapy monitoring of DFO [87,88] and, despite the different protocols of acquisition adopted among the different studies, all authors concordantly agree that hybrid imaging is able to better localize the uptake into bone or soft tissues with an excellent definition of the extent of the infective process. Przybylski et al. reported a sensitivity, specificity, and diagnostic accuracy of ^{99m}Tc WBC scintigraphy with SPECT/CT were 87.5%, 71.4%, and 80% respectively [85]. Heiba et al. examined 272 patients by using a combined approach with ^{111}In WBC scintigraphy and bone scan [66], concluding that dual isotope SPECT/CT was superior than bone scan or WBC scintigraphy with SPECT/CT alone in discriminating STI from OM and, in another paper, they concluded that this combined approach is associated with a reduced length of hospitalization [67]. In the series studied in 2009 by Filippi et al., the interpretation of planar images substantially changed with the addition of SPECT/CT in 52.6% of cases, being able to rule out the infection in 6 cases, to diagnose OM in 1 case and to better define the extent of the process in 3 cases [86].

Therefore, concluding, data in the literature support the use of SPECT/CT in addition to planar images in the evaluation of DFI, in order to better localize the infection into bone or soft tissues and to accurately assess the extent of the process.

5.6. Can [^{18}F]FDG PET/CT Be Used as an Alternative to WBC?

The answer to this specific question is not easy, because it mainly depends on the local center's equipment and facilities. As previously mentioned, the labeling procedures of leukocytes requires classified environments and laboratories and with isolators or class A wood with laminar flow, depending on local regulations. Personnel must be specifically trained to perform this procedure and must attend certified courses, thus impacting the department's costs. Moreover, it is a time-consuming procedure that requires multiple times-point acquisition, and therefore, the patients need to come back to the hospital the day after in order to complete the examination. Aiming to overcome these limitations, several authors suggested the use of alternative approaches and [^{18}F]FDG PET/CT, of course, represents the most attractive one due to higher quality images, shorter length of execution, and the easier and quicker length of handling of radioactive compounds, which does not require the manipulation of potentially infected blood. However, the well-known low specificity of [^{18}F]FDG in differentiating an infection from a sterile inflammation and the lack of unanimous consensus on interpretation criteria make the diagnosis uncertain in most cases.

One paper published in 2011 by Familiari et al. [81] perfectly fits this question. In a small cohort of 13 patients with suspected OM, they compared [^{18}F]FDG PET/CT and planar images of ^{99m}Tc-HMPAO WBC scintigraphy, acquiring both modalities at three times point and using qualitative and semi-quantitative criteria of interpretation with SUVmax and Target/Background ratio (T/B) ratio at each time point. They identified a cutoff of more than 2.0 at late images as the best interpretation criterion for WBC scintigraphy: an increase of this cutoff between 3 and 20 h was suggestive for OM, while a stable or decreased uptake over time was suggestive for STI. Similarly, for [^{18}F]FDG PET/CT, the best criterion for defining an OM was a SUVmax greater than 2.0 at 1 and 2 h p.i. and increasing with time. Whereas, if the uptake remaines stable or decreased over time, the scan was suggestive for STI. By using these criteria, the sensitivity, specificity, and accuracy of radiolabelled WBC scintigraphy were higher compared with [^{18}F]FDG PET/CT. Therefore, they concluded that radiolabelled WBC scintigraphy should not be replaced by [^{18}F]FDG PET/CT.

In accordance with this view, we strongly recommend the use of radiolabelled WBC scintigraphy in suspected pedal OM, as it also emerged from a recently published retrospective multicenter study [89]. [^{18}F]FDG PET/CT could represent a valid alternative if it is not possible to perform this imaging modality due to the limitations of the single center, but the interpretation of a PET scan, at the moment, really relies on personal experience, and therefore, the scans must be evaluated with caution.

5.7. *Is SUVmax Evaluation Useful for the Correct Interpretation of by [^{18}F]FDG PET/CT Scan?*

PET provides better resolution images and allows easier quantification methods than SPECT imaging. With radiolabelled WBC imaging, it is only possible to calculate T/B ratios between delayed and late images and to assess whether there is an increase or decrease of this value. With SUVmax evaluation on PET imaging, it is possible to quantify the uptake of by [^{18}F]FDG at the infectious focus. Therefore, several authors tried to assess whether the use of this SUVmax could be beenficial in order to better differentiate between sterile inflammation, STI, OM, and Charcot.

For example, Basu et al. found higher SUVmax values in patients with OM compared with patients with Charcot and uncomplicated DF (2.9–6.2 versus 0.7–2.4 versus 0.2–0.7), concluding that SUVmax could be a useful parameter for differentiating these conditions [80]. Kagna at al. found a statistically significant difference in SUVmax between OM and STI (6.7 ± 3.7 versus 4.4 ± 2.4) [90]. However, these results were not confirmed by other studies [79,81], which may be because several techinical and practical factors may influence the variation of SUVmax calculations among different centers. Moreover, universally recognised cutoff values to differentiate among Charcot's neuropathy, OM, and STI have not been defined yet.

Therefore, as it also stands for oncologic diseases, there is currently insufficient evidence to recommend that SUVmax could be a reliable tool for discriminating among different foot complications.

5.8. *Is It Possible to Perform Radiolabelled WBC Scintigraphy during an Antibiotic Treatment?*

The issue that ongoing antibiotic treatment could influence the sensitivity of radiolabelled WBC scintigraphy is still a matter of debate, and the opinions are very contrasting. From some papers, it emerges that the diagnostic accuracy of radiolabelled WBC is not significantly affected by the administration of antibiotics [87,88,91,92]. In 2013, Glaudemans et al. retrospectively studied a large population of patients with prosthetic joint infection, and they did not find significant differences in terms of diagnostic performance between patients under antibiotic treatment and patients that were not receiving therapy. Although this study was not focused on DFI, it was in support of the idea that this imaging modality retains a high sensitivity and specificity in detecting residual disease, independently by the administration of antibiotics. [93]. Indeed, as also indicated in recently published EANM guidelines [55], "patients receiving antibiotic treatment should not be excluded a priori since reports regarding their effect on WBC scintigraphy give various results".

However, not all NM physicians place very much trust in performing this exam during antibiotic treatment, because possible false negative scans may be observed. Therefore, despite a perfect timing to perform WBCs scintigraphy following antimicrobial therapy not being clearly indicated in the literature, it is often a common practice to delay the radiolabelled WBC scintigraphy until 2 weeks after therapy withdrawal or to repeat the scan, in case of doubts in patients receiving antibiotics 2 weeks later.

Data in the literature on therapy monitoring in DF are mainly based on small series and do not allow drawing definite conclusions, but preliminary results seem to encourage the use of radiolabelled WBC scintigraphy, especially with SPECT/CT acquisitions, for the assessment of treatment response [87,88]. Similarly, [^{18}F]FDG PET/CT could be used to follow signs of inflammation in the foot that may be still present, although the patient is considered clinically recovered [94], but definitive evidences are still lacking in the literature.

5.9. *Do We Need to Perform a Combined Bone Marrow Scintigraphy in Addition to Radiolabelled WBC Scintigraphy for the Evaluation of Charcot?*

Charcot osteoarthropathy is a condition that further complicates the challenging diagnosis of DFI. Radiolabelled WBC uptake in mid/hind-foot must be always interpreted with caution considering the possible physiologic accumulation into expanded BM that is typically present in a Charcot foot, independently by the presence of an infection or not. Therefore, a BMS is strongly suggested in order to have a scintigraphic map of BM and to compare with WBC images. Palestro described two criteria to diagnose OM in the presence of Charcot's arthropathy: (1) the presence of labeled leukocyte uptake without corresponding activity on marrow images and (2) the spatially incongruent distribution of two radiopharmaceuticals [70,71].

[^{18}F]FDG also shows several limitations in the evaluation of Charcot, because the uptake in this condition is usually very intense and diffuse involving all the tarsal and metatarsal joints, reflecting the evident changes in bony architecture typical of this conditions. Therefore [^{18}F], FDG is not able to discriminate whether Charcot is infected or not.

6. Conclusions

An accurate identification and differentiation among different types of DFI still represent a challenge for the clinician. The appeal to multimodality imaging and a multidisciplinary approach are mandatory in order to plan the most appropriate therapeutic strategy for the single patient. Several radiological and NM approaches are available, being MRI, radiolabelled WBC scintigraphy, and [^{18}F]FDG PET/CT the most appropriate, but larger multicenter studies are still needed in order to create standardized diagnostic flow charts that could be applied worldwide.

Author Contributions: Conceptualization, C.L.; methodology, C.L. and A.S.; resources, C.L., A.L., M.C., A.S., L.G., L.U.; writing—original draft preparation, C.L., A.L., M.C., A.S., L.G., L.U.; writing—review and editing, C.L.; supervision, A.S. All authors have read and agreed to the published version of the manuscript.

References

1. Raspovic, K.M.; Wukich, D.K. Self-reported quality of life and diabetic foot infections. *J. Foot. J. Med.* **2017**, *376*, 2367–2375. [CrossRef]
2. Singh, N.; Armstrong, D.G.; Lipsky, B.A. Preventing foot ulcers in patients with diabetes. *JAMA* **2005**, *293*, 217–228. [CrossRef] [PubMed]
3. Armostrong, D.G.; Lavery, L.A.; Harkless, L.B. Validation of a diabetic wound classification system. The contribution of depth, infection and ischemia to risk of amputation. *Diabetes Care* **1998**, *21*, 855–859. [CrossRef] [PubMed]
4. Prompers, L.; Huijbert, M.; Alpeqvist, J.; Jude, E.; Piaggesi, A.; Bakker, K.; Edmonds, M.; Holstein, P.; Jirkovska, A.; Mauricio, D.; et al. High prevalence of ischaemia, infection and serious comorbidity in patients with diabetic foot disease in Europe. Baseline results from the Eurodiale study. *Diabetologia* **2007**, *50*, 18–25. [CrossRef] [PubMed]
5. Delamaire, M.; Maugendre, D.; Moreno, M.; Le Goff, M.C.; Allannic, H.; Genetet, B. Impaired leucocyte functions in diabetic patients. *Diabet. Med.* **1997**, *14*, 29–34. [CrossRef]
6. Alexiewicz, J.M.; Kumar, D.; Smogorzewski, M.; Klin, M.; Massry, S.G. Polymorphonuclear leukocytes in non-insulin-dependent diabetes mellitus: Abnormalities in metabolism and function. *Ann. Intern. Med.* **1995**, *123*, 919–924. [CrossRef]
7. Lipsky, B.A.; Berendt, A.R.; Cornia, P.B.; Pile, J.C.; Peters, E.J.; Armstrong, D.G.; Deery, H.G.; Embil, J.M.; Joseph, W.S.; Karchmer, A.W.; et al. Infectious Diseases Society of America. 2012 Infectious Diseases Society of America Clinical Practice Guideline for the Diagnosis and Treatment of Diabetic Foot Infections. *Clin. Infect. Dis.* **2012**, *54*, e132–e173. [CrossRef]
8. Lipsky, B.A.; Aragon-Sanchez, J.; Diggle, M.; Embil, J.; Kono, S.; Lavery, L.; Senneville, E.; Urbancic Rovan, V.; van Asten, S.; on behalf of the International Working Group on the Diabetic Foot; et al. IWGDF guidance on the diagnosis and management of foot infections in persons with diabetes. *Diabetes Metab. Res. Rev.* **2016**, *32*, 45–74. [CrossRef] [PubMed]
9. Lavery, L.A.; Armstrong, D.G.; Murdoch, D.P.; Peters, E.J.; Lipsky, B.A. Validation of the Infectious Diseases Society of America's diabetic foot infection classification system. *Clin. Infect. Dis.* **2007**, *44*, 562–565. [CrossRef]

10. Lipsky, B.A.; Senneville, É.; Abbas, Z.G.; Aragón-Sánchez, J.; Diggle, M.; Embil, J.M.; Kono, S.; Lavery, L.A.; Malone, M.; van Asten, S.A.; et al. International Working Group on the Diabetic Foot (IWGDF). Guidelines on the diagnosis and treatment of foot infection in persons with diabetes (IWGDF 2019 update). *Diabetes Metab. Res. Rev.* **2020**, *36*, e3280. [CrossRef]
11. Lipsky, B.A.; Berendt, A.R.; Deery, H.G.; Embil, J.M.; Joseph, W.S.; Karchmer, A.W.; LeFrock, J.L.; Lew, D.P.; Mader, J.T.; Norden, C.; et al. Infectious Diseases Society of America. Diagnosis and treatment of diabetic foot infections. *Clin. Infect. Dis.* **2004**, *39*, 885–910. [CrossRef] [PubMed]
12. Faglia, E.; Clerici, G.; Caminiti, M.; Quarantiello, A.; Gino, M.; Morabito, A. The role of Early Surgical Debridement and Revascularization in Patients with Diabetes and Deep Foot Space Abscess: Retrospective review of 106 patients with Diabetes. *J. Foot Ankle Surg.* **2006**, *45*, 220–226. [CrossRef]
13. Lavery, L.A.; Ryan, E.C.; Ahn, J.; Crisologo, P.A.; Oz, O.K.; La Fontaine, J.; Wukich, D.K. The infected Diabetic Foot: Re-evaluating the infectious Diseases Society of America Diabetic Foot Infection Classification. *Clin. Infect. Dis.* **2020**, *70*, 1573–1579. [CrossRef]
14. Giurato, L.; Meloni, M.; Izzo, V.; Uccioli, L. Osteomyelitis in diabetic foot. A comprehensive overview. *World J. Diabetes* **2017**, *8*, 135–142. [CrossRef]
15. Aragón-Sánchez, J.; Lipsky, B.A.; Lázaro-Martínez, J.L. Diagnosing diabetic foot osteomyelitis: Is the combination of probe-to-bone test and plain radiography sufficient for high-risk inpatients? *Diabet. Med.* **2011**, *28*, 191–194. [CrossRef] [PubMed]
16. Alvaro-Afonso, F.J.; Lazaro-Martinez, J.L.; Aragón-Sánchez, J.; Garcia-Morales, E.; Garcia-Alvarez, Y.; Molines-Barroso, R.J. Inter-observer reproducibility of diagnosis of diabetic foot osteomyelitis based on a combination of probe-to-bone test and simple radiography. *Diabetes Res. Clin. Prac.* **2014**, *105*, e3–e5. [CrossRef] [PubMed]
17. Malone, M.; Bowling, F.L.; Gannass, A.; Jude, E.B.; Boulton, A.J.M. Deep wound cultures correlate well with bone biopsy culture in diabetic foot osteomyelitis. *Diabetes Metab. Res. Rev.* **2013**, *29*, 546–550. [CrossRef] [PubMed]
18. Singer, A. Surgical treatment of mal perforans. *Arch. Surg.* **1976**, *111*, 964–968. [CrossRef]
19. Kelly, P.J.; Coventry, M.B. Neurotrophic ulcers of the feet; review of forty-seven cases. *JAMA* **1958**, *168*, 388–393. [CrossRef]
20. Lavery, L.A. Effectiveness and safety of elective surgical procedures to improve wound healing and reduce re-ulceration in diabetic patients with foot ulcers. *Diabetes Metab. Res. Rev.* **2012**, *28*, 60–63. [CrossRef]
21. Ledoux, W.R.; Shofer, J.B.; Smith, D.G.; Sullivan, K.; Hayes, S.G.; Assal, M.; Reiber, G.E. Relationship between foot type, foot deformity, and ulcer occurrence in the high-risk diabetic foot. *J. Rehabil. Res. Dev.* **2005**, *42*, 665–672. [CrossRef] [PubMed]
22. Fernando, M.E.; Crowther, R.G.; Lazzarini, P.A.; Yogakanthi, S.; Sangla, K.S.; Buttner, P.; Jones, R.; Golledge, J. Plantar pressures are elevated in people with longstanding diabetes-related foot ulcers during follow-up. *PLoS ONE* **2017**, *12*, e018191. [CrossRef] [PubMed]
23. Armstrong, D.G.; Boulton, A.J.M.; Bus, S.A. Diabetic foot ulcers and their recurrence. *N. Engl. J. Med.* **2017**, *376*, 2367–2375. [CrossRef]
24. Frykberg, R.G.; Bevilacqua, N.J.; Habershaw, G. Surgical off-loading of the diabetic foot. *J. Vasc. Surg.* **2010**, *52*, 44S–58S. [CrossRef] [PubMed]
25. Frykberg, R.G.; Wittmayer, B.; Zgonis, T. Surgical management of diabetic foot infections and osteomyelitis. *Clin. Podiatr. Med. Surg.* **2007**, *24*, 469–482. [CrossRef]
26. Armstrong, D.G.; Frykberg, R.G. Classifying diabetic foot surgery: Toward a rational definition. *Diabet. Med.* **2003**, *20*, 329–331. [CrossRef]
27. Cavallini, M. *Gestione Delle Lesioni Cutanee (Wound Care & Cure)*; Cic Edizioni Internazionali: Rome, Italy, 2020; ISBN 978-88-9389-029-8.
28. Harries, R.L.; Bosanquet, D.C.; Harding, K.G. Wound bed preparation: TIME for an update. *Int. Wound J.* **2016**, *13*, 8–14. [CrossRef]
29. Forsberg, J.A.; Potter, B.K.; Cierny, G., III; Webb, L. Diagnosis and management of chronic infection. *J. Am. Acad. Orthop. Surg.* **2011**, *19*, S8–S19. [CrossRef]
30. Simpson, A.H.R.W.; Deakin, M.; Latham, J.M. Chronic osteomyelitis: The Effect of the Extent of Surgical Resection on Infection-Free Survival. *J. Bone Joint Surg. Br.* **2001**, *83*, 403–407. [CrossRef]

31. Costerton, J.W. Biofilm theory can guide the treatment of device-related orthopaedic infections. *Clin. Orthop. Relat. Res.* **2005**, *437*, 7–11. [CrossRef]
32. Percival, S.L.; McCarty, S.M.; Lipsky, B. Biofilms and wounds: An overview of the evidence. *Adv. Wound Care (New Rochelle)* **2015**, *4*, 373–381. [CrossRef]
33. Tiemann, A.H.; Hofmann, G.O. Principles of the therapy of bone infections in adult extremities: Are there any new developments? *Strateg. Trauma Limb Reconstr.* **2009**, *4*, 57–64. [CrossRef]
34. Cavallini, M. Ulcer piercing: Cleansing of complicated diabetic neuropathic foot ulcers by positive pressure irrigation. *J. Wound Care* **2014**, *23*, 60–65. [CrossRef] [PubMed]
35. Butalia, S.; Palda, V.A.; Sargeant, R.J.; Detsky, A.S.; Mourad, O. Does this patient with diabetes have osteomyelitis of the lower extremity? *JAMA* **2008**, *299*, 806–813. [CrossRef]
36. Lam, K.; van Asten, S.A.; Nguyen, T.; La Fontaine, J.; Lavery, L.A. Diagnostic Accuracy of Probe to Bone to Detect Osteomyelitis in the Diabetic Foot: A Systematic Review. *Clin. Infect. Dis.* **2016**, *63*, 944–948. [CrossRef]
37. Wrobel, J.; Schmidt, B. Probe-to-bone testing for osteomyelitis in the diabetic foot: A literature review. *Diabet. Foot J.* **2016**, *19*, 64–68.
38. Walker, E.A.; Beaman, F.D.; Wessell, D.E.; Cassidy, R.C.; Czuczman, G.J.; Demertzis, J.L.; Lenchik, L.; Motamedi, K.; Pierce, J.L.; Sharma, A.; et al. Expert Panel on Musculoskeletal Imaging. ACR Appropriateness Criteria® Suspected Osteomyelitis of the Foot in Patients with Diabetes Mellitus. *J. Am. Coll. Radiol.* **2019**, *16*, S440–S450. [CrossRef] [PubMed]
39. Lim, A.K. Diabetic nephropathy-complications and treatment. *Int. J. Nephrol. Renov. Dis.* **2014**, *7*, 361–381. [CrossRef]
40. Markanday, A. Diagnosing diabetic foot osteomyelitis: Narrative review and a suggested 2-step score-based diagnostic pathway for clinicians. *Open Forum Infect. Dis.* **2014**, *1*, ofu060. [CrossRef]
41. Merashli, M.; Chowdhury, T.A.; Jawad, A.S. Musculoskeletal manifestations of diabetes mellitus. *QJM* **2015**, *108*, 853–857. [CrossRef]
42. Donovan, A.; Schweitzer, M.E. Use of MR imaging in diagnosing diabetes-related pedal osteomyelitis. *Radiographics* **2010**, *30*, 723–736. [CrossRef] [PubMed]
43. Tan, P.L.; Teh, J. MRI of the diabetic foot: Differentiation of infection from neuropathic change. *Br. J. Radiol.* **2007**, *80*, 939–948. [CrossRef] [PubMed]
44. Kapoor, A.; Page, S.; Lavalley, M.; Gale, D.R.; Felson, D.T. Magnetic resonance imaging for diagnosing foot osteomyelitis: A meta-analysis. *Arch. Intern. Med.* **2007**, *167*, 125–132. [CrossRef] [PubMed]
45. Martín Noguerol, T.; Luna Alcalá, A.; Beltrán, L.S.; Gómez Cabrera, M.; Broncano Cabrero, J.; Vilanova, J.C. Advanced MR Imaging Techniques for Differentiation of Neuropathic Arthropathy and Osteomyelitis in the Diabetic Foot. *Radiographics* **2017**, *37*, 1161–1180. [CrossRef] [PubMed]
46. Leone, A.; Vitiello, C.; Gullì, C.; Sikora, A.K.; Macagnino, S.; Colosimo, C. Bone and soft tissue infections in patients with diabetic foot. *Radiol. Med.* **2020**, *125*, 177–187. [CrossRef] [PubMed]
47. Morrison, W.B.; Schweitzer, M.E.; Batte, W.G.; Radack, D.P.; Russel, K.M. Osteomyelitis of the foot: Relative importance of primary and secondary MR imaging signs. *Radiology* **1998**, *207*, 625–632. [CrossRef]
48. Toledano, T.R.; Fatone, E.A.; Weis, A.; Cotten, A.; Beltran, J. MRI evaluation of bone marrow changes in the diabetic foot: A practical approach. *Semin. Musculoskelet. Radiol.* **2011**, *15*, 257–268. [CrossRef]
49. Ledermann, H.P.; Morrison, W.B.; Schweitzer, M.E. MR image analysis of pedal osteomyelitis: Distribution, patterns of spread, and frequency of associated ulceration and septic arthritis. *Radiology* **2002**, *223*, 747–755. [CrossRef]
50. Low, K.T.; Peh, W.C. Magnetic resonance imaging of diabetic foot complications. *Singap. Med. J.* **2015**, *56*, 23–33. [CrossRef]
51. Ahmadi, M.E.; Morrison, W.B.; Carrino, J.A.; Schweitzer, M.E.; Raikin, S.M.; Ledermann, H.P. Neuropathic arthropathy of the foot with and without superimposed osteomyelitis: MR imaging characteristics. *Radiology* **2006**, *238*, 622–631. [CrossRef]
52. Signore, A.; Lauri, C.; Galli, F. Radiolabelled probes targeting infection and inflammation for personalized medicine. *Curr. Pharm. Des.* **2014**, *20*, 2338–2345. [CrossRef]
53. de Vries, E.F.; Roca, M.; Jamar, F.; Israel, O.; Signore, A. Guidelines for the labelling of leucocytes with 99mTc-HMPAO. Inflammation/Infection Taskgroup of the European Association of Nuclear Medicine. *Eur. J. Nucl. Med. Mol. Imaging* **2010**, *37*, 842–848. [CrossRef]

54. Roca, M.; de Vries, E.F.; Jamar, F.; Israel, O.; Signore, A. Guidelines for the labelling of leucocytes with 111In-oxine. Inflammation/Infection Taskgroup of the European Association of Nuclear Medicine. *Eur. J. Nucl. Med. Mol. Imaging* **2010**, *37*, 835–841. [CrossRef]
55. Signore, A.; Jamar, F.; Israel, O.; Buscombe, J.; Martin-Comin, J.; Lazzeri, E. Clinical indications, image acquisition and data interpretation for white blood cells and anti-granulocyte monoclonal antibody scintigraphy: An EANM procedural guideline. *Eur. J. Nucl. Med. Mol. Imaging* **2018**, *45*, 1816–1831. [CrossRef]
56. Glaudemans, A.W.; de Vries, E.F.; Vermeulen, L.E.; Slart, R.H.; Dierckx, R.A.; Signore, A. A large retrospective single-centre study to define the best image acquisition protocols and interpretation criteria for white blood cell scintigraphy with (99) mTc-HMPAO-labelled leucocytes in musculoskeletal infections. *Eur. J. Nucl. Med. Mol. Imaging* **2013**, *40*, 1760–1769. [CrossRef]
57. Erba, P.A.; Glaudemans, A.W.; Veltman, N.C.; Sollini, M.; Pacilio, M.; Galli, F.; Dierckx, R.A.; Signore, A. Image acquisition and interpretation criteria for 99mTc-HMPAO-labelled white blood cell scintigraphy: Results of a multicenter study. *Eur. J. Nucl. Med. Mol. Imaging* **2014**, *41*, 615–623. [CrossRef]
58. Glaudemans, A.W.; Prandini, N.; Di Girolamo, M.; Argento, G.; Lauri, C.; Lazzeri, E.; Muto, M.; Sconfienza, L.M.; Signore, A. Hybrid imaging of musculoskeletal infections. *Q. J. Nucl. Med. Mol. Imaging* **2018**, *62*, 3–13. [CrossRef]
59. Lauri, C.; Tamminga, M.; Glaudemans, A.W.J.M.; Juárez Orozco, L.E.; Erba, P.A.; Jutte, P.C.; Lipsky, B.A.; IJzerman, M.J.; Signore, A.; Slart, R.H.J.A. Detection of Osteomyelitis in the Diabetic Foot by Imaging Techniques: A Systematic Review and Meta-analysis Comparing MRI, White Blood Cell Scintigraphy, and FDG-PET. *Diabetes Care* **2017**, *40*, 1111–1120. [CrossRef]
60. Lauri, C.; Glaudemans, A.W.J.M.; Signore, A. Leukocyte Imaging of the Diabetic Foot. *Curr. Pharm. Des.* **2018**, *24*, 1270–1276. [CrossRef]
61. Maurer, A.H.; Millmond, S.H.; Knight, L.C.; Mesgarzadeh, M.; Siegel, J.A.; Shuman, C.R.; Adler, L.P.; Greene, G.S.; Malmud, L.S. Infection in diabetic osteoarthropathy: Use of indium-labeled leukocytes for diagnosis. *Radiology* **1986**, *161*, 221–225. [CrossRef]
62. Keenan, A.M.; Tindel, N.L.; Alavi, A. Diagnosis of pedal osteomyelitis in diabetic patients using current scintigraphic techniques. *Arch. Intern. Med.* **1989**, *149*, 2262–2266. [CrossRef]
63. Johnson, J.E.; Kennedy, E.J.; Shereff, M.J.; Patel, N.C.; Collier, B.D. Prospective study of bone, indium-111-labeled white blood cell, and gallium-67 scanning for the evaluation of osteomyelitis in the diabetic foot. *Foot Ankle Int.* **1996**, *17*, 10–16. [CrossRef]
64. Newman, L.G.; Waller, J.; Palestro, C.J.; Hermann, G.; Klein, M.J.; Schwartz, M.; Harrington, E.; Harrington, M.; Roman, S.H.; Stagnaro-Green, A. Leukocyte scanning with 111In is superior to magnetic resonance imaging in diagnosis of clinically unsuspected osteomyelitis in diabetic foot ulcers. *Diabetes Care* **1992**, *15*, 1527–1530. [CrossRef]
65. Unal, S.N.; Birinci, H.; Baktiroğlu, S.; Cantez, S. Comparison of Tc- 99m methylene diphosphonate, Tc-99m human immune globulin, and Tc-99m-labeled white blood cell scintigraphy in the diabetic foot. *Clin. Nucl. Med.* **2001**, *26*, 1016–1021. [CrossRef]
66. Heiba, S.I.; Kolker, D.; Mocherla, B.; Kapoor, K.; Jiang, M.; Son, H.; Rangaswamy, B.; Kostakoglu, L.; Savitch, I.; DaCosta, M.; et al. The optimized evaluation of diabetic foot infection by dual isotope SPECT/CT imaging protocol. *J. Foot Ankle Surg.* **2010**, *49*, 529–536. [CrossRef]
67. Heiba, S.; Kolker, D.; Ong, L.; Sharma, S.; Travis, A.; Teodorescu, V.; Ellozy, S.; Kostakoglu, L.; Savitch, I.; Machac, J. Dual-isotope SPECT/CT impact on hospitalized patients with suspected diabetic foot infection: Saving limbs, lives, and resources. *Nucl. Med. Commun.* **2013**, *34*, 877–884. [CrossRef]
68. Ertugrul, M.B.; Baktiroglu, S.; Salman, S.; Unal, S.; Aksoy, M.; Berberoglu, K.; Calangu, S. The diagnosis of osteomyelitis of the foot in diabetes: Microbiological examination vs. magnetic resonance imaging and labelled leucocyte scanning. *Diabet. Med.* **2006**, *23*, 649–653. [CrossRef]
69. Larcos, G.; Brown, M.L.; Sutton, R.T. Diagnosis of osteomyelitis of the foot in diabetic patients: Value of 111In-leukocyte scintigraphy. *Am. J. Roentgenol.* **1991**, *157*, 527–531. [CrossRef]
70. Palestro, C.J.; Mehta, H.H.; Patel, M.; Freeman, S.J.; Harrington, W.N.; Tomas, M.B.; Marwin, S.E. Marrow versus infection in the Charcot joint: Indium-111 leukocyte and technetium-99m sulphur colloid scintigraphy. *J. Nucl. Med.* **1998**, *39*, 346–350.

71. Palestro, C.J.; Roumanas, P.; Swyer, A.J.; Kim, C.K.; Goldsmith, S.J. Diagnosis of musculoskeletal infection using combined In-111 labeled leukocyte and Tc-99m SC marrow imaging. *Clin. Nucl. Med.* **1992**, *17*, 269–273. [CrossRef]
72. Tomas, M.B.; Patel, M.; Marwin, S.E.; Palestro, C.J. The diabetic foot. *Br. J. Radiol.* **2000**, *73*, 443–450. [CrossRef] [PubMed]
73. Auletta, S.; Riolo, D.; Varani, M.; Lauri, C.; Galli, F.; Signore, A. Labelling and clinical performance of human leukocytes with 99mTc-HMPAO using Leukokit® with gelofusine versus Leukokit® with HES as sedimentation agent. *Contrast Media Mol. Imaging* **2019**, 4368342. [CrossRef] [PubMed]
74. Dominguez-Gadea, L.; Martin-Curto, L.M.; de la Calle, H.; Crespo, A. Diabetic foot infections: Scintigraphic evaluation with 99mTc labelled anti-granulocyte antibodies. *Nucl. Med. Commun.* **1993**, *14*, 212–218. [CrossRef] [PubMed]
75. Palestro, C.J.; Caprioli, R.; Love, C.; Richardson, H.L.; Kipper, S.L.; Weiland, F.L.; Tomas, M.B. Rapid diagnosis of pedal osteomyelitis in diabetics with a technetium-99m-labeled monoclonal antigranulocyte antibody. *J. Foot Ankle Surg.* **2003**, *42*, 2–8. [CrossRef]
76. Delcourt, A.; Huglo, D.; Prangere, T.; Benticha, H.; Devemy, F.; Tsirtsikoulou, D.; Lepeut, M.; Fontaine, P.; Steinling, M. Comparison between Leukoscan (Sulesomab) and Gallium-67 for the diagnosis of osteomyelitis in the diabetic foot. *Diabetes Metab.* **2005**, *31*, 125–133. [CrossRef]
77. Jamar, F.; Buscombe, J.; Chiti, A.; Christian, P.E.; Delbeke, D.; Donohoe, K.J.; Israel, O.; Martin-Comin, J.; Signore, A. EANM/SNMMI guideline for 18F-FDG use in inflammation and infection. *J. Nucl. Med.* **2013**, *54*, 647–658. [CrossRef]
78. Treglia, G.; Sadeghi, R.; Annunziata, S.; Zakavi, S.R.; Caldarella, C.; Muoio, B.; Bertagna, F.; Ceriani, L.; Giovannella, L. Diagnostic performance of Fluorine-18-Fluorodeoxyglucose positron emission tomography for the diagnosis of osteomyelitis related to diabetic foot: A systematic review and a meta-analysis. *Foot (Edinb)* **2013**, *23*, 140–148. [CrossRef]
79. Nawaz, A.; Torigian, D.A.; Siegelman, E.S.; Basu, S.; Chryssikos, T.; Alavi, A. Diagnostic performance of FDG-PET, MRI, and plain film radiography (PFR) for the diagnosis of osteomyelitis in the diabetic foot. *Mol. Imaging Biol.* **2010**, *12*, 335–342. [CrossRef]
80. Basu, S.; Chryssikos, T.; Houseni, M.; Scot Malay, D.; Shah, J.; Zhuang, H.; Alavi, A. Potential role of FDG PET in the setting of diabetic neuro-osteoarthropathy: Can it differentiate uncomplicated Charcot's neuroarthropathy from osteomyelitis and soft-tissue infection? *Nucl. Med. Commun.* **2007**, *28*, 465–472. [CrossRef]
81. Familiari, D.; Glaudemans, A.W.; Vitale, V.; Prosperi, D.; Bagni, O.; Lenza, A.; Cavallini, M.; Scopinaro, F.; Signore, A. Can sequential 18F-FDG PET/CT replace WBC imaging in the diabetic foot? *J. Nucl. Med.* **2011**, *52*, 1012–1019. [CrossRef]
82. Glaudemans, A.W.; Uçkay, I.; Lipsky, B.A. Challenges in diagnosing infection in the diabetic foot. *Diabet. Med.* **2015**, *32*, 748–759. [CrossRef]
83. Gariani, K.; Lebowitz, D.; von Dach, E.; Kressmann, B.; Lipsky, B.A.; Uçkay, I. Remission in diabetic foot infections: Duration of antibiotic therapy and other possible associated factors. *Diabetes Obes. Metab.* **2019**, *21*, 244–251. [CrossRef] [PubMed]
84. Erdman, W.A.; Buethe, J.; Bhore, R.; Ghayee, H.K.; Thompson, C.; Maewal, P.; Anderson, J.; Klemow, S.; Oz, O.K. Indexing severity of diabetic foot infection with 99mTc-WBC SPECT/CT hybrid imaging. *Diabetes Care* **2012**, *35*, 1826–1831. [CrossRef] [PubMed]
85. Przybylski, M.M.; Holloway, S.; Vyce, S.D.; Obando, A. Diagnosing osteomyelitis in the diabetic foot: A pilot study to examine the sensitivity and specificity of Tc(99m) white blood cell-labelled single photon emission computed tomography/computed tomography. *Int. Wound J.* **2016**, *13*, 382–389. [CrossRef] [PubMed]
86. Filippi, L.; Uccioli, L.; Giurato, L.; Schillaci, O. Diabetic foot infection: Usefulness of SPECT/CT for 99mTc-HMPAO-labeled leukocyte imaging. *J. Nucl. Med.* **2009**, *50*, 1042–1046. [CrossRef]
87. Vouillarmet, J.; Morelec, I.; Thivolet, C. Assessing diabetic foot osteomyelitis remission with white blood cell SPECT/CT imaging. *Diabet. Med.* **2014**, *31*, 1093–1099. [CrossRef]
88. Lazaga, F.; Van Asten, S.A.; Nichols, A.; Bhavan, K.; La Fontaine, J.; Oz, O.K.; Lavery, L.A. Hybrid imaging with 99mTc-WBC SPECT/CT to monitor the effect of therapy in diabetic foot osteomyelitis. *Int. Wound J.* **2016**, *13*, 1158–1160. [CrossRef]

89. Lauri, C.; Glaudemans, A.W.J.M.; Campagna, G.; Keidar, Z.; Kurash, M.M.; Georga, S.; Arsos, G.; Noriega-Álvarez, E.; Argento, G.; Kwee, T.C.; et al. Comparison of White Blood Cell Scintigraphy, FDG PET/CT and MRI in Suspected Diabetic Foot Infection: Results of a Large Retrospective Multicenter Study. *J. Clin. Med.* **2020**, *9*, 1645. [CrossRef]
90. Kagna, O.; Srour, S.; Melamed, E.; Militianu, D.; Keidar, Z. FDG PET/CT imaging in the diagnosis of osteomyelitis in the diabetic foot. *Eur. J. Nucl. Med. Mol. Imaging* **2012**, *39*, 1545–1550. [CrossRef]
91. Vesco, L.; Boulahdour, H.; Hamissa, S.; Kretz, S.; Montazel, J.L.; Perlemuter, L.; Meignan, M.; Rahmouni, A. The value of combined radionuclide and magnetic resonance imaging in the diagnosis and conservative management of minimal or localized osteomyelitis of the foot in diabetic patients. *Metabolism* **1999**, *48*, 922–927. [CrossRef]
92. Newman, L.G.; Waller, J.; Palestro, C.J.; Schwartz, M.; Klein, M.J.; Hermann, G.; Harrington, E.; Harrington, M.; Roman, S.H.; Stagnaro-Green, A. Unsuspected osteomyelitis in diabetic foot ulcers. Diagnosis and monitoring by leukocyte scanning with indium 111 oxyquinoline. *JAMA* **1991**, *266*, 1246–1251. [CrossRef] [PubMed]
93. Glaudemans, A.W.; Galli, F.; Pacilio, M.; Signore, A. Leukocyte and bacteria imaging in prosthetic joint infections. *Eur. Cell Mater.* **2013**, *25*, 61–77. [CrossRef] [PubMed]
94. Ruotolo, V.; Di Pietro, B.; Giurato, L.; Masala, S.; Meloni, M.; Schillaci, O.; Bergamini, A.; Uccioli, L. A new natural history of Charcot foot: Clinical evolution and final outcome of stage 0 Charcot neuroarthropathy in a tertiary referral diabetic foot clinic. *Clin. Nucl. Med.* **2013**, *38*, 506–509. [CrossRef] [PubMed]

15

Multimodality Imaging in the Diagnostic Work-Up of Endocarditis and Cardiac Implantable Electronic Device (CIED) Infection

Nicola Galea [1,†,*], Francesco Bandera [2,3,†], Chiara Lauri [4], Camillo Autore [5], Andrea Laghi [6] and Paola Anna Erba [7,8]

1 Department of Experimental Medicine, "Sapienza" University of Rome, 00161 Rome, Italy
2 Heart Failure Unit, Cardiology University Department, IRCCS Policlinico San Donato, Piazza Malan, 1, San Donato Milanese, 20097 Milan, Italy; francesco.bandera@unimi.it
3 Department of Biomedical Sciences for Health, University of Milano, Via Luigi Mangiagalli, 31, 20133 Milan, Italy
4 Nuclear Medicine Unit, Department of Medical-Surgical Sciences and of Translational Medicine, "Sapienza" University of Rome, 00161 Rome, Italy; chialau84@hotmail.it
5 Department of Clinical and Molecular Sciences, "Sapienza" University of Rome, 00189 Rome, Italy; camillo.autore@uniroma1.it
6 Radiology Unit, Department of Medical-Surgical Sciences and of Translational Medicine, "Sapienza" University of Rome, 00189 Rome, Italy; andrea.laghi@uniroma1.it
7 Department of Nuclear Medicine, Department of Translational Research and New Technology in Medicine, University of Pisa, 56126 Pisa, Italy; p.erba@med.unipi.it
8 Medical Imaging Center, Department of Nuclear Medicine and Molecular Imaging, University of Groningen, University Medical Center Groningen, 9713 Groningen, The Netherlands
* Correspondence: nicola.galea@uniroma1.it
† Galea and Bandera equally contributed.

Abstract: Infective endocarditis (IE) is a serious cardiac condition, which includes a wide range of clinical presentations, with varying degrees of severity. The diagnosis is multifactorial and a proper characterization of disease requires the identification of the primary site of infection (usually the cardiac valve) and the search of secondary systemic complications. Early depiction of local complications or distant embolization has a great impact on patient management and prognosis, as it may induce to aggressive antibiotic treatment or, in more advanced cases, cardiac surgery. In this setting, the multimodality imaging has assumed a pivotal role in the clinical decision making and it requires the physician to be aware of the advantages and disadvantages of each imaging technique. Echocardiography is the first imaging test, but it has several limitations. Therefore, the integration with other imaging modalities (computed tomography, magnetic resonance imaging, nuclear imaging) becomes often necessary. Different strategies should be applied depending on whether the infection is suspected or already ascertained, whether located in native or prosthetic valves, in the left or right chambers, or if it involves an implanted cardiac device. In addition, detection of extracardiac IE-related lesions is crucial for a correct management and treatment. The aim of this review is to illustrate strengths and weaknesses of the various methods in the most common clinical scenarios.

Keywords: Infective endocarditis; echocardiography; multimodality imaging; computed tomography; magnetic resonance imaging; nuclear imaging; positron emission tomography; endocarditis team

1. Introduction

Infective endocarditis (IE) is a complex pathological entity with various clinical presentations, whose diagnosis may be challenging as based on a combination of multiple clinical, biological, and imaging criteria [1,2]. Similar difficulties are encountered when the infection is suspected in patients with prosthetic valve (PV) or cardiac implantable electronic device (CIED).

The key elements for disease characterization are to identify the pathogen in the blood, to detect vegetation on the cardiac valves (native or prosthetic) or adhering to CIED, and to assess local complication or distant embolization.

In this perspective, the choice of the most appropriate diagnostic imaging tool can play a crucial role in both confirming the diagnosis and guiding the treatment.

Results of imaging need to be multidisciplinarily discussed within the Endocarditis Team to optimize its value, thus guiding proper therapeutic strategies, eventually improving patient care.

The aim of the present review was to provide an overview of the pros and cons of the different imaging techniques to answer specific questions in the most common clinical scenarios.

2. Clinical Diagnosis: From the Duke Criteria to the European Society of Cardiology (ESC) 2015 Criteria and the Novel 2019 International CIED Infection Criteria

Imaging plays a key role in both the diagnosis and management of IE. Imaging-derived parameters are also useful for the prognostic assessment of patients with IE, for its follow-up under therapy, and during and after surgery. Imaging findings are part of the diagnostic criteria used in clinical practice to reach a diagnosis. The diagnostic strategy proposed by Durack et al. [3] (the Duke criteria) combined echocardiographic findings with clinical and microbiological data. Three echocardiographic findings were considered to be major criteria for the diagnosis of IE: (a) Presence of vegetations, (b) presence of abscesses, or (c) presence of a new dehiscence of a valvular prosthesis. Other abnormal echocardiographic findings not fulfilling these definitions were considered minor criteria. This classification has an overall sensitivity of approximately 80% when the criteria are evaluated at the end of patient follow-up in epidemiological studies. However, the Duke criteria show a lower accuracy for early diagnosis in clinical practice, especially in the case of prosthetic valve endocarditis (PVE) and CIED-related infective endocarditis (CIED-IE), for which echocardiography is normal or inconclusive in up to 30% of cases [4].

Therefore, more recent guidelines [2] incorporate the use of multimodality imaging, including molecular imaging techniques, to integrate the traditional diagnostic criteria in order to fill in such uncertainty gap with information on the biochemical burden of these infections.

Abnormal activity around the prosthetic valve detected by fluoro-18-fluorodeoxyglucose ((^{18}F)FDG) positron emission tomography/computed tomography (PET/CT) or radiolabeled white blood cells (WBC) scintigraphy with single-photon emission computed tomography/computed tomography (SPECT/CT) is considered a major criterion for the diagnosis of IE according to ESC guidelines published in 2015. Both techniques are currently applied in the diagnostic workup of IE and CIED with two main indications: Confirming the presence of infection and identification of septic emboli. By this approach, a substantial reduction in the rate of misdiagnosed IE has been demonstrated. In general, (^{18}F)FDG PET/CT is characterized by higher spatial resolution and sensitivity, better image quality, and shorted acquisition times compared to WBC scan. In contrast, WBC scintigraphy is more specific than (^{18}F)FDG PET/CT, being able to achieve a differential diagnosis between a sterile inflammation, as observed early after surgery. Therefore, WBC imaging should be preferred in all the situations that require higher specificity or in case of inconclusive (^{18}F)FDG PET/CT. Major drawbacks of WBC include the relatively complex and time-consuming labeling procedure that requires a particular equipment, the handling of potentially infected blood, and longer acquisition times. At the moment, no sufficient literature exists in support of one of these imaging modalities rather than another. Therefore, the choice mainly depends on local center availability and expertise, including the presence of SPECT/CT equipment, which is the gold standard for this application, waiting list, and isolated strains (*Candida* spp. and *Enterococcus* spp. may provide false negatives scan due to their ability to create biofilm that impairs granulocytes accumulation in the infected site). In addition, the choice between WBC scintigraphy and (^{18}F)FDG PET/CT remains a prerogative of the Endocarditis Team's discussion. Important parameters to be considered for a proper positron emission tomography (PET) reading are the location, pattern, and intensity of the (^{18}F)FDG. The uptake can be classified as intravalvular (in the leaflets), valvular, or perivalvular [5], even though it should be noted that the intravalvular location is rare. Focal and heterogeneous uptake is consistent with an infected valve. A typical location for abscesses in PVE is the aorto-mitral intervalvular fibrosa, but abscesses can develop in any region in contact with prosthetic material. The probability of infection increases with the intensity of the (^{18}F)FDG uptake; however, several factors may influence (^{18}F)FDG avidity and, therefore, they must be carefully considered for the correct interpretation of a PET/CT scan. For example, prolonged antibiotic therapy, and consequently reduced inflammatory burden, or small vegetations may result in a false negative PET/CT scan. Conversely, recent implantation, especially of mechanical valves, some types of surgical adhesives, or inadequate myocardial suppression usually shows enhanced (^{18}F)FDG uptake. Moreover, active thrombi, vasculitis, primary cardiac tumors, or cardiac metastasis could mimic a focal uptake, thus representing additional confounding factors [5]. In these cases, a WBC scintigraphy could be nullifying. If PET/CT acquisition is combined with a cardiac computed tomography angiography (CCTA), the metabolic findings provided by the (^{18}F)FDG uptake distribution and intensity might be added to the anatomic findings already described for CCTA within a single imaging procedure [6]. The advantages of combining (^{18}F) FDG PET/CT with CCTA include the identification of a larger number of anatomic lesions and clarification of the indeterminate studies by echocardiography [6,7]; furthermore, it assumes a great value in specific clinical situations such as in patients with aortic grafts or with congenital heart disease who have complex anatomy, as their surgical treatment often requires implantation of a large amount of prosthetic material.

In case of CIED-IE, which includes pacemakers and implantable cardioverter defibrillators, the presence of (^{18}F)FDG uptake located on or alongside a lead and that persists on non-attenuation-corrected (NAC) images, is considered consistent for an infectious process according to the very recently published Novel 2019 International CIED Infection Criteria [8].

3. Multidisciplinary Approach of Endocarditis Team

Given the complexity of both diagnosis and therapeutic approach of IE and CIED-IE, no practitioner would be able to manage alone such diseases, being that they are characterized by a wide panel of signs and symptoms and clinical presentations. Therefore, the collaboration between different specialists that look at the same problem from different points of view is crucial for the successful treatment of such infections. A multidisciplinary approach had already shown several advantages in other clinical contexts, for example, in valve diseases, as also recommended by American Heart Association/American College of Cardiology [9]. Following this view, ESC guidelines on IE published in 2015 [2] underlined the need to refer such kind of patients to specialized centers with immediate access to diagnostic procedures and surgical facilities. A pivotal aspect of this approach is represented by the "Endocarditis Team" that involves cardiologists, cardiac surgeons, imaging specialists, microbiologists, infective diseases specialists, neurosurgeons, and other specialists involved in a case-by-case scenario, each one with his or her specific expertise and competence, aiming to ensure best management for the patients, especially in complicated scenarios. Communication among these different specialists plays an important role and, therefore, cases should be regularly discussed during meetings in order to achieve a consensus on the most appropriate treatment for each patient and to define the type and duration of follow-up.

Beside "multidisciplinarity", "multimodality" and "multitracers" are the other two key words that are becoming increasingly important for the management of IE and CIED-IE, thus configuring the so-called "3M" approach to cardiovascular infections [10]. It underlines the importance to appeal to several imaging modalities and strategies that are able to study different aspects of the same problem and to provide relevant information for the clinicians.

4. Left Heart Native Valve IE

4.1. Main Clinical Characteristics

IE of the left heart valves is an infective process affecting the endothelial surface of the aortic or mitral valve. In the general population, the incidence is 3–10 per 100,000 patients per year, but it can reach 20–60 per 1000 patients/year in the case of recurrence [11]. In the last decades, the peak of age has been shifted toward the elderly [12]. The great clinical impact of IE relies on the high in-hospital and six months' mortality rate of 20% and 25–30%, respectively [13,14].

The main valve-related risk factor is the presence of degenerative (fibro-calcific disease in high-income countries or rheumatic disease in low-income countries) or congenital (mitral prolapse, bicuspid aortic valve) abnormalities, determining abnormal flow and increased shear stress on the endothelial surface. The host-related risk factors are the clinical conditions determining systemic immunodepression, such as diabetes and cancer [2].

Clinical presentation is typically characterized by the signs and symptoms incorporated in Duke criteria (fever, vascular and immunological phenomena). Nevertheless, elderly patients can have atypical presentations characterized by the absence of fever, pre-existing heart murmurs, or blunted rise of inflammatory markers, resulting in more difficult diagnostic work-up.

The microbiological isolation, by means of repeated blood cultures, and the demonstration of vegetation at echocardiography are the cornerstones of diagnosis, according to Duke criteria [1]. The overall criteria provide a definite, possible, or rejected diagnosis, according with the clinical probability defined by the combination of them. Left heart valves are generally well explored by ultrasound; however, conditions such as age-related, fibro-calcific degeneration, low-quality acoustic window, or pre-existing valve disease can challenge the identification of vegetation. Nevertheless, in the case of possible IE (according with Duke criteria) or high suspicious IE, further diagnostic work-up is indicated using CCTA scan [2].

The main complications of left-sided IE are heart failure (HF), systemic embolism, and uncontrolled infection [15]. HF is the most frequent complication and can be observed in up to 60% of patients with aortic valve IE, being a predictor of in-hospital, six and 12 months' mortality [16]. HF represents an indication for early surgery also in case of hemodynamic instability. The perivalvular extension and the presence of difficult-to-treat organisms are the main causes of uncontrolled infection, representing an additional indication for early surgery [17]. Finally, systemic embolism is a very common and disregarded complication (up to 50% of cases) requiring specific diagnostic work-up when it is suspected, especially in patients with persistent or recurrent fever and bacteremia or symptomatic patients with recent neurological events. The vegetation size and mobility, age, diabetes, infection by *Staphilococcus aureus*, atrial fibrillation, and previous embolism are the main risk factors for embolism occurrence. During the first two weeks of antibiotic treatment, the risk of embolism is higher, requiring a strict clinical monitoring [18].

4.2. When to Ask for Transthoracic Echocardiography (TTE) and When to Ask for Transoesophageal Echocardiography (TOE)

All patients with a diagnostic suspicion of left heart IE should receive transthoracic echocardiography (TTE). TTE is the first-line diagnostic step and is aimed at the direct identification of the vegetation and of the related damages of the valves (Class of recommendations I, Level of evidence B) [2]. The presence of abscess or pseudoaneurysm and new dehiscence of prosthesis are additional major Duke criteria. In both aortic and mitral IE, acute regurgitation can develop, especially when the causative germs are *Staphilococci* (Figure 1).

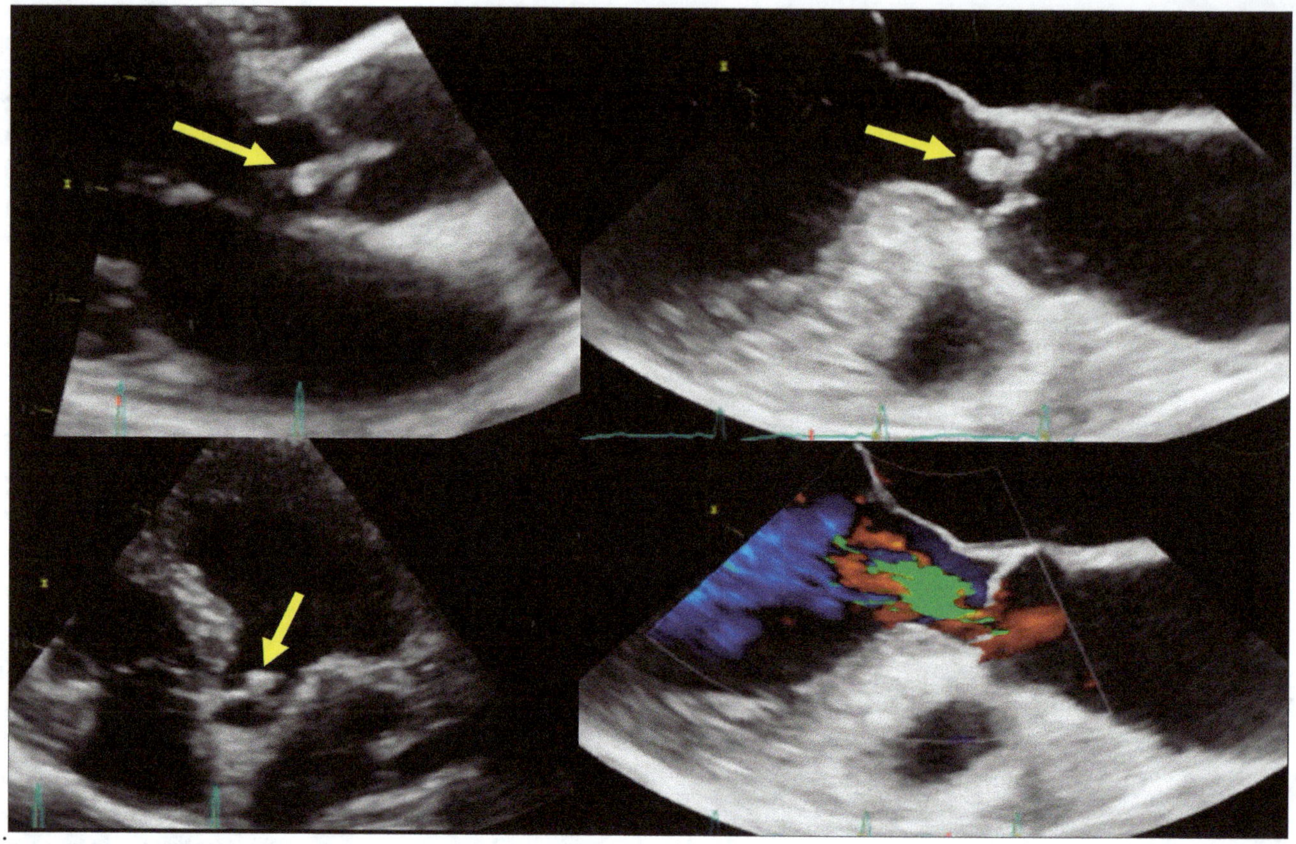

Figure 1. Infective endocarditis (IE) on aortic valve. Top and bottom left: Parasternal long axis and apical four-chamber transthoracic echocardiography (TTE) showing vegetation (arrows) in the left ventricle outflow tract. Top and bottom right: Transoesophageal echocardiography (TOE) showing the vegetation and the related valvular regurgitation.

Serial monitoring is required, even when the diagnosis has been achieved [19].

TTE has a limited sensitivity (ranging from 50 to 60%) mainly related to the anatomical or technical limitations; therefore, transoesophageal echocardiography (TOE) is strongly indicated in case of nondiagnostic or negative TTE (Class of recommendations I, Level of evidence B) [2]. TOE should also be considered in case of positive TTE to obtain a more accurate characterization of the vegetation, to exclude the complications, and to evaluate the vegetation sizes. Globally, the diagnostic sensitivity of TOE is about 85–90% [20]. According to the Euro-Endo registry, TTE has been performed in 91% of cases, while TOE in 53% of native valves' IE [21]. However, some heterogeneity in the diagnostic workup has been reported, with some countries having a more extensive use of imaging, possibly associated with a relatively low mortality [22]. Globally, the data confirm the current role of TTE as a first-line test, while TOE is still limited to selected cases.

Both TTE and/or TOE are indicated during the follow up to identify clinically evident (Class of recommendations I, Level of evidence B) or silent (class Class of recommendations IIa, Level of evidence B) complications, as well as to re-evaluate the patient at the completion of antibiotic therapy (Class of recommendations I, Level of evidence C, Figure 2) [2].

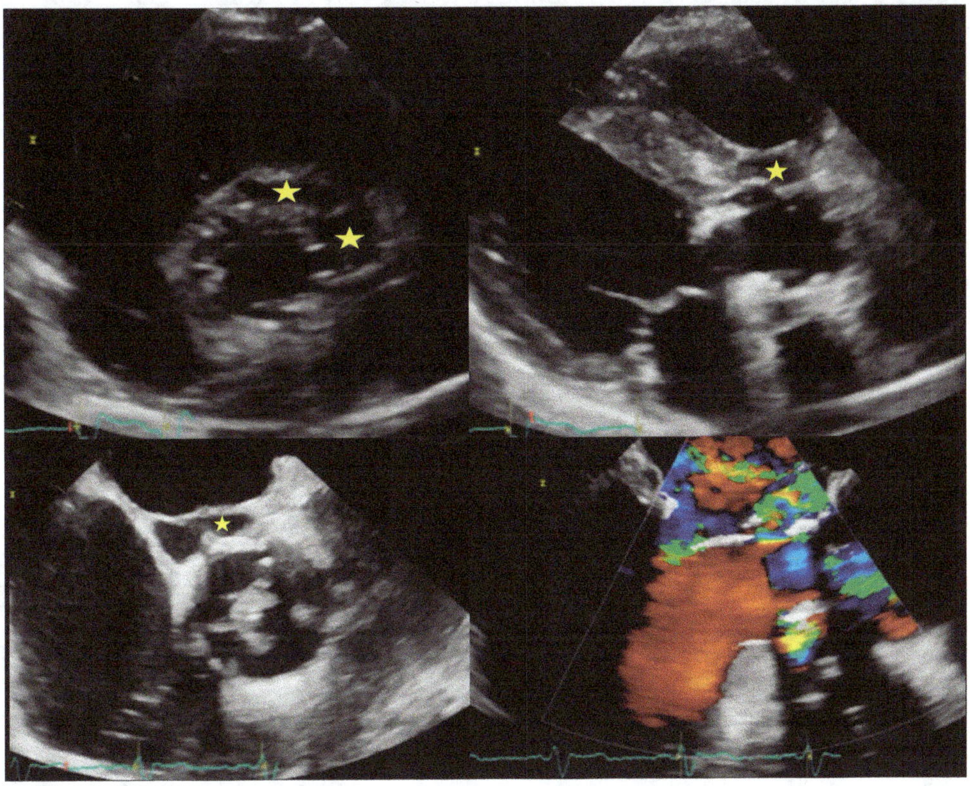

Figure 2. Complications of IE. Top: Example of peri-aortic abscess (stars) with large anechoic cavity surrounding the biological prosthesis (left: TTE with parasternal short axis view, right: TTE with parasternal long axis view). Bottom: Example of peri-aortic pseudoaneurysm (star) with large cavity communicating with cardiovascular lumen (left: TOE short axis view showing large vegetation on prosthesis cusps, right: TOE log axis view with color Doppler showing flow into the perivalvular cavity).

4.3. Role of CCTA in Diagnosing IE and Local Complications

CCTA offers valve imaging with high spatial and temporal resolution and has been established as a valid imaging option when TTE is not definitive or is limited (e.g., poor acoustic window, unclear findings, extensive calcification) [2] or when it does not show any abnormality even though IE is clinically suspected.

On CCTA images, vegetations may appear as leaflet thickening or irregularly shaped soft-tissue oscillating masses, adherent to the valve or endomyocardial surface (Figure 3) [23].

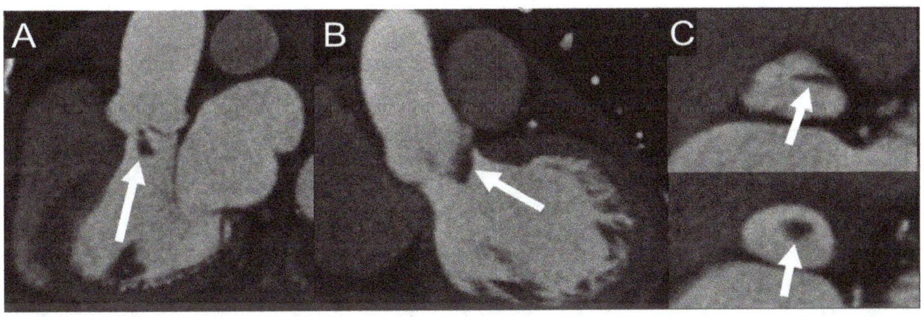

Figure 3. Vegetation on cardiac computed tomography angiography (CCTA) images. A 69-year-old man with fever and IE. Multiplanar CCTA reconstructions on three-chamber (**A**) and coronal (**B**) views show a 2-cm, hypodense, club-shaped, soft-tissue oscillating mass (arrows) attached to the ventricular side of aortic valve leaflets, which appear floating in the lumen of the left ventricular outflow tract in reconstructed axial valve planes (**C**). Sensitivity of CCTA in detecting vegetation ranges from 52.8% for small lesion to 94.4% for larger ones (>10 mm) [24].

CCTA can play a role in assessing the embolic risk as several factors, in particular vegetation size >10 mm and mobility, are predictors of embolic events [2].

CCTA is inferior to TOE in detecting small vegetations (<2 mm) and valve perforations, but is superior in the assessment of the perivalvular extent of the disease such as abscesses, pseudoaneurysms, and fistulas [25], with a sensitivity of 100% using surgery as a reference standard [26].

Abscesses are seen on CCTA images as a perivalvular, low-attenuated fluid collection, bordered by thickened inflammatory tissue, which typically enhance after contrast administration or irregular inhomogeneous tissue adjacent to the fluid. CCTA imaging may identify the abscess extension into surrounding structures, such as into the interatrial septum or mitral-aortic intervalvular fibrous body, which may have implications in surgical planning.

Pseudoaneurysms appear on CCTA as contrast-containing outpouchings of endocardial wall, freely communicating with cardiac chambers or the aortic root, usually located at the paravalvular or periannular regions, possibly extending to the myocardium or pericardium (Figure 4).

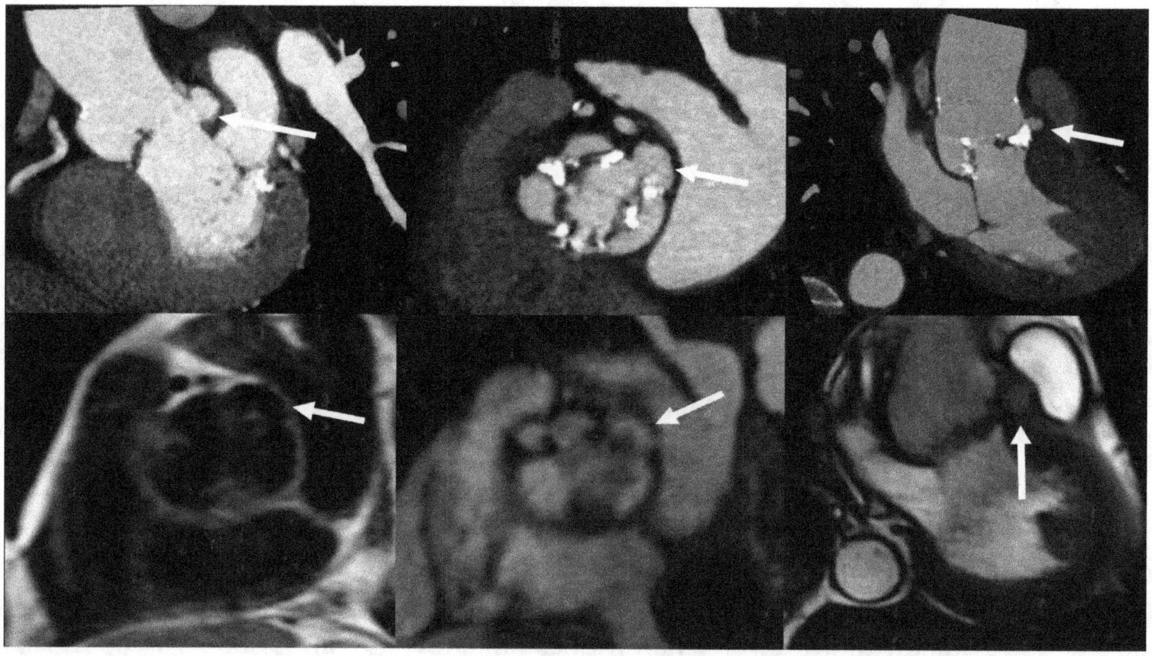

Figure 4. Paravalvular abscesses. CCTA (top images) multiplanar reconstructions and Cardiovascular Magnetic Resonance (CMR) images (bottom images: T1-weighted Turbo Spin Echo on the left, contrast-enhanced T1-weighted Gradient Echo 3D image in the middle and cine-CMR on the right) show a diffuse, partially calcified, thickening of the aortic valve leaflets in a 58-year-old man with *Staphilococcus aureus* IE and bicuspid valve. IE was complicated by the formation of small perivalvular abscesses, which, following the opening of their contents in the lumen, appear as little saccular outpouchings (arrows).

Perforation of the aortic or mitral valve leaflets is visible on CCTA as focal defect and its detection may be helped by the application of 3D volume-rendering reconstructions [27].

Furthermore, CCTA can non-invasively rule out coronary artery disease before surgery by avoiding invasive coronary angiography, which has an intrinsic procedural risk of systemic embolism of valve vegetations or aortic wall perforation, especially in patients with extensive involvement of the aortic valve by IE [25].

4.4. When to Ask for Nuclear Imaging

The value of (^{18}F)FDG PET/CT and WBC imaging is limited in native valve IE, in which the sensitivity is too poor to recommend its routine use [28–30]. However, in the case of native valve

IE, (^{18}F)FDG PET/CT is useful for the detection of distant embolic events, a condition currently considered a minor criterion in the 2015 ESC guidelines [2]. Indeed, whole body (^{18}F)FDG PET/CT offers the possibility to evaluate, with a single imaging modality, both cardiac and extra-cardiac foci, thus allowing the identification of eventual "metastatic" sites of infection with high sensitivity (see below). In addition, (^{18}F)FDG PET/CT imaging is also useful in the identification of the portal of entry (POE), fundamental to minimize the risk of recurrence.

4.5. How to Search for Embolisms

As embolic events complicate a large number of IE patients [2,18], especially during the first week of therapy, and may have a dramatic impact on patient prognosis, their prompt recognition is required. Septic emboli or vascular phenomena may be totally silent in 20–50% of cases [2,31], especially those affecting the splenic or cerebral circulation, which are the most frequent sites of embolism in left-sided IE.

The evidence of septic emboli or vascular phenomena on imaging is included as minor Duke criterion for IE diagnosis [1,2]. Thus, systematic, whole-body contrast-enhanced computed tomography (CT) and/or [^{18}F]FDG PET/CT and cerebral CT or magnetic resonance imaging (MRI) should be considered in both suspected and definite IE.

Cerebral imaging is mandatory for any suspicion of neurological complication and brain MRI is more sensitive than CT for detection of cerebral lesions (mostly ischemic and, less frequently, abscessual or hemorrhagic). However, in unstable or uncooperative patients, CT may be preferable because it is faster and easily feasible. MRI or nongated, contrast-enhanced CT angiography should be included in the imaging protocol in order to rule out vascular lesions such as embolic occlusion or mycotic aneurysm [31].

Contrast-enhanced, whole-body CT and (^{18}F)FDG PET/CT scan have high diagnostic accuracy for splenic abscesses, metastatic infection of other abdominal parenchymal organs, and vascular lesions (splanchnic or peripheral septic emboli). Nevertheless, the administration of iodinated contrast media should be avoided or limited in patients with renal impairment, especially when antibiotic with nephrotoxic effect is used.

4.6. Role of Cardiovascular Magnetic Resonance (CMR) in Diagnosing IE and Local Complications

Although CMR may detect vegetations, abscesses, or pseudoaneurysms in IE, its role in the initial diagnosis is limited and it is not included in ESC 2015 modified diagnostic criteria.

In particular, CMR could be preferred to CCTA in the presence of renal insufficiency as vegetations and local complications may be well depicted on noncontrast CMR images (Figure 4) or in pediatric patients, to avoid radiation exposure. Vegetations, in particular, appear as low signal nodules or floating filaments adherent to the leaflets surface or endocardium.

CMR with late, enhanced imaging may help to detect myocarditis, which is frequently associated with abscess formation or immune reaction [2].

4.7. Diagnostic Workflow Summary

- The initial assessment of suspected left-sided native IE is based on Duke criteria.
- The patient must receive TTE, TOE, and blood cultures.
- If IE is rejected and the suspicious is low, no more investigations are needed.
- If the diagnosis is definite, the patient should be investigated for silent embolism using CT or PET/CT scan, as well as MRI for cerebral involvement (embolism or hemorrhage), according with clinical status.
- In the case of possible IE or rejected IE but high suspicion there is indication for repeating new TTE/TEE and blood cultures, further investigations, such as whole-body, contrast-enhanced CT

or PET/CT scan, should be considered to detect silent embolism or metastatic infections and, therefore, to reclassify the patient, according with ESC 2015 modified diagnostic criteria [2].

5. Right Heart Native Valve IE

5.1. Main Clinical Characteristics

Right heart IE represents 5–10% of all IE and is typically associated with intravenous drug use, congenital heart disease, intravascular catheters, and immunodepression states (such as HIV infection) [32]. The tricuspid valve is predominantly involved, especially in active intravenous drug users, whose 5-year survival is 50% in case of surgical treatment [33].

The clinical presentation is frequently characterized by respiratory symptoms resulting from pulmonary emboli, pneumonia, and abscess formation. Anemia and microscopic hematuria can typically be present when the tricuspid valve is involved [34]. Systemic emboli and sepsis are potential complications accounting for a worse prognosis. The overall mortality has been reported to be as high as 10.2%, with a surgical mortality of 7.8%, both related to the risk factors, vegetation size, and location [35].

In intravenous drug users, *Staphylococcus aureus* is the most common germ for IE, localizing on the tricuspid valve and accounting for a 16% mortality rate [36]. IE related to the presence of central venous catheter is predominantly caused by *Staphylococcus aureus* (54.6%), coagulase-negative *Staphylococcus* (37.5%), *Candida* species (16.6%), and *Enterococcus* (12.5%) [37].

A specific subgroup of IE is represented by the infections affecting people with congenital heart disease (CHD). The incidence is 15–140 times higher than in the general population and the reported mortality ranges between 4 to 10% [38,39]. The diagnostic management is substantially similar to that of native valve IE but it is challenged by the morphological complexity of some CHD. A specific risk factor for both early and late IE is the presence of valve-containing prosthetics, a condition frequently encountered in complex CHD that predisposes a patient to a greater long-term risk [40].

5.2. When to Ask for TTE and When to Ask for TOE

As for left-side IE, TTE is the first-line diagnostic tool allowing for a good evaluation of the tricuspid valve, especially when using off-axis plans. The pulmonary and Eustachian valves are more challenging to explore with TTE and, therefore, they frequently require trans-esophageal approach. The vegetation size (highly correlated with the risk of recurrent embolism), the worsening of regurgitation, the degree of congestion, and the presence of HF represent a class IIaC indication for surgical treatment and require systematic echocardiographic assessment during follow up [2]. In case of suspected IE in CHD adult patients, TTE is often inadequate for a complete visualization of cardiac structures, especially in complex malformations and, therefore, TOE is required to provide a complete assessment [39]. In children, TTE generally allows for a correct assessment.

5.3. Role of CCTA in Diagnosing IE and Local Complications

Similarly to what is described for the left valves, CCTA play a role in detecting the vegetations and local complications, such as perivalvular extension of infection, transvalvular fistula, perivalvular abscess, and pseudoaneurysm [41]. In particular, the evaluation of the pulmonary and tricuspid valves by TTE is limited by the poor acoustic window; therefore, CCTA can offer an added value when echocardiography is not definitive [31].

The CCTA protocol should guarantee an adequate contrast enhancement of the right chambers, whereas the standard CCTA protocol for the assessment of the coronary tree and left chambers comprises the complete washing of the right cavities with iodine.

5.4. When to Ask for Nuclear Imaging

As for left side native valve IE, the use of nuclear imaging in native valve IE is limited and mainly addressed to the detection of pulmonary embolism and for the identification of POE (see below).

5.5. How to Search for Embolisms

Right-side IE and CIED-IE are associated to lung metastatic infection. Pulmonary infectious emboli should always be sought when the IE diagnosis is possible, according to modified Duke criteria, or rejected despite the high clinical suspicion, as it is considered a minor diagnostic criterion [2]. Noncontrast chest CT is generally sufficient in the detection of small septic emboli within the lung parenchyma. Contrast-enhanced CT, (^{18}F)FDG PET/CT, and WBC SPECT/CT well may detect pulmonary consolidations and discriminate septic infarcts and abscesses from neoplastic lesions. The use of ventilation-perfusion scintigraphy has been replaced by other techniques, particularly (^{18}F)FDG PET/CT and WBC SPECT/CT, which have the clear advantage to combine the detection of distant embolism, the assessment of valve-involvement, and identification of POE [31].

5.6. Role of CMR in Diagnosing IE and Local Complications

As for the left valves, the role of CMR in the diagnosis of IE and local complications is poorly codified and limited to selected cases, where the other imaging techniques are not sufficient or contraindicated (e.g., renal failure or pediatric population in substitution of CCTA).

Nevertheless, CMR may offer a superior evaluation of right transvalvular flows compared to TEE by using phase contrast imaging, which is particularly useful to quantify pulmonary valve regurgitation caused by perforations or destruction of the cusps or the abnormal flow of paravalvular leakage [41].

5.7. Diagnostic Workflow Summary

- Similarly to left-sided native IE, the workflow of suspected right-sided IE is based on TTE, TEE, and blood cultures to stratify patients according with Duke criteria. TTE has a central role in exploring tricuspid valve, while TOE is generally required in the case of pulmonary valve involvement.
- Second-line imaging (CT, PET/CT, WBC SPECT/CT) is indicated to search for perivalvular and pulmonary complications, to detect distal embolisms, and to identify POE.

6. Early and Late Prosthetic Valve Infective Endocarditis (PVE)

6.1. Main Clinical Characteristics

IE is one of the most challenging complications after heart valve surgery, often requiring complex diagnostic work-up and affecting up to 6% of patients with prosthetic valves [42]. PVE or post-repair endocarditis accounts for the 30% of cases in Euro-Endo registry [21], with 18.1% of patients having a history of previous endocarditis. Traditionally, PVE is classified as early PVE if infection occurs within 12 months from surgery and late PVE if it occurs thereafter [2]. In early PVE, patients are generally infected perioperatively and, more frequently, can present complications involving the sewing ring (abscess, dehiscence, pseudoaneurysms, and fistulae), with Staphylococci, fungi, and Gram-negative bacilli as the main responsible germs [43]. Late PVE generally occurs with valve regurgitation if a bioprosthesis is involved, while mechanical valves may present with large vegetations causing valve stenosis [44]. The germs responsible for late PVE are substantially the same involved in native valve IE.

PVE presents the highest in-hospital mortality (20–40%) among IE [45]. Older age, diabetes mellitus, healthcare-associated infections, staphylococcal or fungal infection, early PVE, HF, stroke, and intracardiac abscess are the main risk factors associated with poor prognosis [46]. The high mortality and the complex diagnostic work-up require an early treatment strategy, eventually including surgery, to control the disease burden. Surgery is mandatory in case of HF, severe prosthetic dysfunction, abscess, or persistent fever [2]. A conservative strategy with close follow up is indicated for the low-risk cases.

6.2. When to Ask for TTE and When to Ask for TOE

As for native IE, the suspicion of PVE requires TTE and TOE evaluation. Unfortunately, false negative examinations are more frequent and limit the accuracy of the echocardiography [4]. The TOE is generally preferred as a first-line evaluation and it is also indicated in case of negative TTE, in both early and late PVE, and for the identification of periprosthetic abscess and leak (both major Duke criteria, Figure 5).

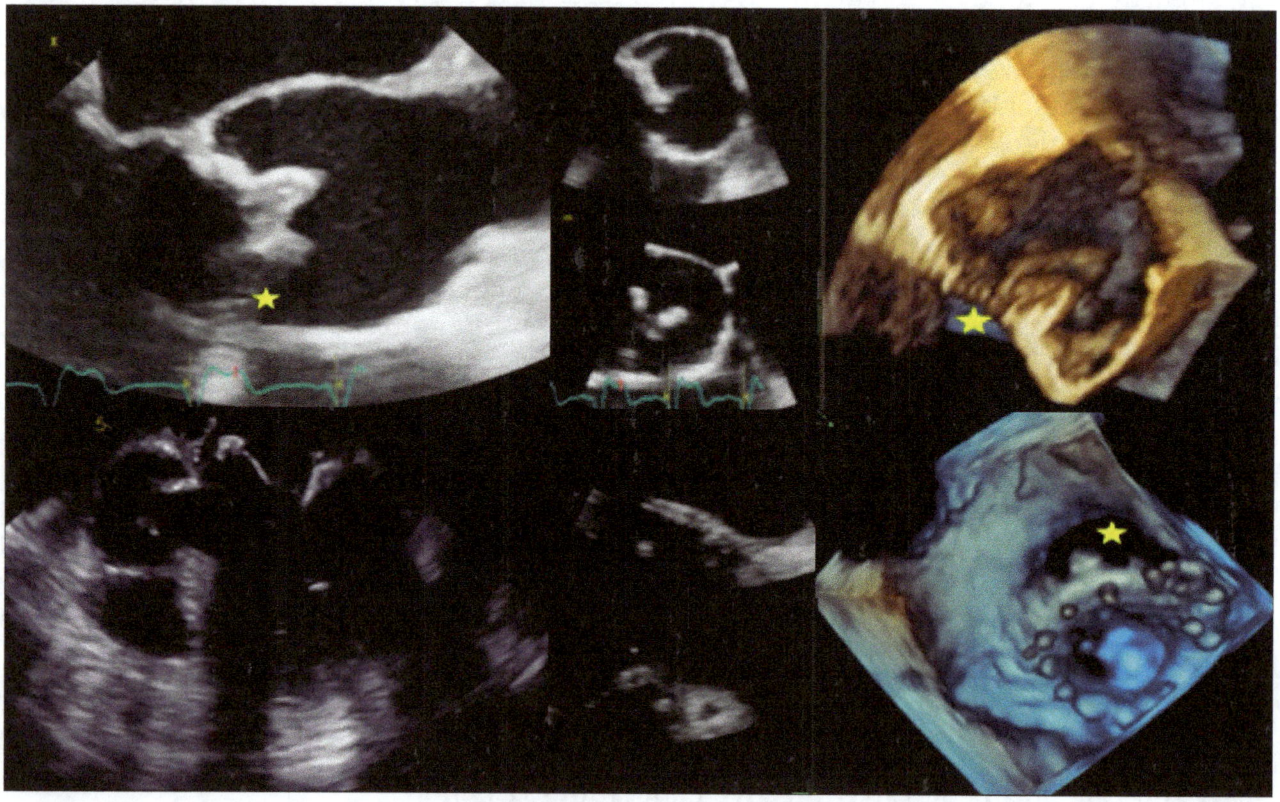

Figure 5. Complications of prosthetic valve endocarditis (PVE). Top: Biological prosthesis dehiscence in aortic position with large perivalvular leak (left: TOE long-axis view, right: 3D TOE view). Bottom: Biological prosthesis dehiscence in mitral position with large perivalvular leak (left: TOE long-axis view showing the direct communication between atrium and ventricle, right: 3D TOE view). Stars indicate the place of maximal prosthesis dehiscence.

The Euro-Endo Registry showed that TOE is generally performed in the 66% of subjects, showing a significant percentage of abscesses (19%), pseudoaneurysm (6%), and prosthetic dehiscence (11%) [21]. The limited sensitivity of Duke criteria in PVE supports the indication to repeat TOE when the clinical suspicion is high, according with the clinical evolution [47].

6.3. Role of CCTA in Diagnosing PVE and Local Complication

CCTA imaging helps diagnose PVE when results of TTE or TOE are indeterminate or to assess paravalvular complications if the PVE diagnosis has already been established [2]. In PVE, the infection usually spreads from the sewing ring or adjacent thrombi and may result in complications such as paravalvular leakage, abscess, pseudoaneurysm, dehiscence, and extension to adjacent structures [44].

Despite the beam-hardening artifacts, due to the metal component of the prosthesis, which affect image quality and may hinder the visualization of small vegetations (<4 mm), vegetations larger than

10 mm are usually detected with high accuracy by CCTA. They typically appear as round, mobile, hypodense masses on the valve leaflet or sewing ring, typically on the ventricular side of aortic or mitral leaflets [48].

CCTA is more sensitive than TOE in detecting paravalvular and extracardiac infection involvement [48] and should be acquired with retrospective gating with subsequent reconstruction of every 10% RR interval of the entire cardiac cycle to enable cinetic CT visualization.

Paravalvular abscesses are well recognized by CCTA as a thickened, hypoattenuating area or irregular, inhomogeneous mass surrounding the PV or the aortic root, inconstantly associated to rim delayed enhancement and gas bubbles, reflecting infected cavities adjacent to the PV.

Extent of inflammation to surrounding tissues is depicted by adjacent fat stranding or, exceptionally, by myocardial thickening and enhancement, or mediastinal gas and fluid collections when the infection spreads outside the pericardial sac.

Pseudoaneurysms are a typical late complication after valve surgery during aortic root graft replacement or Bentall procedure and they can occur when a perivalvular cavitating abscess drains into the adjacent cardiac chamber, with the formation of wall outpouching containing circulating blood (Figure 6).

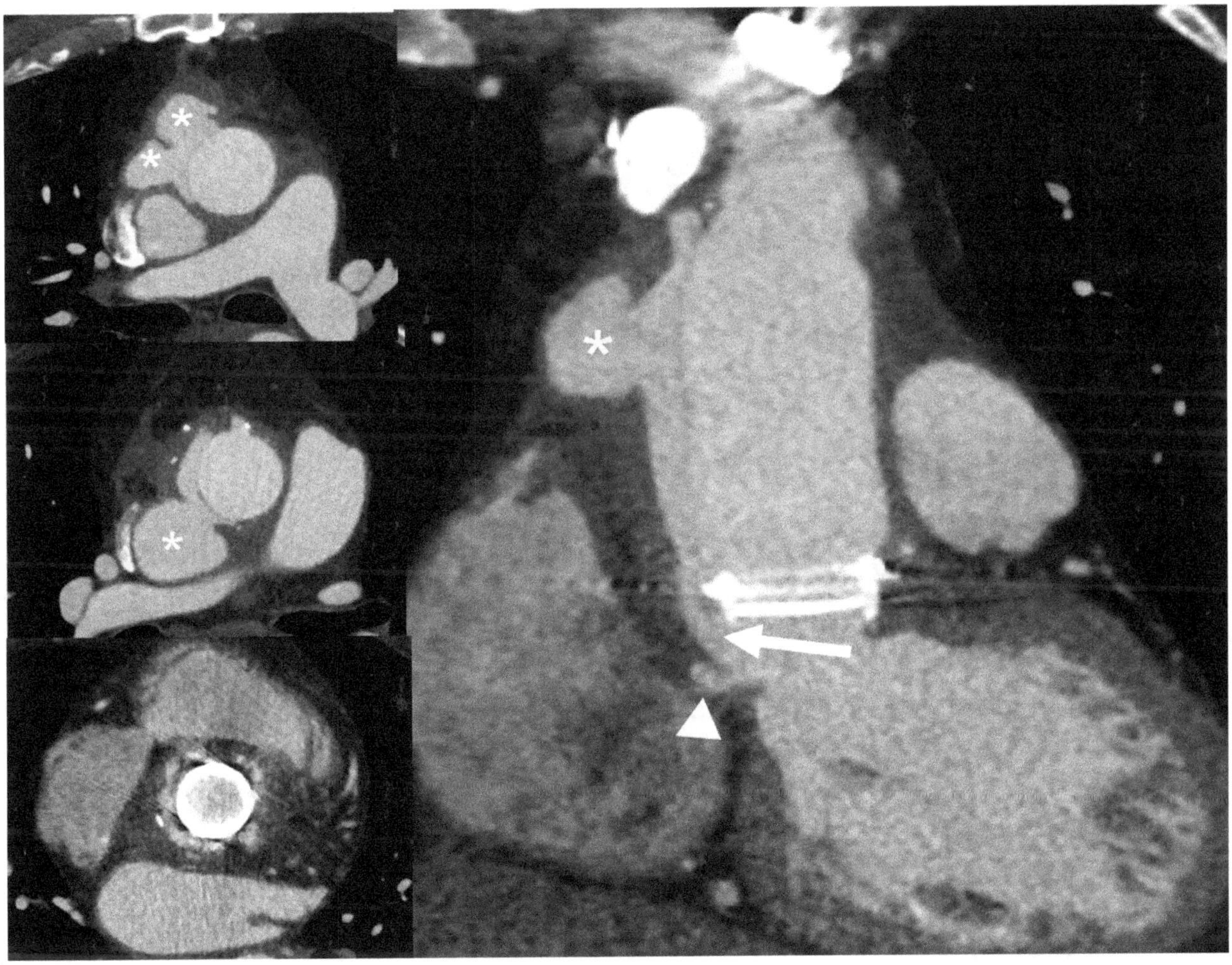

Figure 6. Infective late complication in a patient with Bentall prosthesis: Dehiscence and periprosthetic pseudoaneurysm. CCTA multiplanar reconstructions show a large dehiscence of the surgical suture at the proximal anastomosis of the prosthesis with large communication (arrow) of the left ventricular cavity with a large false lumen (asterisks) recanalized from perivalvular communication (arrow); a little periannular pseudoaneurysm (arrowhead) is seen adjacent to the ventriculo-aortic junction.

PVE may be complicated by perforation of leaflets (exclusively in biological prostheses) or dehiscence, defined detachment of the PV from its annulus due to rupture of the suture line between the sewing ring and annular tissue. CCTA imaging, including cine-CT reconstruction, may visualize the rocking motion from a severely detached prosthesis. PVE-related dehiscence may also cause paravalvular leakage with abnormal communication between two different chambers through the hole at the undocking point.

Another potential complication, which can be demonstrated by CCTA, is the formation of fistula connecting two neighboring cavities (such as a Valsalva sinus with right ventricle or left atrium or between the left ventricle and right atrium); in this setting CCTA offers a detailed morphological visualization of the abnormal connections.

Finally, CCTA improves the precision of radionuclide imaging study by providing an anatomical map co-registered with functional information provided by metabolic imaging [49].

6.4. When to Ask for Nuclear Imaging

In the case of prosthetic valves, "abnormal activity around the site of implantation" detected by (^{18}F)FDG PET/CT is a major criteria for IE according to ESC 2015 guidelines [4]. Therefore, all patients with possible or even rejected IE by Duke criteria, but with high clinical suspicion, should be assessed by (^{18}F)FDG PET/CT and/or WBC imaging or CCTA to confirm/rule out IE (Figure 7) [31]. Conversely, patients with rule-out IE according to Duke criteria and with low clinical suspicion do not require further examinations.

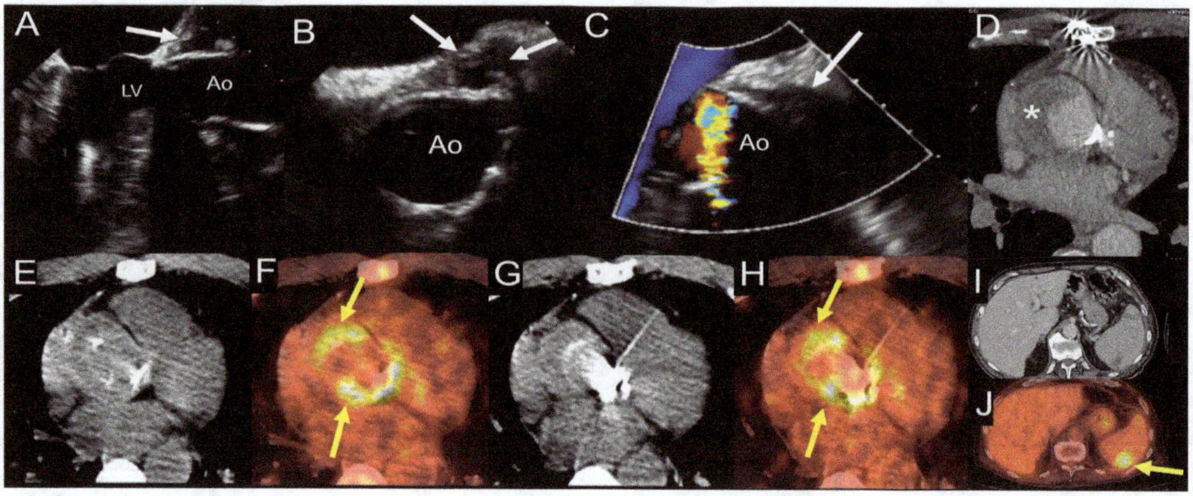

Figure 7. Example of the use of multimodality imaging. A patient with history of aortic valve replacement with mechanical prosthesis and ascending aorta graft presented four years later with acute right lower limb ischemia due to occlusion of proximal fibular, anterior tibial, and posterior tibial arteries treated with revascularization attempts and finally leg amputation. During hospitalization, the patient had fever with increased erythrocyte sedimentation rate and C-reactive protein. TTE (**A**) and at TOE (**B**,**C**) show the presence of hyperechogenic periprosthetic area (white arrows), most likely consistent with abscess. Blood culture was negative. The fluoro-18-fluorodeoxyglucose positron emission tomography/computed tomography ((^{18}F)FDG PET/CT) exam including CCTA (**D**–**J**) was performed showing an organized fluid perigraft collection surrounded by thick walls (asterisk) that enhance after iodinated contrast injection on CCTA images (**D**), which is associated to intense uptake of (^{18}F)FDG around the aortic valve prosthesis, as shown by the yellow arrows ((**E**,**G**) show noncontrast CT transaxial images while (**F**,**H**) show the fused PET/CT images). Myocardial suppression of (^{18}F)FDG uptake is achieved by high-fat, low-carb diet. In addition, the whole-body images showed an area of spleen uptake, consistent with septic embolism ((**I**,**J**), noncontrast CT and fused PET/CT transaxial images, respectively), as indicated by the yellow arrow. Ao: ascending aorta; LV: left ventricle.

Several recent meta-analyses indicated that the overall pooled sensitivity of (^{18}F)FDG PET/CT in PVE is about 73–81% [50] with an overall accuracy with an area under curve (AUC) of 0.897 when including only studies reporting adequate cardiac preparation. Even in the case of negative PET results (that includes also a whole-body evaluation for embolism detection), a thorough interpretation of the echocardiography and CCTA scan is essential. Indeed, in the absence of infection, PV generally shows mild, diffuse, and homogeneous uptake that usually remains stable for at least one year after surgery, most likely resulting from persistent host reaction against the biomaterial coating the sewing ring of PV and chronic tension or friction exerted on these anchor points [51–53]. Such (^{18}F)FDG uptake seems to be slightly greater in mechanical versus biological prostheses.

Very recent data proved the prognostic value of (^{18}F)FDG PET/CT in PVE. In a large retrospective study on 173 patients with left-sided IE and examined after seven days from the first antibiotic administration, a moderate to intense valvular (^{18}F)FDG uptake was predictive of major adverse cardiac events defined as in-hospital death, one-year death, recurrence of IE, acute cardiac insufficiency, symptomatic embolism under antibiotics, and nonscheduled rehospitalization for cardiovascular indication [54]. These results reinforce the utility of (^{18}F)FDG PET/CT in PVE and justify its use in this population, not only for diagnostic purposes, but also for prognostic assessment. Therefore, (^{18}F)FDG PET/CT should be used in clinical practice for optimal patient management and therapy decision making, particularly in PVE.

6.5. *How to Search for Embolisms*

Notable advantages of PET/CT and WBC SPECT/CT are their ability to perform the extra-cardiac workup within a single imaging procedure and to reveal the concomitant presence of extra-cardiac infection sites as the consequence of both septic embolism as well as primary infective processes (with the exception of the brain location, since brain uptake is always high due to its specific metabolism) [28,55,56]. Detection of metastatic infection by (^{18}F)FDG PET/CT leads to change of treatment in up to 35% of patients [57]. PET/CT has demonstrated to be able to reveal the source of infection, including cases where the sustaining POE was a neoplasia (colonic cancer) [6]. As for IE of native valves, with distant septic embolization a minor criterion for PVE diagnosis, their search depends on the left or right side of the prosthetic valve and includes also cerebral MRI and whole-body, contrast-enhanced CT, as previously described for native valves.

6.6. *Role of CMR in Diagnosing PVE and Local Complications*

CMR is affected by metal artifacts especially from mechanical prostheses and offers similar information to the CCTA (including detection of paravalvular leakage, abscess, pseudoaneurysm, and dehiscence) but with lower spatial resolution and lower anatomical definition. It is typically used when CCTA is contraindicated or to assess complex hemodynamic, such as to ascertain or evaluate intracardiac fistula where CMR is able also to quantify the shunt.

6.7. *Diagnostic Workflow Summary*

- As for native valve IE, in case of suspected PVE the initial assessment is based on Duke criteria, with the specific indication to perform both TTE and TOE for the higher accuracy of transesophageal approach.
- If IE is rejected and the suspicious is low, no more investigations are needed.
- If the diagnosis is definite, the patient should be investigated for silent embolism or metastatic infections using CT or PET/CT scan and with CCTA to detect periprosthetic extension. MRI to detect cerebral involvement (embolism or hemorrhage) is also indicated according with the clinical status.
- In case of possible IE or rejected IE but high suspicion, there is indication for repeating new TTE/TEE and blood cultures. CCTA or PET/CT are recommended to detect periprosthetic extension. A whole-body, contrast-enhanced CT or PET/CT or WBC SPECT/CT is indicated to

detect silent embolism or metastatic infections. All these methods contribute to reclassify the patient according with ESC 2015-modified diagnostic criteria [2].

7. CIED-Related Infective Endocarditis

7.1. Main Clinical Characteristics

CIED-IE represents about 10% of total IE, with an in-hospital mortality of 15.3%, according with Euro-Endo Registry [21]. A wider use of CIEDs in the elderly contributes to the increased rate of CIED-IE, with an incidence of 1.9 per 1000 device/year reported in a population-based study [58]. Clinically, CIED-IE can be divided into infections limited to the pocket of the skin and infections extended to the electrode leads, cardiac valve leaflets, or endocardial surface. This difference is challenging to define and can require the use of advanced imaging, such as WBC scintigraphy or (^{18}F)FDG PET/CT [59].

The infection can primarily involve the pocket, after direct manipulation (i.e., change of generator) and spread to the leads producing multiple vegetations or it can directly originate on the leads during bacteremia, secondary to a distant site of infection. In addition to the typical risk factors for IE (renal failure, corticosteroid use, congestive HF, and diabetes mellitus), other factors related to the surgical procedure may play a role in CIED-IE (i.e., type of intervention, device revision, use of temporary pacing, use of antimicrobial prophylaxis, and use of anticoagulation) [60]. *Staphilococci* accounts for 60–80% of the cases, with a significant proportion of *S. aureus* (about 50%), according with the Euro-Endo registry [21].

From a clinical perspective, it is important to differentiate superficial incisional infection, which does not require CIED system extraction [61,62], from infection limited to the pocket, extending to the leads potentially associated with systemic infections and/or IE.

7.2. When to Ask for TTE and When to Ask for TOE

The clinical manifestation of CIED-IE can be variable and misleading, with acute manifestations or chronic evolution, especially in the elderly. As for other specific conditions of IE, the TTE and TOE play a first-line role for searching vegetation in the intracardiac and intravascular portions of the leads. The diagnostic usefulness of echocardiography is limited to the infections involving the explorable portions of the leads (i.e., the intracardiac and superior vena cava initial segments), having a negligible role in pocket-related infections. TOE has higher sensitivity than TTE in identifying the tricuspid involvement, the presence of vegetation on the leads, and the involvement of left-sided valves [63]. TTE allows for a better assessment of pulmonary pressures, pericardial effusion, and left ventricle function. Both approaches are, therefore, recommended in case of suspected CIED-IE. The echocardiography should be used to identify the vegetation and its localization, but a negative examination does not rule out the presence of infection. The Euro-Endo Registry showed that a high proportion (67%) of patients with CIED-IE received TOE, but a significant percentage of subjects (26% and 37%, respectively) also required PET/CT or chest CT [21]. This observation confirms the need for multidisciplinary work-up in CIED-IE.

7.3. Role of CCTA in Diagnosing CIED-IE and Local Complications

In CIED-IE, CCTA has poorer sensitivity in detection of vegetations on pacemaker leads compared to TTE or TOE, due to blooming and beam-hardening artifacts and should be limited to situations when radionuclide imaging is not available [31].

Electrocardiographic (ECG)-gating embedded in CCTA refines the anatomical map co-registered during radionuclide imaging study, improving the diagnostic accuracy of hybrid exams [64].

Moreover, CCTA can be followed by a nongated, contrast-enhanced CT scan, which plays a role in assessing infection of the pacemaker pocket by depicting local inflammatory tissue changes or abscess collection around the device, which should be distinguished from non-infected hematomas, superficial cellulitis, or infection that commonly occurs at the surgical site in the postoperative phase [65].

Contrast-enhanced CT is also required in the detection of distant septic emboli and predominantly pulmonary and vascular complications such as mycotic aneurysms. This represents additional criteria for CIED-IE diagnosis with direct impact on patient management and treatment strategy.

7.4. When to Ask for Nuclear Imaging

(^{18}F)FDG PET/CT provides added diagnostic value to the Duke criteria, particularly in the subset of possible CIED-IE [66–71] and it has the capability to explore the whole device. Therefore, (^{18}F)FDG PET/CT and WBC SPECT/CT might be used in all the cases when CIED involvement is suspected [8]. In CIED-IE the presence of (^{18}F)FDG uptake should be described as pertinent to generator pocket (superficial or deep) and/or to the leads (intravascular or intracardiac portion of the leads). In addition, signs of cardiac (valvular or pericardial) involvement as well as systemic signs of infections (septic embolism, in particular in the lung parenchyma and POE) should be carefully assessed and reported. The (^{18}F)FDG PET/CT is useful in patients with evidence of pocket infection and negative microbiologic and echocardiographic examination and in patients with positive blood cultures but negative echocardiographic examination. All the related studies have shown an almost 100% accuracy for infection of the generator pocket and for the extracardiac portion of the lead (sensitivity, specificity, and accuracy for the diagnoses of pocket infection were 93%, 98%, and 98%, respectively) [31,50,72]. The presence of (^{18}F)FDG uptake along pacing leads, in particular, in the same location as mobile elements on echocardiography and in association with septic pulmonary emboli appearing as multiple focal (^{18}F)FDG spots, is highly suggestive of pacing lead infection [67] (Figure 8). Of notice, in the Euro-Endo registry extracardiac uptake was found in 43.8% of patients with CIED-IE [14].

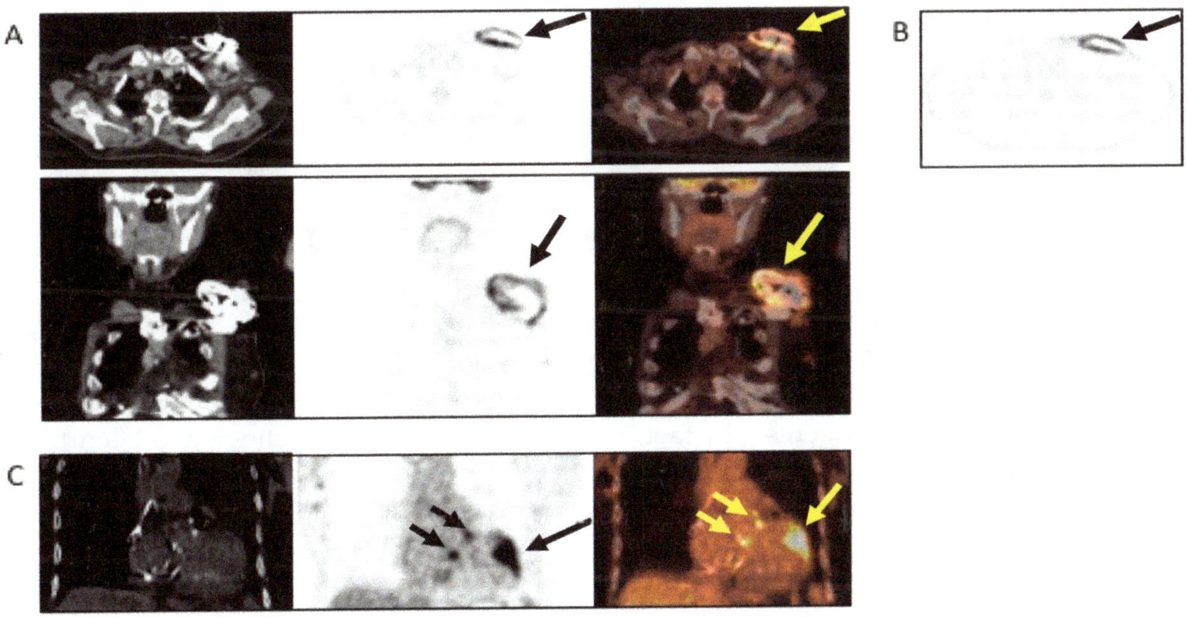

Figure 8. Example of the use of (^{18}F)FDG PET/CT in a patient with non-Hodgkin's lymphoma and sudden onset of fever and a positive blood culture for *Streptococcus dysgalactiae*. The patient underwent TTE and TEE, which were negative. Antimicrobial treatment was started. Due to the lack of clinical response, the patient underwent (^{18}F)FDG PET/CT, which revealed infection, as indicated by the black and yellow arrows, involving the pocket of the device ((**A**), from left to right, CT, PET, and superimposed PET/CT transaxial (upper panel) and coronal (lower panel and (**B**) non-attenuated corrected transaxial images) as well as the intracardiac portion of the lead extending to the tricuspid valve ((**C**), from left to right, noncontrast CT, PET, and fused PET/CT coronal images). Based to the PET/CT findings, the device was extracted and replaced.

In the case of lead-related IE, (^{18}F)FDG PET/CT is very specific when tracer uptake is visualized. However, its sensitivity is low, and a negative result does not completely exclude the presence of small vegetations with low metabolic activity [68]. Every positive blood culture should be carefully evaluated, with prompt, active exclusion of CIED-IE with other diagnostic techniques [8].

7.5. Diagnostic Workflow Summary

- In case of suspected CIED-IE, the physician should address the Duke criteria, being aware of the significantly limited diagnostic accuracy. However, blood cultures, TTE, and eventually TOE should be considered also in case of suspected infection limited to the pocket.
- In case of possible CIED-IE or rejected CIED-IE but persistent high clinical suspicion there is indication to repeat TTE/TOE and blood cultures.
- Chest CT has a specific role in searching for pulmonary embolism, infarct or abscess. The (^{18}F)FDG PET/CT and WBC SPECT/CT have a central role in detecting pocket infection, lead infection, and pulmonary embolism.

8. Current Challenges and Future Perspectives

The diagnosis of IE and CIED-IE still remains sometimes a challenge for the clinicians for both diagnostic and therapeutic points of view. As previously shown, each imaging modality has its own pros and cons (Table 1) and, therefore, the appeal to an integrated and multimodal approach in the diagnostic workup of IE and CIED-IE is mandatory. It has already demonstrated to be effective for the early identification of the infection. But, at the moment, the role of imaging as tool to follow-up after antibiotic therapy or in decision making between a surgical rather than a medical approach is still debated and the lack of a reference standard represents one of the most critical aspects that should be faced in the near future.

Novel trends in radiopharmaceuticals' developments as well as significant progresses in technology and new insights on the various mechanisms that play a role in cardiovascular infections will likely provide in the future new diagnostic and therapeutic targets for further developments in the field.

As for the radiopharmaceutical perspective, while radiolabeled granulocytes are a common clinical practice with SPECT applications, tracking WBC in vivo with PET using the positron emitting is still in the research phase [73–75]. A very interesting innovative strategy, based on the development of selective metabolic probes that are substrate for specific strains, has recently renewed the interest in pathogen-specific imaging agents. In fact, while traditional approaches have been based on radiolabeling existing antibiotics (i.e., ciprofloxacin) or antimicrobial peptides (i.e., ubiquicidin), researchers have recently tested almost 1000 radiolabeled small molecules as substrates for essential metabolic pathways in bacteria, demonstrating (^{18}F)fluorodeoxysorbitol [76,77] holds tremendous potential for identifying and monitoring known or suspected infection caused by *Enterobacteriaceae*. On the other hand, in addition to technological developments, new equipment such as PET/MRI and total-body PET/CT will provide new opportunities to extend clinical diagnosis in specific scenarios (i.e., myocarditis) as well as to implement the use of quantitative imaging analysis. All together, this synergy arising from the combination of clinical and technological aspects represents the next challenge to unravel the full potential of multimodality imaging into daily clinical practice of patients with cardiovascular infections.

Table 1. Multimodality imaging in the assessment of patient with IE, PVE, or CIED infection.

	Echocardiography		CCTA		PET/CT		WBC SPECT/CT		CMR	
	Pro	Cons	Pro	Cons	Pro	Cons	Pro	Cons	Pro	Cons
General Comments	The first-line diagnostic tool. Diagnostic significance: providing information major Duke/ESC criteria. Prognostic significance: complication and prediction of the risk of embolism. Able to assess treatment response. Widely available and unexpensive. TTE can be easily repeated	Diagnostic accuracy of TTE/TOE is operator-related. TOE requires patient sedation, not always feasible. Limiting factors: poor acoustic window (COPD, thorax conformation), artifacts due to calcium/metals.	Diagnostic significance: major ESC criteria. Possibility to study coronary arteries at the same time. Prognostic assessment: embolisms detection with whole body contrast enhanced CT scan. Wide availability	Radiation exposure. Risk of contrast-induced nephropathy.	Combination of metabolic evaluation and anatomic assessment. Diagnostic significance: major ESC criteria. Prognostic assessment: Simultaneous detection of embolism, metastatic lesions, portal of entry. Good availability. Easy to perform. Possibility to combine with CCTA evaluation of coronary tree at the same time.	Radiation Exposure. Patient preparation for myocardial suppression. If iodinate contrast is not administrated limited value for brain assessment. Prolonged antimicrobial treatment reduce intensity of [18F]FDG uptake. Pattern of uptake is important.	Combination of metabolic and anatomic assessment. High specificity for infection. Diagnostic significance: major ESC criteria. Prognostic assessment: simultaneous detection of embolism, metastatic lesions, portal of entry.	Radiation Exposure. Need of blood manipulation. Limited sensitivity for small lesions. Relative complex procedure. Low availability. Long acquisition time.	Absence of ionizing radiation. It can offer diagnostic images even without using contrast medium (can replace CCTA in patients with renal failure). It offers morphological and functional information (i.e., valve dysfunction, shunt quantification)	Sensitive to breath artifacts (good patient compliance required). Intermediate availability. Long acquisition time.
Left-sided IE	Good visualization of mitral and aortic valve. Valvular dysfuction assessment. Identification of complication (i.e., valvular regurgitation).	Difficult differential diagnosis in presence of marantic vegetations or high calcification.	Detection of vegetations and valve perforation. Assessment of perivalvular extent of disease (abscesses, pseudoaneursysm, fistula).	Inferior to TTE/TOE in detecting small vegetations (<2 mm).	Prognostic assessment: simultaneous detection of embolism, metastatic lesions and portal of entry.	Limited sensitivity for small vegetations.	Evaluation of distant emboli and portal of entry.	Limited role because of low sensitivity for small vegetations.	Capability to assess vegetations (inferior to TTE/TOE). Capability to assess local complications. Independent by acoustic window May detect concomitant myocardial inflammation.	Not included in current guidelines for IE diagnosis.
Right-sided IE	TTE generally provides good visualization of tricuspid valve TOE is useful in the assessment of IE related to CHD.	Pulmonary valve is difficult to assess.								
PVE	Routinely used for follow up; it allows sequential assessment of prosthesis function. TOE is often required to correctly assess the prosthesis.	Limited by prosthetic material artifacts (i.e., acoustic shadow). Early complication (i.e., abscess) can be difficult to identify.	Identification of complications (paravalvular leakage, abscesses, pseudoaneurysm, dehiscence, and extension to adjacent structures). Capability to visualize large vegetations (>10 mm).	Low image quality for beam hardening artifacts. Limited in assessing small vegetations (<4 mm).	High diagnostic accuracy. Good assessment of perivalvular/ periprosthetic complications. Reduction of rate of misdiagnosed PVE. Role in prediction of MACEs. Prognostic significance.	Host reaction may reduce specificity (risk of false-positive studies until 3 months after surgery).	High specificity for infection. Reduction of rate of misdiagnosed PVE. Differential diagnosis between septic and sterile vegetations.	Limited sensitivity for small lesions.		Image quality severely hampered by susceptibility artifacts (especially from mechanical prostheses).
CIED-IE	Useful to assess intracardiac lead segments. TTE can be integrated by ultrasound evaluation of device pocket, to assessing inflamation or fluid collection.	Limited role in the assessment of unexplorable lead segments. Differential diagnosis of vegetation vs. lead fibrosis/thrombi can be challenging.	Possibility to combine the CT assessment of generator pocket.	Blooming and beam hardening artefacts. Poor sensitivity in detecting vegetations on leads.	Very high sensitivity and specificity for generator/pocket and extracardiac or extravascular lead infection.	Low sensitivity for small vegetations along the leads.	Good sensitivity and specificity for generator/ pocket and extracardiac or extravascular lead infection.	Limited diagnostic sensitivity for intracardiac and intravascular lead infection.		Image quality severely hampered by susceptibility artifacts from lead and device. Limited to patients with MRI conditional devices and with numerous precautions.

IE: Infective Endocarditis; PVE: Prosthetic Valve Endocarditis; CIED-IE: Cardiac Implantable Electronic Device-related infective endocarditis; CCTA: Cardiac Computed Tomography; PET/TC: Fluoro-18-fluorodeoxyglucose positron emission tomography/computed tomography; WBC SPECT/CT: radiolabelled white blood cells scintigraphy with single-photon emission computed tomography/computed tomography; CMR: Cardiac Magnetic Resonance; TTE: trans-thoracic echocardiography; TOE: trans-oesophageal echocardiography; CT: computed tomography; IE: infective endocarditis; COPD: Chronic obstructive pulmonary disease; CHD: congenital heart disease; MACEs: major adverse cardiac events; CIED-IE: cardiac implantable electronic device-related infective endocarditis; MRI: magnetic resonance imaging.

9. Conclusions

A modern and updated management of IE and CIED-IE requires a correct and synergistic integration of diagnostic tools and therapeutic strategies. Multimodality imaging is a crucial part of diagnostic work-up where different techniques provide additional and unique information. Clinicians and imaging specialists should be aware of strengths and limitations of every approach in order to correctly interact with other specialists and, therefore, to optimize the management of patients and to improve the outcome.

Author Contributions: Conceptualization, N.G., F.B., and P.A.E.; writing—original draft preparation, N.G., F.B., and P.A.E.; writing—review and editing, N.G., F.B., C.L., C.A., A.L., P.A.E. All authors have read and agreed to the published version of the manuscript.

References

1. Li, J.S.; Sexton, D.J.; Mick, N.; Nettles, R.; Fowler, V.G., Jr.; Ryan, T.; Bashore, T.; Corey, G.R. Proposed modifications to the duke criteria for the diagnosis of infective endocarditis. *Clin. Infect. Dis.* **2000**, *30*, 633–638. [CrossRef]
2. Habib, G.; Lancellotti, P.; Antunes, M.J.; Bongiorni, M.G.; Casalta, J.P.; Del Zotti, F.; Dulgheru, R.; El Khoury, G.; Erba, P.A.; Iung, B.; et al. 2015 ESC guidelines for the management of infective endocarditis: The task force for the management of infective endocarditis of the European Society of Cardiology (ESC). Endorsed by: European Association for Cardio-Thoracic Surgery (EACTS), the European Association of Nuclear Medicine (EANM). *Eur. Heart J.* **2015**, *36*, 3075–3128.
3. Durack, D.T.; Lukes, A.S.; Bright, D.K. New criteria for diagnosis of infective endocarditis: Utilization of specific echocardiographic findings. Duke endocarditis service. *Am. J. Med.* **1994**, *96*, 200–209. [CrossRef]
4. Habib, G.; Derumeaux, G.; Avierinos, J.F.; Casalta, J.P.; Jamal, F.; Volot, F.; Garcia, M.; Lefevre, J.; Biou, F.; Maximovitch-Rodaminoff, A.; et al. Value and limitations of the duke criteria for the diagnosis of infective endocarditis. *J. Am. Coll. Cardiol.* **1999**, *33*, 2023–2029. [CrossRef]
5. Swart, L.E.; Scholtens, A.M.; Tanis, W.; Nieman, K.; Bogers, A.; Verzijlbergen, F.J.; Krestin, G.P.; Roos-Hesselink, J.W.; Budde, R.P.J. 18F-fluorodeoxyglucose positron emission/computed tomography and computed tomography angiography in prosthetic heart valve endocarditis: From guidelines to clinical practice. *Eur. Heart J.* **2018**, *39*, 3739–3749. [CrossRef]
6. Pizzi, M.N.; Roque, A.; Fernandez-Hidalgo, N.; Cuellar-Calabria, H.; Ferreira-Gonzalez, I.; Gonzalez-Alujas, M.T.; Oristrell, G.; Gracia-Sanchez, L.; Gonzalez, J.J.; Rodriguez-Palomares, J.; et al. Improving the diagnosis of infective endocarditis in prosthetic valves and intracardiac devices with 18F-fluordeoxyglucose positron emission tomography/computed tomography angiography: Initial results at an infective endocarditis referral center. *Circulation* **2015**, *132*, 1113–1126. [CrossRef] [PubMed]
7. Roque, A.; Pizzi, M.N.; Cuellar-Calabria, H.; Aguade-Bruix, S. 18F-FDG-PET/CT angiography for the diagnosis of infective endocarditis. *Curr. Cardiol. Rep.* **2017**, *19*, 15. [CrossRef] [PubMed]
8. Blomstrom-Lundqvist, C.; Traykov, V.; Erba, P.A.; Burri, H.; Nielsen, J.C.; Bongiorni, M.G.; Poole, J.; Boriani, G.; Costa, R.; Deharo, J.C.; et al. European Heart Rhythm Association (EHRA) international consensus document on how to prevent, diagnose, and treat cardiac implantable electronic device infections-endorsed by the Heart Rhythm Society (HRS), the Asia Pacific Heart Rhythm Society (APHRS), the Latin American Heart Rhythm Society (LAHRS), International Society for Cardiovascular Infectious Diseases (ISCVID) and the European Society of Clinical Microbiology and Infectious Diseases (ESCMID) in collaboration with the European Association for Cardio-Thoracic Surgery (EACTS). *EP Eur.* **2020**, *22*, 515–549.
9. Nishimura, R.A.; Otto, C.M.; Bonow, R.O.; Carabello, B.A.; Erwin, J.P., 3rd; Guyton, R.A.; O'Gara, P.T.; Ruiz, C.E.; Skubas, N.J.; Sorajja, P.; et al. 2014 AHA/ACC guideline for the management of patients with valvular heart disease: A report of the american college of cardiology/american heart association task force on practice guidelines. *J. Am. Coll. Cardiol.* **2014**, *63*, e57–e185. [CrossRef]

10. Sollini, M.; Berchiolli, R.; Delgado Bolton, R.C.; Rossi, A.; Kirienko, M.; Boni, R.; Lazzeri, E.; Slart, R.; Erba, P.A. The "3M" approach to cardiovascular infections: Multimodality, multitracers, and multidisciplinary. *Semin. Nucl. Med.* **2018**, *48*, 199–224. [CrossRef]
11. Cahill, T.J.; Prendergast, B.D. Infective endocarditis. *Lancet* **2016**, *387*, 882–893. [CrossRef]
12. Correa de Sa, D.D.; Tleyjeh, I.M.; Anavekar, N.S.; Schultz, J.C.; Thomas, J.M.; Lahr, B.D.; Bachuwar, A.; Pazdernik, M.; Steckelberg, J.M.; Wilson, W.R.; et al. Epidemiological trends of infective endocarditis: A population-based study in olmsted county, minnesota. *Mayo Clin. Proc.* **2010**, *85*, 422–426. [CrossRef] [PubMed]
13. Chu, V.H.; Cabell, C.H.; Benjamin, D.K., Jr.; Kuniholm, E.F.; Fowler, V.G., Jr.; Engemann, J.; Sexton, D.J.; Corey, G.R.; Wang, A. Early predictors of in-hospital death in infective endocarditis. *Circulation* **2004**, *109*, 1745–1749. [CrossRef] [PubMed]
14. Habib, G.; Erba, P.A.; Iung, B.; Donal, E.; Cosyns, B.; Laroche, C.; Popescu, B.A.; Prendergast, B.; Tornos, P.; Sadeghpour, A.; et al. Clinical presentation, aetiology and outcome of infective endocarditis. Results of the esc-eorp euro-endo (european infective endocarditis) registry: A prospective cohort study. *Eur. Heart J.* **2019**, *40*, 3222–3232. [CrossRef] [PubMed]
15. Tornos, P.; Iung, B.; Permanyer-Miralda, G.; Baron, G.; Delahaye, F.; Gohlke-Barwolf, C.; Butchart, E.G.; Ravaud, P.; Vahanian, A. Infective endocarditis in europe: Lessons from the euro heart survey. *Heart* **2005**, *91*, 571–575. [CrossRef]
16. Nadji, G.; Rusinaru, D.; Remadi, J.P.; Jeu, A.; Sorel, C.; Tribouilloy, C. Heart failure in left-sided native valve infective endocarditis: Characteristics, prognosis, and results of surgical treatment. *Eur. J. Heart Fail.* **2009**, *11*, 668–675. [CrossRef]
17. Kang, D.H.; Kim, Y.J.; Kim, S.H.; Sun, B.J.; Kim, D.H.; Yun, S.C.; Song, J.M.; Choo, S.J.; Chung, C.H.; Song, J.K.; et al. Early surgery versus conventional treatment for infective endocarditis. *N. Engl. J. Med.* **2012**, *366*, 2466–2473. [CrossRef]
18. Vilacosta, I.; Graupner, C.; San Roman, J.A.; Sarria, C.; Ronderos, R.; Fernandez, C.; Mancini, L.; Sanz, O.; Sanmartin, J.V.; Stoermann, W. Risk of embolization after institution of antibiotic therapy for infective endocarditis. *J. Am. Coll. Cardiol.* **2002**, *39*, 1489–1495. [CrossRef]
19. Eudailey, K.; Lewey, J.; Hahn, R.T.; George, I. Aggressive infective endocarditis and the importance of early repeat echocardiographic imaging. *J. Thorac. Cardiovasc. Surg.* **2014**, *147*, e26–e28. [CrossRef]
20. Habib, G.; Badano, L.; Tribouilloy, C.; Vilacosta, I.; Zamorano, J.L.; Galderisi, M.; Voigt, J.U.; Sicari, R.; Cosyns, B.; Fox, K.; et al. Recommendations for the practice of echocardiography in infective endocarditis. *Eur. J. Echocardiogr.* **2010**, *11*, 202–219. [CrossRef]
21. Habib, G.; Lancellotti, P.; Erba, P.A.; Sadeghpour, A.; Meshaal, M.; Sambola, A.; Furnaz, S.; Citro, R.; Ternacle, J.; Donal, E.; et al. The esc-eorp euro-endo (european infective endocarditis) registry. *Eur. Heart J. Qual. Care Clin. Outcomes* **2019**, *5*, 202–207. [CrossRef] [PubMed]
22. El Kadi, S.; van den Buijs, D.M.F.; Meijers, T.; Gilbers, M.D.; Bekkers, S.; van Melle, J.P.; Riezebos, R.K.; Blok, W.L.; Tanis, W.; Wahadat, A.R.; et al. Infective endocarditis in the netherlands: Current epidemiological profile and mortality: An analysis based on partial esc eorp collected data. *Neth. Heart J.* **2020**. [CrossRef] [PubMed]
23. Grob, A.; Thuny, F.; Villacampa, C.; Flavian, A.; Gaubert, J.Y.; Raoult, D.; Casalta, J.P.; Habib, G.; Moulin, G.; Jacquier, A. Cardiac multidetector computed tomography in infective endocarditis: A pictorial essay. *Insights Imaging* **2014**, *5*, 559–570. [CrossRef]
24. Kim, I.C.; Chang, S.; Hong, G.R.; Lee, S.H.; Lee, S.; Ha, J.W.; Chang, B.C.; Kim, Y.J.; Shim, C.Y. Comparison of cardiac computed tomography with transesophageal echocardiography for identifying vegetation and intracardiac complications in patients with infective endocarditis in the era of 3-dimensional images. *Circ. Cardiovasc. Imaging* **2018**, *11*, e006986. [CrossRef]
25. Bruun, N.E.; Habib, G.; Thuny, F.; Sogaard, P. Cardiac imaging in infectious endocarditis. *Eur. Heart J.* **2014**, *35*, 624–632. [CrossRef] [PubMed]
26. Feuchtner, G.M.; Stolzmann, P.; Dichtl, W.; Schertler, T.; Bonatti, J.; Scheffel, H.; Mueller, S.; Plass, A.; Mueller, L.; Bartel, T.; et al. Multislice Computed Tomography in Infective Endocarditis. *J. Am. Coll. Cardiol.* **2009**, *53*, 436–444. [CrossRef] [PubMed]
27. Entrikin, D.W.; Gupta, P.; Kon, N.D.; Carr, J.J. Imaging of infective endocarditis with cardiac CT angiography. *J. Cardiovasc. Comput. Tomogr.* **2012**, *6*, 399–405. [CrossRef]

28. Kestler, M.; Garcia-Pavia, P.; Rodríguez-Créixems, M.; Rotger, A.; Jimenez-Requena, F.; Mari, A.; Orcajo, J.; Hernández, L.; Alonso, J.C.; Bouza, E.; et al. Role of 18F-FDG PET in patients with infectious endocarditis. *J. Nucl. Med.* **2014**, *55*, 1093–1098. [CrossRef]
29. Kouijzer, I.J.; Vos, F.J.; Janssen, M.J.; van Dijk, A.P.; Oyen, W.J.; Bleeker-Rovers, C.P. The value of 18F-FDG PET/CT in diagnosing infectious endocarditis. *Eur. J. Nucl. Med. Mol. Imaging* **2013**, *40*, 1102–1107. [CrossRef]
30. Granados, U.; Fuster, D.; Pericas, J.M.; Llopis, J.L.; Ninot, S.; Quintana, E.; Almela, M.; Pare, C.; Tolosana, J.M.; Falces, C.; et al. Diagnostic accuracy of 18F-FDG PET/CT in infective endocarditis and implantable cardiac electronic device infection: A cross-sectional study. *J. Nucl. Med.* **2016**, *57*, 1726–1732. [CrossRef]
31. Erba, P.A.; Pizzi, M.N.; Roque, A.; Salaun, E.; Lancellotti, P.; Tornos, P.; Habib, G. Multimodality imaging in infective endocarditis: An imaging team within the endocarditis team. *Circulation* **2019**, *140*, 1753–1765. [CrossRef] [PubMed]
32. Frontera, J.A.; Gradon, J.D. Right-side endocarditis in injection drug users: Review of proposed mechanisms of pathogenesis. *Clin. Infect. Dis.* **2000**, *30*, 374–379. [CrossRef] [PubMed]
33. Carozza, A.; De Santo, L.; Romano, G.; Della Corte, A.; Ursomando, F.; Scardone, M.; Caianiello, G.; Cotrufo, M. Infective endocarditis in intravenous drug abusers: Patterns of presentation and long-term outcomes of surgical treatment. *J. Heart Valve Dis.* **2006**, *15*, 125–131. [PubMed]
34. Nandakumar, R.; Raju, G. Isolated tricuspid valve endocarditis in nonaddicted patients: A diagnostic challenge. *Am. J. Med Sci.* **1997**, *314*, 207–212. [PubMed]
35. Yuan, S.M. Right-sided infective endocarditis: Recent epidemiologic changes. *Int. J. Clin. Exp. Med.* **2014**, *7*, 199–218.
36. De Rosa, F.G.; Cicalini, S.; Canta, F.; Audagnotto, S.; Cecchi, E.; Di Perri, G. Infective endocarditis in intravenous drug users from Italy: The increasing importance in HIV-infected patients. *Infection* **2007**, *35*, 154–160. [CrossRef] [PubMed]
37. Chrissoheris, M.P.; Libertin, C.; Ali, R.; Ghantous, A.; Bekui, A.; Donohue, T. Endocarditis complicating central venous catheter bloodstream infections: A unique form of health care associated endocarditis. *Clin. Cardiol.* **2009**, *32*, E48–E54. [CrossRef]
38. Moller, J.H.; Anderson, R.C. 1000 consecutive children with a cardiac malformation with 26- to 37-year follow-up. *Am. J. Cardiol.* **1992**, *70*, 661–667. [CrossRef]
39. Niwa, K.; Nakazawa, M.; Tateno, S.; Yoshinaga, M.; Terai, M. Infective endocarditis in congenital heart disease: Japanese national collaboration study. *Heart* **2005**, *91*, 795–800. [CrossRef]
40. Kuijpers, J.M.; Koolbergen, D.R.; Groenink, M.; Peels, K.C.; Reichert, C.L.; Post, M.C.; Bosker, H.A.; Wajon, E.M.; Zwinderman, A.H.; Mulder, B.; et al. Incidence, risk factors, and predictors of infective endocarditis in adult congenital heart disease: Focus on the use of prosthetic material. *Eur. Heart J.* **2017**, *38*, 2048–2056. [CrossRef]
41. Saremi, F.; Gera, A.; Ho, S.Y.; Hijazi, Z.M.; Sánchez-Quintana, D. CT and MR imaging of the pulmonary valve. *Radiogrphics* **2014**, *34*, 51–71. [CrossRef]
42. Vongpatanasin, W.; Hillis, L.D.; Lange, R.A. Prosthetic heart valves. *N. Engl. J. Med.* **1996**, *335*, 407–416. [CrossRef]
43. Tuñón, V.P.; Gutiérrez, C.; Curiel, L.; Baruque, B.; Tárrago, C.P.; Corchado, E.; Rodríguez, M.A.M.; Ibáñez, A.F.; Lasso, M.C.; Abad, S.M.; et al. Genetic algorithms to simplify infective endocarditis outcome. *Eur. J. Intern. Med.* **2011**, *22*, S76–S77. [CrossRef]
44. Piper, C.; Körfer, R.; Horstkotte, D. Prosthetic valve endocarditis. *Heart* **2001**, *85*, 590–593. [CrossRef] [PubMed]
45. Habib, G.; Thuny, F.; Avierinos, J.-F. Prosthetic Valve Endocarditis: Current Approach and Therapeutic Options. *Prog. Cardiovasc. Dis.* **2008**, *50*, 274–281. [CrossRef] [PubMed]
46. Kiefer, T.; Park, L.; Tribouilloy, C.; Cortés, C.; Casillo, R.; Chu, V.; Delahaye, F.; Durante-Mangoni, E.; Edathodu, J.; Falces, C.; et al. Association between valvular surgery and mortality among patients with infective endocarditis complicated by heart failure. *JAMA* **2011**, *306*, 2239–2247. [CrossRef] [PubMed]
47. Pérez-Vázquez, A.; Fariñas, M.C.; García-Palomo, J.D.; Bernal, J.M.; Revuelta, J.M.; González-Macías, J. Evaluation of the Duke criteria in 93 episodes of prosthetic valve endocarditis: Could sensitivity be improved? *Arch. Intern. Med.* **2000**, *160*, 1185–1191. [CrossRef]
48. Rajiah, P.; Moore, A.; Saboo, S.; Goerne, H.; Ranganath, P.; MacNamara, J.; Joshi, P.; Abbara, S. Multimodality imaging of complications of cardiac valve surgeries. *Radiographics* **2019**, *39*, 932–956. [CrossRef]

49. Tanis, W.; Scholtens, A.; Habets, J.; Brink, R.B.V.D.; Van Herwerden, L.A.; Chamuleau, S.A.; Budde, R.P. CT Angiography and 18F-FDG-PET Fusion Imaging for Prosthetic Heart Valve Endocarditis. *JACC Cardiovasc. Imaging* **2013**, *6*, 1008–1013. [CrossRef]
50. Cantoni, V.; Sollini, M.; Green, R.; Berchiolli, R.N.; Lazzeri, E.; Mannarino, T.; Acampa, W.; Erba, P.A. Comprehensive meta-analysis on [18F] FDG PET/CT and radiolabelled leukocyte SPECT–SPECT/CT imaging in infectious endocarditis and cardiovascular implantable electronic device infections. *Clin. Transl. Imaging* **2018**, *6*, 3–18. [CrossRef]
51. Swart, L.; Gomes, A.; Scholtens, A.; Sinha, B.; Tanis, W.; Lam, M.G.; Van Der Vlugt, M.J.; Streukens, S.A.F.; Aarntzen, E.H.; Bucerius, J.; et al. Improving the diagnostic performance of 18 F-Fluorodeoxyglucose Positron-Emission tomography/computed tomography in prosthetic heart valve endocarditis. *Circulation* **2018**, *138*, 1412–1427. [CrossRef] [PubMed]
52. Mathieu, C.; Mikaïl, N.; Benali, K.; Iung, B.; Duval, X.; Nataf, P.; Jondeau, G.; Hyafil, F.; Le Guludec, D.; Rouzet, F. Characterization of 18F-Fluorodeoxyglucose Uptake Pattern in Noninfected Prosthetic Heart Valves. *Circ. Cardiovasc. Imaging* **2017**, *10*, e005585. [PubMed]
53. Roque, A.; Pizzi, M.N.; Fernández-Hidalgo, N.; Permanyer, E.; Cuellar-Calabria, H.; Romero-Farina, G.; Ríos, R.; Almirante, B.; Castell-Conesa, J.; Escobar, M.; et al. Morpho-metabolic post-surgical patterns of non-infected prosthetic heart valves by [18F]FDG PET/CTA: "normality" is a possible diagnosis. *Eur. Heart J. Cardiovasc. Imaging* **2019**, *21*, 24–33. [CrossRef] [PubMed]
54. San, S.; Ravis, E.; Tessonier, L.; Philip, M.; Cammilleri, S.; Lavagna, F.; Norscini, G.; Arregle, F.; Martel, H.; Oliver, L.; et al. Prognostic value of (18)F-Fluorodeoxyglucose positron emission tomography/computed tomography in infective endocarditis. *J. Am. Coll. Cardiol.* **2019**, *74*, 1031–1040. [CrossRef] [PubMed]
55. Vos, F.J.; Bleeker-Rovers, C.P.; Sturm, P.D.; Krabbe, P.F.M.; Van Dijk, A.; Cuijpers, M.L.H.; Adang, E.M.M.; Wanten, G.J.A.; Kullberg, B.J.; Oyen, W. 18F-FDG PET/CT for detection of metastatic infection in Gram-positive bacteremia. *J. Nucl. Med.* **2010**, *51*, 1234–1240. [CrossRef]
56. Gomes, A.; Glaudemans, A.W.J.M.; Touw, D.J.; Van Melle, J.P.; Willems, T.P.; Maass, A.H.; Natour, E.; Prakken, N.H.J.; Borra, R.J.H.; Van Geel, P.P.; et al. Diagnostic value of imaging in infective endocarditis: A systematic review. *Lancet Infect. Dis.* **2017**, *17*, e1–e14. [CrossRef]
57. Orvin, K.; Goldberg, E.; Bernstine, H.; Groshar, D.; Sagie, A.; Kornowski, R.; Bishara, J. The role of FDG-PET/CT imaging in early detection of extra-cardiac complications of infective endocarditis. *Clin. Microbiol. Infect.* **2015**, *21*, 69–76. [CrossRef]
58. Uslan, D.Z.; Sohail, M.R.; Sauver, J.L.S.; Friedman, P.A.; Hayes, D.L.; Stoner, S.M.; Wilson, W.R.; Steckelberg, J.M.; Baddour, L.M. Permanent pacemaker and implantable cardioverter defibrillator infection. *Arch. Intern. Med.* **2007**, *167*, 669. [CrossRef]
59. Erba, P.A.; Sollini, M.; Conti, U.; Bandera, F.; Tascini, C.; De Tommasi, S.M.; Zucchelli, G.; Doria, R.; Menichetti, F.; Bongiorni, M.G.; et al. Radiolabeled WBC scintigraphy in the diagnostic workup of patients with suspected device-related infections. *JACC Cardiovasc. Imaging* **2013**, *6*, 1075–1086. [CrossRef]
60. Klug, D.; Balde, M.; Pavin, D.; Hidden-Lucet, F.; Clementy, J.; Sadoul, N.; Rey, J.L.; Lande, G.; Lazarus, A.; Victor, J.; et al. Risk factors related to infections of implanted pacemakers and cardioverter-defibrillators. *Circulation* **2007**, *116*, 1349–1355. [CrossRef]
61. Klug, D.; Wallet, F.; Lacroix, D.; Marquié, C.; Kouakam, C.; Kacet, S.; Courcol, R. Local symptoms at the site of pacemaker implantation indicate latent systemic infection. *Heart* **2004**, *90*, 882–886. [CrossRef] [PubMed]
62. Bongiorni, M.G.; Burri, H.; Deharo, J.C.; Starck, C.; Kennergren, C.; Saghy, L.; Rao, A.; Tascini, C.; Lever, N.; Kutarski, A.; et al. 2018 EHRA expert consensus statement on lead extraction: Recommendations on definitions, endpoints, research trial design, and data collection requirements for clinical scientific studies and registries: Endorsed by APHRS/HRS/LAHRS. *EP Eur.* **2018**, *20*, 1217. [CrossRef] [PubMed]
63. Vilacosta, I.; Sarriá, C.; Roman, J.A.S.; Jiménez, J.; Castillo, J.A.; Iturralde, E.; Rollan, M.J.; Elbal, L.M. Usefulness of transesophageal echocardiography for diagnosis of infected transvenous permanent pacemakers. *Circulation* **1994**, *89*, 2684–2687. [CrossRef] [PubMed]
64. Erba, P.A.; Lancellotti, P.; Vilacosta, I.; Gaemperli, O.; Rouzet, F.; Hacker, M.; Signore, A.; Slart, R.H.; Habib, G. Recommendations on nuclear and multimodality imaging in IE and CIED infections. *Eur. J. Nucl. Med. Mol. Imaging* **2018**, *45*, 1795–1815. [CrossRef] [PubMed]
65. Baddour, L.M.; Cha, Y.-M.; Wilson, W.R. Infections of Cardiovascular Implantable Electronic Devices. *N. Engl. J. Med.* **2012**, *367*, 842–849. [CrossRef]

66. Bensimhon, L.; Lavergne, T.; Hugonnet, F.; Mainardi, J.L.; Latremouille, C.; Maunoury, C.; Lepillier, A.; Le Heuzey, J.Y.; Faraggi, M. Whole body [18F]fluorodeoxyglucose positron emission tomography imaging for the diagnosis of pacemaker or implantable cardioverter defibrillator infection: A preliminary prospective study. *Clin. Microbiol. Infect.* **2011**, *17*, 836–844. [CrossRef]
67. Sarrazin, J.-F.; Philippon, F.; Tessier, M.; Guimond, J.; Molin, F.; Champagne, J.; Nault, I.; Blier, L.; Nadeau, M.; Charbonneau, L.; et al. Usefulness of Fluorine-18 positron emission tomography/computed tomography for identification of cardiovascular implantable electronic device infections. *J. Am. Coll. Cardiol.* **2012**, *59*, 1616–1625. [CrossRef]
68. Cautela, J.; Alessandrini, S.; Cammilleri, S.; Giorgi, R.; Richet, H.; Casalta, J.-P.; Habib, G.; Raoult, D.; Mundler, O.; Deharo, J.-C. Diagnostic yield of FDG positron-emission tomography/computed tomography in patients with CEID infection: A pilot study. *EP Eur.* **2012**, *15*, 252–257. [CrossRef]
69. Graziosi, M.; Nanni, C.; Lorenzini, M.; Diemberger, I.; Bonfiglioli, R.; Pasquale, F.; Ziacchi, M.; Biffi, M.; Martignani, C.; Bartoletti, M.; et al. Role of 18F-FDG PET/CT in the diagnosis of infective endocarditis in patients with an implanted cardiac device: A prospective study. *Eur. J. Nucl. Med. Mol. Imaging* **2014**, *41*, 1617–1623. [CrossRef]
70. Tlili, G.; Amraoui, S.; Mesguich, C.; Riviere, A.; Bordachar, P.; Hindié, E.; Bordenave, L. High performances of 18F-fluorodeoxyglucose PET-CT in cardiac implantable device infections: A study of 40 patients. *J. Nucl. Cardiol.* **2015**, *22*, 787–798. [CrossRef]
71. Ahmed, F.Z.; James, J.; Cunnington, C.; Motwani, M.; Fullwood, C.; Hooper, J.; Burns, P.; Qamruddin, A.; Al-Bahrani, G.; Armstrong, I.; et al. Early diagnosis of cardiac implantable electronic device generator pocket infection using 18F-FDG-PET/CT. *Eur. Hear. J. Cardiovasc. Imaging* **2015**, *16*, 521–530. [CrossRef]
72. Juneau, D.; Golfam, M.; Hazra, S.; Erthal, F.; Zuckier, L.S.; Bernick, J.; Wells, G.A.; Beanlands, R.S.; Chow, B.J. Molecular Imaging for the diagnosis of infective endocarditis: A systematic literature review and meta-analysis. *Int. J. Cardiol.* **2018**, *253*, 183–188. [CrossRef] [PubMed]
73. Wu, C.; Ma, G.; Li, J.; Zheng, K.; Dang, Y.; Shi, X.; Sun, Y.; Li, F.; Zhu, Z. In vivo cell tracking via 18F-fluorodeoxyglucose labeling: A review of the preclinical and clinical applications in cell-based diagnosis and therapy. *Clin. Imaging* **2013**, *37*, 28–36. [CrossRef] [PubMed]
74. Fairclough, M.; Prenant, C.; Ellis, B.; Boutin, H.; McMahon, A.; Brown, G.; Locatelli, P.; Jones, A.K. A new technique for the radiolabelling of mixed leukocytes with zirconium-89 for inflammation imaging with positron emission tomography. *J. Label. Compd. Radiopharm.* **2016**, *59*, 270–276. [CrossRef]
75. Li, Z.; Chen, K.; Wu, Z.; Wang, H.; Niu, G.; Chen, X. 64Cu-Labeled PEGylated Polyethylenimine for cell trafficking and tumor imaging. *Mol. Imaging Boil.* **2009**, *11*, 415–423. [CrossRef] [PubMed]
76. Ordonez, A.A.; Weinstein, E.A.; Bambarger, L.E.; Saini, V.; Chang, Y.S.; Demarco, V.P.; Klunk, M.H.; Urbanowski, M.E.; Moulton, K.L.; Murawski, A.M.; et al. A Systematic Approach for Developing Bacteria-Specific Imaging Tracers. *J. Nucl. Med.* **2016**, *58*, 144–150. [CrossRef] [PubMed]
77. Weinstein, E.A.; Ordonez, A.A.; Demarco, V.P.; Murawski, A.M.; Pokkali, S.; Macdonald, E.M.; Klunk, M.; Mease, R.C.; Pomper, M.G.; Jain, S.K. Imaging Enterobacteriaceae infection in vivo with 18F-fluorodeoxysorbitol positron emission tomography. *Sci. Transl. Med.* **2014**, *6*, 259ra146. [CrossRef]

Permissions

All chapters in this book were first published by MDPI; hereby published with permission under the Creative Commons Attribution License or equivalent. Every chapter published in this book has been scrutinized by our experts. Their significance has been extensively debated. The topics covered herein carry significant findings which will fuel the growth of the discipline. They may even be implemented as practical applications or may be referred to as a beginning point for another development.

The contributors of this book come from diverse backgrounds, making this book a truly international effort. This book will bring forth new frontiers with its revolutionizing research information and detailed analysis of the nascent developments around the world.

We would like to thank all the contributing authors for lending their expertise to make the book truly unique. They have played a crucial role in the development of this book. Without their invaluable contributions this book wouldn't have been possible. They have made vital efforts to compile up to date information on the varied aspects of this subject to make this book a valuable addition to the collection of many professionals and students.

This book was conceptualized with the vision of imparting up-to-date information and advanced data in this field. To ensure the same, a matchless editorial board was set up. Every individual on the board went through rigorous rounds of assessment to prove their worth. After which they invested a large part of their time researching and compiling the most relevant data for our readers.

The editorial board has been involved in producing this book since its inception. They have spent rigorous hours researching and exploring the diverse topics which have resulted in the successful publishing of this book. They have passed on their knowledge of decades through this book. To expedite this challenging task, the publisher supported the team at every step. A small team of assistant editors was also appointed to further simplify the editing procedure and attain best results for the readers.

Apart from the editorial board, the designing team has also invested a significant amount of their time in understanding the subject and creating the most relevant covers. They scrutinized every image to scout for the most suitable representation of the subject and create an appropriate cover for the book.

The publishing team has been an ardent support to the editorial, designing and production team. Their endless efforts to recruit the best for this project, has resulted in the accomplishment of this book. They are a veteran in the field of academics and their pool of knowledge is as vast as their experience in printing. Their expertise and guidance has proved useful at every step. Their uncompromising quality standards have made this book an exceptional effort. Their encouragement from time to time has been an inspiration for everyone.

The publisher and the editorial board hope that this book will prove to be a valuable piece of knowledge for researchers, students, practitioners and scholars across the globe.

List of Contributors

Chiara Giraudo, Anna Sara Fraia, Amalia Lupi and Emilio Quaia
Department of Medicine-DIMED,Institute of Radiology, University of Padova, 35100 Padova, Italy

Laura Evangelista
Nuclear Medicine Unit, Department of Medicine-DIMED, University of Padova, 35128 Padova, Italy

Diego Cecchin
Nuclear Medicine Unit, Department of Medicine-DIMED, University of Padova, 35128 Padova, Italy
Padova Neuroscience Center (PNC), University of Padova, 35131 Padova, Italy

Massimiliano Casali
Azienda Unità Sanitaria Locale–IRCCS di Reggio Emilia, 42121 Reggio Emilia, Italy

Christel H. Kamani, Gilles Allenbach, Mario Jreige, Marie Meyer, Nathalie Testart, Maria Firsova, Victor Fernandes Vieira, Sarah Boughdad and Marie Nicod Lalonde
Department of Nuclear Medicine and Molecular Imaging, Lausanne University Hospital, CH-1011 Lausanne, Switzerland

Anna G. Pavon
Department of Cardiology, Lausanne University Hospital, CH-1011 Lausanne, Switzerland

Niklaus Schaefer and John O. Prior
Department of Nuclear Medicine and Molecular Imaging, Lausanne University Hospital, CH-1011 Lausanne, Switzerland
University of Lausanne, CH-1011 Lausanne, Switzerland

Benoit Guery
University of Lausanne, CH-1011 Lausanne, Switzerland
Department of Infectious Diseases, Lausanne University Hospital, CH-1011 Lausanne, Switzerland

Pierre Monney
Department of Cardiology, Lausanne University Hospital, CH-1011 Lausanne, Switzerland
University of Lausanne, CH-1011 Lausanne, Switzerland

Giorgio Treglia
Clinic of Nuclear Medicine and Molecular Imaging, Imaging Institute of Southern Switzerland, Ente Ospedaliero Cantonale, CH-6500 Bellinzona, Switzerland
Health Technology Assessment Unit, Academic Education, Research and Innovation Area, Ente Ospedaliero Cantonale, CH-6500 Bellinzona, Switzerland
Nuclear Medicine and PET/CT Center, Imaging Institute of Southern Switzerland, Ente Ospedaliero Cantonale Via Lugano 4F, CH-6500 Bellinzona, Switzerland
Department of Nuclear Medicine and Molecular Imaging, Lausanne University Hospital and University of Lausanne, 1011 Lausanne, Switzerland

Anne Skovsbo Clausen and Andreas Kjaer
Department of Clinical Physiology, Nuclear Medicine & PET, Rigshospitalet, DK-2100 Copenhagen, Denmark
Cluster for Molecular Imaging, Department of Biomedical Sciences, University of Copenhagen, DK-2200 Copenhagen, Denmark

Mathilde Ørbæk
Department of Infectious Diseases, Copenhagen University Hospital, Rigshospitalet, DK-2100 Copenhagen, Denmark

Regitze Renee Pedersen
Costerton Biofilm Center, Department of Immunology and Microbiology, University of Copenhagen, DK-2200 Copenhagen, Denmark

Peter Oestrup Jensen
Costerton Biofilm Center, Department of Immunology and Microbiology, University of Copenhagen, DK-2200 Copenhagen, Denmark
Department of Clinical Microbiology, Copenhagen University Hospital, Rigshospitalet, DK-2100 Copenhagen, Denmark
Center for Rheumatology and Spine Diseases, Institute for Inflammation Research, Copenhagen University Hospital, Rigshospitalet, DK-2100, Copenhagen, Denmark

Anne-Mette Lebech
Department of Infectious Diseases, Copenhagen University Hospital, Rigshospitalet, DK-2100 Copenhagen, Denmark
Institute of Clinical Medicine, University of Copenhagen, DK-2100 Copenhagen, Denmark

Geertruida W. Dijkstra and Luc W. M. van der Sluis
Center for Dentistry and Oral Hygiene, University Medical Center Groningen, University of Groningen, The Netherlands

Andor W. J. M. Glaudemans and David Vállez García
Department of Nuclear Medicine and Molecular Imaging, University Medical Center Groningen, University of Groningen, Groningen, The Netherlands

Paola A. Erba
Department of Nuclear Medicine and Molecular Imaging, University Medical Center Groningen, University of Groningen, Groningen, The Netherlands
Department of Nuclear Medicine, Department of Translational Research and New Technology in Medicine, University of Pisa, 56128 Pisa, Italy

Marjan Wouthuyzen-Bakker and Bhanu Sinha
Department of Medical Microbiology and Infection Prevention, University Medical Center Groningen, University of Groningen, Groningen, The Netherlands

Riemer H. J. A. Slart
Department of Nuclear Medicine and Molecular Imaging, University Medical Center Groningen, University of Groningen, Groningen, The Netherlands
Department of Biomedical Photonic Imaging, University of Twente, 7522 NB Enschede, The Netherlands

Alexander Braun, Thomas Germann, Felix Wünnemann, Hans-Ulrich Kauczor and Christoph Rehnitz
Department of Diagnostic and Interventional Radiology, University Hospital Heidelberg, 69120 Heidelberg, Germany

Marc-André Weber
Institute of Diagnostic and Interventional Radiology, Pediatric Radiology and Neuroradiology, University Medicine Rostock, 18057 Rostock, Germany

Marcus Schiltenwolf and Michael Akbar
Department of Orthopedics and Trauma Surgery, University Hospital Heidelberg, 69118 Heidelberg, Germany

Iris Burkholder
Department of Nursing and Health, University of Applied Sciences of the Saarland, 66117 Saarbruecken, Germany

Stamata Georga, Paraskevi Exadaktylou, Ioannis Petrou, Dimitrios Katsampoukas, Vasilios Mpalaris, Efstratios-Iordanis Moralidis and Georgios Arsos
3rd Department of Nuclear Medicine, Aristotle University of Thessaloniki Medical School, Papageorgiou General Hospital, 56403 Thessaloniki, Greece

Kostoula Arvaniti
ICU and Antimicrobial Stewardship Unit, Papageorgiou General Hospital, 56403 Thessaloniki, Greece

Christos Papastergiou
Department of Radiology, Papageorgiou General Hospital, 56403 Thessaloniki, Greece

Roberto Iezzi, Alessandro Posa and Alessandro Tanzilli
Radiology Unit, Fondazione Policlinico Universitario A. Gemelli IRCCS, Roma-Università Cattolica de Sacro Cuore, 00168 Rome, Italy

Michele Rossi
Radiology Unit, Department of Medical-Surgical Sciences and Translational Medicine, Faculty of Medicine and Psychology, Sant'Andrea Hospital, "Sapienza" University of Rome, 00161 Rome, Italy

Giovanni Tinelli, Simona Sica and Yamume Tshomba
Unit of Vascular Surgery, Fondazione Policlinico Universitario Gemelli IRCCS, Roma-Università Cattolica del Sacro Cuore, 00168 Rome, Italy

Chiara Panzera and Maurizio Taurino
Vascular Surgery Unit, Department of Clinical and Molecular Medicine, Faculty of Medicine and Psychology, Sant'Andrea Hospital, "Sapienza" University of Rome, 00161 Rome, Italy

Paola Anna Erba
Department of Nuclear Medicine and Molecular Imaging, University of Groningen, University Medical Center Groningen, 9700 Groningen, The Netherlands
Nuclear Medicine, Department of Translational Research and New Technology in Medicine, University of Pisa, 56123 Pisa, Italy
Department of Nuclear Medicine, Department of Translational Research and New Technology in Medicine, University of Pisa, 56126 Pisa, Italy
Medical Imaging Center, Department of Nuclear Medicine and Molecular Imaging, University of Groningen, University Medical Center Groningen, 9713 Groningen, The Netherlands

Corinna Altini, Valentina Lavelli, Alessia Branca and Giulia Santo
Nuclear Medicine Unit, Interdisciplinary Department of Medicine, University of Bari Aldo Moro, Piazza Giulio Cesare, 11–70124 Bari, Italy

Artor Niccoli-Asabella
Nuclear Medicine Unit, AOU Policlinic "A. Perrino", 72100 Brindisi, Italy

Angela Sardaro
Radiation Oncology Unit, Interdisciplinary Department of Medicine - University of Bari "Aldo Moro", Piazza Giulio Cesare, 11, 70124 Bari, Italy

Michela Varani, Filippo Galli and Gabriela Capriotti
Nuclear Medicine Unit, Department of Medical-Surgical Sciences and of Translational Medicine, Faculty of Medicine and Psychology, "Sapienza" University of Rome, 00189 Roma, Italy

Alberto Signore
Nuclear Medicine Unit, Department of Medical-Surgical Sciences and of Translational Medicine, Faculty of Medicine and Psychology, Sapienza University of Rome, 00189 Rome, Italy
Department of Nuclear Medicine and Molecular Imaging, University of Groningen, University Medical Center Groningen, 9700 Groningen, The Netherlands
Nuclear Medicine Unit Department of Medical-Surgical Sciences and of Translational Medicine, Faculty of Medicine and Psychology, "Sapienza" University of Rome, 00161 Rome, Italy

Maurizio Mattei and Rosella Cicconi
Department of Biology and Centro di Servizi Interdipartimentale-Stazione per la Tecnologia Animale, "Tor Vergata" University of Rome, 00189 Roma, Italy

Francesco Panzuto
Digestive Disease Unit, Sant'Andrea University Hospital, ENETS Center of Excellence Rome, 00189 Roma, Italy

Giuseppe Campagna
Nuclear Medicine Unit, Department of Medical-Surgical Sciences and of Translational Medicine, "Sapienza" University of Rome, 00161 Rome, Italy
Nuclear Medicine Unit, Department of Medical-Surgical Sciences and of Translational Medicine, Faculty of Medicine and Psychology, "Sapienza" University of Rome, 00189 Roma, Italy

Andor W.J.M. Glaudemans and Thomas C. Kwee
Department of Nuclear Medicine and Molecular Imaging, University of Groningen, University Medical Center Groningen, 9700 Groningen, The Netherlands

Zohar Keidar and Marina Muchnik Kurash
Department of Nuclear Medicine, Rambam Health Care Campus, 3109601 Haifa, Israel

Edel Noriega-Álvarez
Department of Nuclear Medicine, University Hospital of Ciudad Real, 13005 Ciudad Real, Spain

Giuseppe Argento
Radiology Unit, Sant'Andrea University Hospital, 00189 Rome, Italy

Riemer H.J.A. Slart
Department of Nuclear Medicine and Molecular Imaging, University of Groningen, University Medical Center Groningen, 9700 Groningen, The Netherlands
Department of Biomedical Photonic Imaging, Faculty of Science and Technology, University of Twente, 7500 Enschede, The Netherlands

Martina Conserva
Nuclear Medicine Unit, Department of Medical-Surgical Sciences and of Translational Medicine, Faculty of Medicine and Psychology, Sapienza University of Rome, 00189 Rome, Italy

Vera Artiko
Center for Nuclear Medicine, Clinical Center of Serbia, Faculty of Medicine, University of Belgrade, 101801 Beograd, Serbia

Guillermina Ferro-Flores
Department of Radioactive Materials, Instituto Nacional de Investigaciones Nucleares, Carretera Mexico-Toluca S/N, La Marquesa, Ocoyoacac 52750, Estado de Mexico, Mexico

Mick M. Welling
Interventional Molecular Imaging Laboratory, Department of Radiology, Leiden University Medical Center, 2333 ZA Leiden, The Netherlands

Sanjay K. Jain
Center for Infection and Inflammation Imaging Research, Johns Hopkins University School of Medicine, Baltimore, MD 21205, USA

Søren Hess
Department of Radiology and Nuclear Medicine, Hospital South West Jutland, University Hospital of Southern Denmark, 6700 Esbjerg, Denmark

Mike Sathekge
Nuclear Medicine Department, University of Pretoria, Pretoria 0001, South Africa

Carlo Luca Romanò
Gruppo di Studio SIOT Infezioni-Clinica San Gaudenzio-Novara-Gruppo Policlinico di Monza, University of Milan, 20100 Milan, Italy

Nicola Petrosillo
Clinical and Research Department for Infectious Diseases, National Institute for Infective Diseases "L. Spallanzani", 00144 Rome, Italy

Luca Maria Sconfienza
IRCCS Istituto Ortopedico Galeazzi, 20161 Milan, Italy
Department of Biomedical Sciences for Health, University of Milan, 20123 Milan, Italy

Abass Alavi
Division of Nuclear Medicine, Department of Radiology, Hospital of the University of Pennsylvania, Philadelphia, PA 1904, USA

Andor W.J.M. Glaudemans
Department of Nuclear Medicine and Molecular Imaging, University of Groningen, University Medical Center Groningen, 9713 GZ Groningen, The Netherlands

Olivier Gheysens
Department of Nuclear Medicine, Cliniques Universitaires Saint-Luc, 1200 Brussels, Belgium

Alex Maes
Department of Nuclear Medicine, AZ Groeninge, Kortrijk Belgium and Department of Imaging and Pathology @ KULAK, KU Leuven campus Kulak, 8500 Kortrijk, Belgium

Christopher J. Palestro
Department of Radiology Donald and Barbara Zucker School of Medicine at Hofstra/Northwell, Hempstead, NY 11549, USA

Giuseppe Rubini, Cristina Ferrari, Rossella Ruta, Francesca Iuele and Nunzio Merenda
Nuclear Medicine Unit, Interdisciplinary Department of Medicine - University of Bari "Aldo Moro", Piazza Giulio Cesare, 11, 70124 Bari, Italy

Domenico Carretta and Carlo D'Agostino
CardioThoracic Department - Policlinic of Bari, Piazza Giulio Cesare, 11, 70124, Bari, Italy

Luigi Santacroce
Ionian Department, Microbiology and Virology Lab - University of Bari "Aldo Moro", Piazza Giulio Cesare, 11, 70124 Bari, Italy

Artor Niccoli Asabella
Nuclear Medicine Unit, A. O. Policlinic "A. Perrino", Strada Statale 7 per Mesagne, 72100 Brindisi, Italy

Chiara Lauri
Department of Nuclear Medicine and Molecular Imaging, University of Groningen, University Medical Center Groningen, 9700 Groningen, The Netherlands
Nuclear Medicine Unit Department of Medical-Surgical Sciences and of Translational Medicine, Faculty of Medicine and Psychology, "Sapienza" University of Rome, 00161 Rome, Italy

Antonio Leone
Department of Radiological and Haematological Sciences, Fondazione Policlinico Universitario A. Gemelli, ISCSS—Università Cattolica del Sacro Cuore, 00168 Rome, Italy

Marco Cavallini
Wound Care Department of Medical-Surgical Sciences and of Translational Medicine, "Sapienza" University of Rome, 00161 Rome, Italy

Laura Giurato and Luigi Uccioli
Diabetic Foot Unit, Department of Systems Medicine, University of Rome Tor Vergata, 00133 Rome, Italy

Nicola Galea
Department of Experimental Medicine, "Sapienza" University of Rome, 00161 Rome, Italy

Francesco Bandera
Heart Failure Unit, Cardiology University Department, IRCCS Policlinico San Donato, Piazza Malan, 1, San Donato Milanese, 20097 Milan, Italy
Department of Biomedical Sciences for Health, University of Milano, Via Luigi Mangiagalli, 31, 20133 Milan, Italy

Camillo Autore
Department of Clinical and Molecular Sciences, "Sapienza" University of Rome, 00189 Rome, Italy

Andrea Laghi
Radiology Unit, Department of Medical-Surgical Sciences and of Translational Medicine, "Sapienza" University of Rome, 00189 Rome, Italy

Index

www.ingramcontent.com/pod-product-compliance
Lightning Source LLC
LaVergne TN
LVHW081025210926
848485LV00004B/950

* 9 7 8 1 6 3 9 2 7 6 4 8 6 *